EMERGENT MANAGEMENT OF TRAUMA

	DATE DUE		
OCT 0 3 2001			

EMERGENT MANAGEMENT OF TRAUMA

Second Edition

Thomas A. Scaletta, M.D., F.A.A.E.M.

Chairman
Department of Emergency Medicine
West Suburban Hospital Medical Center
Oak Park, Illinois

Jeffrey J. Schaider, M.D., F.A.C.E.P.

Associate Chairman and Associate Professor
Department of Emergency Medicine
Cook County Hospital/Rush Medical College
Chicago, Illinois

Boston Burr Ridge, IL Dubuque, IA Madison, WI New York
San Francisco St. Louis Bangkok Bogotá Caracas Kuala Lumpur
Lisbon London Madrid Mexico City Milan Montreal New Delhi
Santiago Seoul Singapore Sydney Taipei Toronto

McGraw-Hill

*A Division of The **McGraw-Hill** Companies*

EMERGENT MANAGEMENT OF TRAUMA, Second Edition

1234567890   DOCDOC   09876543210

ISBN 0-07-134568-X

This book was set in Times Medium by Carlisle Communications.
The editors were Andrea Seils, Kathleen McCullough, and Scott Kurtz.
The production supervisor was Richard Ruzycka.
The cover designer was Aimee Nordin.
The index was prepared by Edwin Durbin.
RR Donnelly/Crawfordsville was printer and binder.

This book is printed on acid-free paper.

Library of Congress Cataloging-in-Publication Data
Cataloging-in-Publication Data for this title is on file at the Library of Congress.

Contents

PART III: EXTREMITY TRAUMA

PART IV: SPECIAL GROUPS

PART V: ENVIRONMENTAL ISSUES

PART VI: USEFUL RESOURCES

PREFACE TO THE SECOND EDITION

We created *Emergent Management of Trauma* simply because we felt there was no effective handbook on trauma evaluation and management covering the breadth of injuries. Our book incorporates a crisp outline approach, abundant illustrations, and careful organization. Consequently, it has become a useful tool amidst the chaos of busy emergency departments. We hope that all trauma care practitioners—physicians, residents, medical students, nurses, and paramedics—find it indispensable.

We refined the book significantly with this second edition. Three new terrorism preparation chapters include specific information on chemical and biologic weapons. The extremity trauma section was completely reorganized and expanded. Updated management recommendations reflect the increased availability of helical CT and of FAST scanning. New agents were added to the drug formulary.

The book is divided into six major sections:

▶ resuscitation concepts
  ▶ comprises prehospital issues, hospital organization, patient evaluation, and "ABC" interventions
▶ anatomic areas of injury
  ▶ includes important management algorithms and covers major traumatic injuries literally from top to bottom
▶ extremity trauma
  ▶ oriented from hand to shoulder and then from hip to foot
▶ special groups
  ▶ focuses on trauma in children, pregnancy, and the elderly
▶ environmental issues
  ▶ covers temperature extremes as well as weapons of mass destruction
▶ useful resources
  ▶ concludes with detailed procedure instructions, radiograph interpretation pearls, and a pertinent drug formulary

As with the first edition, mainstream concepts are presented devoid of institutional biases. When management options exist, each reasonable pathway is described. Throughout the book, consistency of style and depth provide the reader with easy and reliable access to the vast array of information needed to manage trauma patients from head to toe and start to finish.

Trauma strikes unexpectedly, frequently, and with preference for the young and healthy. This book is dedicated to all trauma care practitioners and the patients that benefit from their expertise and commitment.

Thomas A. Scaletta, M.D., F.A.A.E.M.
Jeffrey J. Schaider, M.D., F.A.C.E.P.

ACKNOWLEDGMENTS

We would like to thank Tony Jones who added a second round of expert illustrations to the book. Thanks also go to reviewers, Vasant Acharya, MD, Kim Davis, MD, Kirk Dufty, MD, Phuong-Dung Lê, PharmD, Lawrence Hochman, DDS, Glenn Murphy, MD, Alicia Pufundt, RN EMTP, Carlo Rosen, MD, and David Springer, MD.

Our encouragement came from our wonderful wives Karen and Anna and our energetic boys Jack, Jacob, Peter, and Isaac.

Part I

RESUSCITATION CONCEPTS

1

Prehospital Issues

Trauma Center Considerations

▶ standing medical orders must be in place and approved by a qualified medical director
▶ medical control (over a radio or telephone) of individual cases is most commonly performed by an emergency physician

Physiologic Criteria

General Principles

▶ the following physiologic signs predict significant traumatic injury and mandate transport to a regional trauma center whenever possible

Individual Vital Signs

▶ SBP under 90 mm Hg
▶ HR under 50 or over 120 beats/min
▶ RR under 10 or over 30/min

Glasgow Coma Scale (GCS) (Table 1–1)

▶ add the best score from each of the categories
▶ scores range from 3 to 15
▶ consider transport of those with scores below 13 to a regional trauma center

Table 1–1 GCS: Adults

	Score					
	6	5	4	3	2	1
Eye opening			Spontaneous	To voice	To pain	None
Verbal		Full oriented	Confused but conversant	Inappropriate	Sounds only	None
Motor	Follows commands	Localizes pain	Withdraws to painful stimuli	Decorticate posturing	Decerebrate posturing	None

Table 1–2 CRAMS Scale

	Score		
	2	**1**	**0**
Circulation SBP (mm Hg) Capillary refill	> 100 Normal	< 100 Delayed	<85 Absent
Respirations	Normal	Labored or shallow	Absent
Abdomen or Thorax	Non-tender	Tender	Rigid abdomen or flail chest
Motor	Normal	Responds to pain	None or posturing
Speech	Normal	Confused	Unintelligible

CRAMS Scale (Table 1–2)

▶ score ranges from 0 to 10
▶ consider transport of those with scores below 9 to a regional trauma center

Table 1–3 Revised Trauma Score (RTS)

	Score				
	4	**3**	**2**	**1**	**0**
GCS (total)	13–15	9–12	6–8	4–5	3
SBP (mm Hg)	≥90	≥75	≥50	1–50	0
RR (per min)	10≥30	10–29	6–9	1–5	0

Revised Trauma Score (RTS) (Table 1–3)

▶ the raw RTS score ranges from 0 to 12
  ▶ function of RTS_{GCS}, RTS_{SBP}, and RTS_{RR}, which each range from 0 to 4
▶ consider transport of those with raw RTS_{total} below 12 to a regional trauma center
  ▶ raw $RTS_{total} = RTS_{GCS} + RTS_{SBP} + RTS_{RR}$
  ▶ anything less than a perfect score mandates transport to a trauma center
▶ survival rates are estimated by weighted score
  ▶ weighted $RTS_{total} = 0.94 RTS_{GCS} + 0.73 RTS_{SBP} + 0.29 RTS_{RR}$
    ▷ maximum is 7.84
    ▷ minimum is 0
  ▶ survival correlation
    ▷ 80% with RTS of 5
    ▷ 50% with RTS of 3.5
    ▷ 20% with RTS of 2

Table 1–4 Pediatric Trauma Score

	Score		
	+2	**+1**	**−1**
Weight (kg)	>20	10–20	<10
Airway	Normal	Maintained	Unstable
SBP (mm Hg)	>90	50–90	<50
Mental status	Awake	Altered	Coma
Skeletal	None	Closed fracture	Open or multiple fractures
Open wound	None	Minor	Major or penetrating

Pediatric Trauma Score (Table 1–4)

▶ score ranges from −6 to 12
▶ consider transport all children with score below 9 to a trauma center
▶ survival rates by total score
  ▶ nearly 100% survival with score over 9
  ▶ nearly 100% mortality with score of 0 or less
  ▶ scores between 1 and 8 have linear relationship to mortality

Anatomic Criteria

General Principles

▶ the following are anatomic predictors of significant traumatic injury and mandate transport to a regional trauma center whenever possible

Penetrating Trauma

▶ proximal to the knees or elbows

Blunt Trauma

▶ flail chest
▶ rigid abdomen
▶ pelvic fracture
▶ paralysis
▶ multiple proximal long bone fractures

Amputation

▶ proximal to the wrist or ankle

Burns

- ▶ unlike with other types of trauma, many regional EMS systems do not recommend transport to a trauma center for severe burns
- ▶ primary life-threat most commonly relates to airway, so transport to the closest comprehensive emergency department is preferred
- ▶ criteria defining major burns include
  - ▶ partial thickness burns over 15% total body surface area
  - ▶ full thickness burns over 5% total body surface area
  - ▶ smoke inhalation with respiratory distress
  - ▶ high-voltage electrical injuries
  - ▶ associated blunt trauma or blast trauma

Mechanistic Criteria

General Principles

- ▶ the following mechanistic predictors of significant traumatic injury should provoke consideration for transport to a regional trauma center
  - ▶ contact medical control to determine the most appropriate destination
- ▶ when such patients show no physiologic and anatomic criteria, the paramedic should guide the decision on whether to transport to a regional trauma center
- ▶ in general one should overtriage to a regional trauma center rather than undertriage

Falls

- ▶ over 20 feet

Motor Vehicle Collisions (MVC)

- ▶ speed over 35 mph at impact
- ▶ vehicle characteristics
  - ▶ major damage/rollover
  - ▶ steering wheel deformation
  - ▶ passenger compartment intrusion over 12 inches
- ▶ occupant characteristics
  - ▶ ejection from vehicle
  - ▶ extrication over 20 min
  - ▶ death of another occupant

Pedestrian Hit by Vehicle

- ▶ thrown or run over
- ▶ impact over 5 mph

Motorcycle Collision

▶ speed over 20 mph at impact
▶ separated from cycle

Premorbid Conditions

General Principles

▶ certain preexisting conditions will increase the risk of a significant injury following trauma
▶ when these conditions are present, the threshold for transporting to a regional trauma center should be somewhat lower
  ▶ contact medical control to determine the most appropriate destination

Age Extremes

▶ under 5 years or over 55 years old

Past Medical History

▶ underlying cardiac or pulmonary disease
▶ serious chronic health problems
  ▶ obesity
  ▶ diabetes
  ▶ malignancy
  ▶ coagulopathy
    ▶ cirrhosis
    ▶ hemophilia
    ▶ anticoagulant medication use

Death Pronouncement

General Principles

▶ adhere to regional guidelines for pronouncement of death in the field
▶ appropriate prehospital pronouncement of death results in
  ▶ decreased risk to paramedics and citizens performing unnecessary "lights and siren" transports
  ▶ decreased risk to healthcare workers of body substance exposure from contaminated needle sticks
  ▶ preservation of the crime scene
  ▶ increased resources for salvageable patients

Accepted Criteria

Author Recommendations

▶ blunt trauma patients pulseless at the scene
▶ penetrating trauma patients asystolic and without signs of life at the scene

American College of Surgeons (ACS)

▶ dependent lividity, rigor mortis, or decomposition
▶ decapitation or hemicorporectomy
▶ no signs of life for over 10 min
  ▶ no spontaneous ventilatory effort
  ▶ no pulse or blood pressure
  ▶ no electrical cardiac activity

National Association of EMS Physicians (NAEMSP)

▶ in addition to the ACS criteria, the NAEMSP include the following when associated with no signs of life
  ▶ brain matter extruding from a head wound
  ▶ underwater submersion for over 2 h
  ▶ evisceration of the heart
  ▶ complete incineration
  ▶ multiple extremity amputations

Restraint Devices

Lap Seat Belts

▶ mesenteric or hollow viscus injury
▶ illiac artery or abdominal aortic injury
▶ "Chance" lumbar fracture (see p. 122)

Shoulder Belts

▶ injuries to major branches of the thoracic aorta including the carotid artery
▶ rib fractures and pulmonary contusion

Air Bags

▶ abrasions and burns to the face, cornea, neck, chest
▶ blunt cardiac injury
▶ cervical spine fracture

Ballistics

Energy

▶ kinetic energy is proportional to mass times velocity squared
  ▶ thus velocity of the missile is far more important than its mass with regard to the energy imparted to tissue
▶ most civilian handguns fire low-velocity missiles
  ▶ under 1000 ft/s
▶ military rifles fire high-velocity missiles
  ▶ over 2000 ft/s

Yaw

▶ end-on-end tumbling of the missile, which causes a greater degree of tissue damage (Figure 1–1)

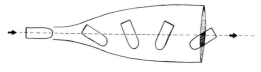

Figure 1–1

Sonic Pressure Wave

▶ low-magnitude pressure wave along the missile path
▶ can cause injury to gas-filled organs

Cavitation

▶ high-velocity missiles produce a large temporary cavity when passing through tissue and generally a huge exit wound (Figure 1–2)
▶ thus, the zone of injury is larger than anticipated and includes a "blunt" component

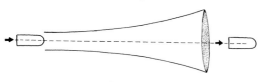

Figure 1–2

Jacketed Bullets

▶ bullet made of a soft lead center covered by a "jacket" of hard copper alloy
▶ originally designed for high-velocity weapons to preserve the rifle barrel
▶ "soft point" or "partially jacketed" bullets have the soft lead exposed at the tip and will expand or "mushroom" on impact
▶ hollowing out the tip causes even more expansion on impact

Shotgun Wounds

▶ degree of injury is related to the range, which is proportional to the spread and impact velocity (Figure 1–3)
   ▶ spread is diameter of area of pellet dispersal
   ▶ "sawn-off" barrels result in widely dispersed but high-velocity pellet wounds when fired at close range so the estimates (below) for injury type do not apply

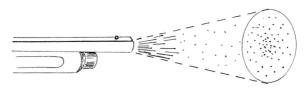

Figure 1–3

▶ low energy
   ▶ range over 12 m and correlating to spread over 24 cm
   ▶ shallow penetration
   ▶ treated like pellet gun injury
▶ moderate energy
   ▶ range 6–12 m and correlating to spread 6–24 cm
   ▶ deep tissue penetration
▶ high energy
   ▶ range under 6 m and correlating to spread under 6 cm
   ▶ extensive tissue destruction

Protective Vests

Kevlar

▶ capable of stopping low-velocity missiles (e.g., bullets from most hand-guns)
▶ made of a light comfortable fabric
▶ stopped missiles still have injury potential
  ▶ dissipation of kinetic energy in a focused area produces significant underlying blast effect despite innocuous skin appearance
  ▶ initiate workup for underlying blunt injury and, at the least, admit for observation

Military Vests

▶ heavy and uncomfortable because they contain ceramic plates
▶ better dissipation of kinetic energy and reduction of blast injury

Stabilization

ABCs

Airway

▶ clear airway and intubate if necessary
▶ the esophageal obturator airway (EOA) is not recommended since it ventilates poorly
▶ the Combitube and laryngeal mask airway are gaining favor as alternatives in adults when ETT is unsuccessful
▶ in some EMS jurisdictions, cricothyrotomy is allowed for failed intubation when ventilation cannot be achieved through a bag-valve-mask
▶ if the patient is still wearing motorcycle or sports helmet, remove only if necessary to secure the airway or treat other immediate life threats

Breathing

▶ perform needle decompression of suspected tension pneumothorax
  ▶ associated with severe hypotension or arrest, absent breath sounds, and deviated trachea
▶ in some rural areas with prolonged transport times, paramedics are trained to insert chest tubes when there is clinical evidence of a hemo- or pneumothorax

Circulation and Cervical Spine Stabilization

▶ establish large-bore intravenous access
▶ in some areas paramedics are trained to access central veins
▶ control all external hemorrhage with direct pressure
  ▶ tourniquets may be used only as a last resort
▶ stabilize the cervical spine through in-line immobilization (Figure 1–4)

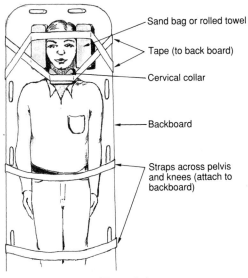

Figure 1–4

Fluid Resuscitation

Guidelines

▶ in urban areas with short transport times
  ▶ "scoop and run" and perform procedures on the way to the hospital
  ▶ while intravenous access is usually successful during the transport, only a small amount of crystalloid generally infuses
▶ aggressive fluid resuscitation can be detrimental when bleeding is not yet definitively controlled
  ▶ the resulting increased arterial pressure disrupts any hemostatic tamponade, increases intracavitary blood loss, and dilutes clotting factors
  ▶ the goal should be "permissive hypotension" (see p. 63) with an SBP of 80–90 mm Hg in patients without severe head injury
  ▶ if the patient becomes pulseless, begin rapid crystalloid infusion

Pneumatic Anti-Shock Garment (PASG)

General Principles

▶ also referred to as military anti-shock trousers (MAST) and originally developed for U.S. Air Force pilots

Pros

▶ splint pelvic or femur fractures to minimize hemorrhage rate
  ▷ many now believe this is the only rationale for PASG use

Cons

▶ studies show worse outcomes with PASG use for uncontrolled intracavitary hemorrhage
  ▷ similarly to limiting crystalloid infusion in the "permissive hypotension" approach, withholding PASG can improve outcomes
▶ movement of unstable pelvic fractures increases pelvic bleeding that can occur while applying the device
▶ makes ventilation difficult and is associated with ischemic complications

Contraindications

▶ pulmonary edema or cardiogenic shock
▶ chest injury
  ▷ worsens intrathoracic hemorrhage
  ▷ more difficult to ventilate, especially with diaphragm rupture
▶ advanced pregnancy
▶ impalement or evisceration
▶ head injury

Procedure

▶ pressure
  ▷ minimum is 40 mm Hg
  ▷ maximum is when the Velcro slips
  ▷ inflate each leg section and then the abdomen section
▶ remove once patient hemodynamically stable
  ▷ slowly deflate one section at a time (abdomen first) watching the BP carefully
  ▷ if the SBP drops more than 5 mm Hg, stop the deflation until volume replacement compensates before continuing to deflate
  ▷ once applied by paramedics, removal should only occur under the direction of a physician

▶ complications
  ▶ duration over 2 h associated with lower-extremity ischemic injuries and compartment syndrome
  ▶ increases the work of breathing
  ▶ unable to examine the entire body when in place

Disasters

Field Triage

General Principles

▶ the goal is to save as many victims as possible
▶ must appreciate and work within the limits of available resources including
  ▶ number of healthcare providers
  ▶ equipment and supplies
  ▶ amount of blood products available
▶ assign a triage officer who appropriately triages into the following treatment groups

Priority Group

▶ immediate transport is necessary for seriously injured individuals with a chance of survival given currently available resources
▶ usually color-coded *red*

Delayed Group

▶ the number in the delayed group generally exceeds that in the priority group by over 5:1
▶ physiologically stable patients for whom delayed treatment would not be expected to endanger life or limb
▶ usually color-coded *yellow* (moderate injury) and *green* (minor injury)

Expectant Group

▶ dead or expected to die given currently available resources
▶ pain should be treated
▶ usually color-coded *black*

Major Disasters

▶ very long delays in definitive care often result in re-triage of patients among the treatment groups
▶ patients must be continually reevaluated in the field and status changes taken into consideration

Systems

Disaster Planning

▶ a disaster plan must be a part of every community EMS system and incorporate paramedics, hospital personnel, police, fire department, coast guard, and other necessary entities
▶ periodic disaster drills should be undertaken to familiarize participants with the plan and to find and solve uncovered problems
▶ a field triage area should be set up and all patients moved to this area
▶ tag patients using the standard color code system correlating to their triage assignment
  ▶ *red*—immediate transport to trauma center by ambulance
  ▶ *yellow*—urgent transport to non-trauma center by ambulance
  ▶ *green*—delayed transport to non-trauma center, often sent in groups
  ▶ *black*—delayed transport to morgue
▶ initiate a communication system between the scene and receiving hospitals
  ▶ this is often cited as the most critical aspect in achieving success
▶ divert traffic and control crowds

Extrication

▶ may need assistance of the fire department or utility companies
▶ consider sending an emergency physician or surgeon to the scene when extrication extremely prolonged
▶ never risk the safety of healthcare workers when the following dangers exist
  ▶ live electrical wires
  ▶ smoke inhalation or thermal injury
  ▶ explosion
  ▶ hostile crowd
▶ tools
  ▶ "jaws of life"
  ▶ jack or winch
  ▶ be careful not to produce sparks in the presence of flammable materials

Hospital Notification

Typical Report

General Principles

▶ the report should be brief and be made en route to the hospital, allowing enough warning for hospital preparation to occur

Demographics

▶ ambulance identification
▶ age and sex of patient

Assessment

▶ mechanism of injury
▶ chief complaint or problem
▶ vital signs
▶ pertinent physical findings
▶ important medical history, medications, and allergies
▶ important scene issues
    ▸ prolonged extrication time
    ▸ hostile crowd
    ▸ need for patient restraint or security standby
    ▸ physician on scene

Management

▶ treatment
    ▸ spinal immobilization
    ▸ airway maneuvers
    ▸ intravenous access
    ▸ medications (given or requested)
▶ response
    ▸ change in vital signs after treatment

Disposition

▶ destination
▶ transport time
▶ need for helicopter

Report of Mass Casualties

General Principles

▶ initial request for information regarding currently available hospital resources
    ▸ ICU beds
    ▸ blood supply
    ▸ available operating rooms
    ▸ medical/surgical beds
    ▸ emergency department clinical space
▶ report of number of patients to be transported within each triage color category
    ▸ no further information necessary

2

Hospital Organization

Emergency Departments

General Information

- ▶ most states define what staffing and services are required for the various levels of trauma center and comprehensive emergency departments
- ▶ the American College of Surgeons publishes criteria for trauma center recognition and adheres to a stringent verification process

Level 1 Trauma Center

- ▶ mainstay of trauma care in most dense urban areas
- ▶ qualified emergency physician always on duty
- ▶ trauma surgeon immediately available at all times
  - ▶ trauma residents typically respond to the emergency department as the first line
- ▶ operating personnel immediately available at all times
  - ▶ surgical assistants
  - ▶ anesthesiologist
  - ▶ surgical nursing team
- ▶ able to deliver definitive care to all types of trauma patients
- ▶ surgical subspecialties are promptly available
  - ▶ neurosurgeon
  - ▶ orthopedic surgeon
  - ▶ plastic surgeon
  - ▶ urologist
- ▶ radiographic capabilities immediately available at all times
  - ▶ CT scan
  - ▶ angiography

Comprehensive Emergency Department

- ▶ mainstay of trauma care in most suburban areas
  - ▶ level 2 trauma center status is common
- ▶ qualified emergency physician always on duty
- ▶ trauma or general surgeon and operating personnel promptly available

► most surgical subspecialties represented
► radiographic capabilities urgently available
► transfer to a level 1 trauma center necessary for certain problems

Limited Emergency Department

► mainstay of trauma care in most rural areas
► emergency physician in attendance at all times
► anesthesiologist in hospital
► general surgeon and limited surgical subspecialists on call
► radiographic capabilities available
► transfers to trauma center occur for many patients requiring immediate operative intervention

Specialty Centers

Burn

► offer burn intensive care with highly experienced staff
► helpful with massive burn injuries or patients at age extremes

Spinal Cord Injury

► offer spinal cord injury intensive care with highly experienced staff
► associated with specialized rehabilitation programs

Pediatric Trauma

► offer neonatal and pediatric intensive care with highly experienced staff
► all surgical subspecialists primarily practice pediatric surgery
► common in major urban areas with a high volume of pediatric trauma

Team Members

Team Captain

► qualified and dedicated physician with experience in trauma management
  ► attending emergency physician
  ► attending trauma surgeon
  ► a senior emergency medicine or surgery resident physician under direct attending supervision
► makes all the decisions and is solely responsible for orders
► should be the only person speaking except when directing others to report information
► maintains control and order of the resuscitation
► performs or supervises the primary and secondary survey

- ideally delegates technical tasks to other personnel
  - repeat vital signs
  - medication and fluid orders
  - necessary procedures

Other Physicians

Trauma Team

- in a level 1 center there are generally sufficient numbers of physicians and medical students ready to assist in the resuscitation, so much can be accomplished simultaneously
  - all take direction from the team captain
  - one individual becomes responsible for airway maintenance and cervical spine control
  - personnel available to perform necessary procedures appropriate for level of training and experience
- in other hospitals the team captain may be the only physician immediately present and must perform the evaluation and procedures in series before assistants arrive

Consultants

- notify appropriate consultants prior to patient arrival whenever possible
- specialists frequently needed include
  - radiologist to perform and interpret certain studies
  - neurosurgeon for head or spinal cord injuries
  - orthopedic surgeon for fractures/dislocations
  - cardiothoracic surgeon for heart or great vessel injuries
  - vascular surgeon for neck, abdominal, or extremity vascular injuries or amputations
  - internist or pediatrician for underlying medical illness management
  - anesthesiologist with particularly difficult airways or when more assistance than usual is needed

Nurses

Ideal Qualifications

- critical care experience
- appropriate training and certification—e.g., Trauma Nursing Core Course (TNCC) offered by the Emergency Nurses Association (ENA)

Assignments

- set up equipment
- completely undress the patient

- obtain peripheral intravenous access and acquire laboratory specimens
- administer fluids and medications
- place uncomplicated nasogastric tubes and urinary catheters
- monitor vital signs frequently
- record the resuscitation
  - this should be the sole responsibility of one nurse
- assist the physician team
- monitor seriously injured patients taken to other departments (i.e., radiology)

Ancillary Personnel

Technical Staff

- clean and dress minor wounds
- obtain vital signs
- assist with nursing tasks
- transport patients to and from procedures
- messenger specimens to the laboratory and return results

Other Technical Staff

- respiratory
- radiology
- laboratory

Clerical Staff

- register new patients
- initiate necessary paperwork
- page consultants
- perform order entry

Security Staff

- limit access to the clinical area
- control crowds
- restrain combative individuals

Chaplain/Social Workers

- support grieving family members and friends after a critical injury or death

Preparation

Personnel

▶ when prehospital notification of a trauma patient is announced, the emergency department staff should immediately prepare
  ▶ notify the trauma team if the patient is unstable or will likely need an immediate operative procedure
    ▹ two-tier systems are becoming popular due to their time and cost efficiencies and involve setting an institutional protocol for which cases are evaluated by the emergency department team and which require the immediate assistance of a trauma team
  ▶ don full barrier precautions
    ▹ gloves
    ▹ mask with eye shield
    ▹ impermeable gown
    ▹ leggings and shoe covers
▶ alert supporting staff of potential needs
  ▶ appropriate consultants
  ▶ operating room team
  ▶ radiology/CT technicians
  ▶ security officers
  ▶ chaplain/social workers

Facility

▶ anticipate and locate all necessary equipment
  ▶ procedure trays
  ▶ pressure infusion device
  ▶ blood/fluid warmer
▶ type O-negative donor blood should be immediately available at all times in the clinical area

3

Patient Evaluation

Primary Survey

General Principles

▶ the "ABCDEs," standing for airway (and cervical spine), breathing, circulation, disability, and exposure/environment, refer to a priority order and elements of the examination that should be done immediately before any history taking or other aspect of the physical examination
  ▶ ideally performed in under 1 minute (excluding interventions)
  ▶ interventions to reverse immediately life-threatening conditions should commence as their need is appreciated
▶ always assume the worst possible injuries based on the mechanism or clinical examination until definitively excluded
▶ the more unstable the patient, the less necessary to confirm life-threatening diagnoses before treatment
  ▶ for instance, the *suspicion* of a tension pneumothorax in a severely hypotensive patient mandates immediate needle thoracostomy before the secondary survey or a chest radiograph
▶ any worsening in the physiologic status of a patient at any point in the evaluation and management course mandates an immediate reevaluation of the "ABCDEs"

Airway and Cervical Spine Control

Goals and Interventions

▶ initially assume a cervical spine injury exists and protect the cervical spine from further injury
▶ inspect and palpate the face, oropharynx, and neck
▶ detect and clear any form of airway obstruction
  ▶ if the patient can verbalize, the airway is generally safe
  ▶ in unconscious patients
    ▶ utilize chin lift or jaw thrust to lift the tongue off the posterior pharynx
    ▶ suction blood, secretions, vomitus, avulsed teeth, or other forms of debris from the oropharynx

▶ utilize oral or nasopharyngeal airway whenever necessary
　▷ the nasopharyngeal airway is contraindicated in patients with severe facial trauma

Management

▶ for patients with injuries above the clavicles or significant mechanism for cervical spine injury
　▶ initiate cervical spine immobilization
　▶ maintain until injury is excluded clinically or radiographically (p. 129)
▶ immediately intubate when
　▶ obstructed airway cannot be adequately cleared
　▶ expanding neck hematoma or a thermal/caustic airway burn is present
　　▷ as delayed airway obstruction can occur and intubation becomes a progressively more difficult procedure
　▶ evidence of severe shock
　▶ GCS is below 11
　　▷ maintain a low threshold to intubate any patient with head injury and decreasing responsiveness
　▶ patient has life- or limb-threatening injury and is too combative to control otherwise
　▶ patient is unable to self-maintain or protect the airway
▶ intubation is generally facilitated by rapid sequence induction of general anesthesia (see p. 41)
▶ an awake intubation may be attempted when
　▶ the patient is spontaneously breathing
　▶ a technically difficult orotracheal intubation is anticipated
　▶ a cervical spine injury is likely
　▶ there is no head injury or open globe
▶ if unable to intubate
　▶ perform a cricothyrotomy (see p. 50) and pass an endotracheal (or tracheostomy) tube into the trachea
　▶ in young children perform a needle cricothyrotomy and start jet ventilation as surgical cricothyrotomy is contraindicated

Breathing

Management

▶ evaluate
　▶ listen for breath sounds or air movement and count the respiratory rate
　▶ observe chest excursion and inspect for a flail segment

▶ palpate for subcutaneous emphysema, rib fractures, and asymmetric chest expansion
▶ cyanosis
  ▷ this is a very late sign of preterminal hypoxia and requires at least 5 g/dl of hemoglobin to appreciate
▶ bag-valve-mask (BVM) ventilation followed by immediate intubation when
  ▶ hypoxia despite supplemental oxygen
  ▶ apnea or inadequate ventilation
▶ other immediate treatment
  ▶ give supplemental oxygen by nonrebreather mask in all major trauma patients
  ▶ perform needle decompression when tension pneumothorax suspected
  ▶ seal an open pneumothorax by creating a flutter valve with a Vaseline gauze bandage taped on three sides (see Figure 13–5, p. 185)
  ▶ place chest tube if clinical hemo-/pneumothorax

Circulation and Hemorrhage Control

Management

▶ if pulseless, either perform immediate thoracotomy or pronounce the patient dead
  ▶ see criteria for death pronouncement (p. 7)
▶ control external bleeding
  ▶ apply pressure over the bleeding point or at a proximal artery
  ▶ a compressive bandage is often effective
    ▷ on an extremity use a gauze pack covered by an elastic bandage wrapped firmly from distal to proximal
  ▶ never use a tourniquet or clamp blindly in the depths of a wound
  ▶ bleeding may become more significant during fluid resuscitation
▶ appreciate likely sources of uncontrolled intracavitary bleeding based on clinical findings
▶ establish multiple, large-bore intravenous access sites
  ▶ place two 14 or 16-gauge catheters in any patient with a significant mechanism
  ▶ further IV access is determined by the degree of hemodynamic instability
  ▶ for patients with advanced hemorrhagic shock any venous access site is permissible and a large-bore line (e.g., 8 Fr cordis) is ideal

- ▶ the following guidelines may be helpful
  - ▷ when patients are pulseless, venous cutdown is often the fastest and most reliable means of access
  - ▷ in young children, consider the intraosseous route when peripheral access is not immediately successful
  - ▷ establish an internal jugular or subclavian venous line when primary injuries are below the diaphragm
  - ▷ establish a femoral venous line or saphenous cutdown when primary injuries are above the diaphragm
- ▶ rapidly assess signs of severe shock (see Table 5–1, p. 58)
  - ▶ note the presence, quality, and rate of pulses
    - ▷ rapid, thready pulse
    - ▷ presence of a carotid pulse implies a minimum SBP (mm Hg) of 60; femoral, 70; radial, 80; pedal, 100
  - ▶ skin signs demonstrate
    - ▷ coolness over patellae or feet
    - ▷ capillary refill delayed over 2 seconds
  - ▶ mental status
    - ▷ disorientation or unresponsiveness
    - ▷ agitation or combativeness
- ▶ consider aggressive fluid resuscitation when benefits outweigh risks
  - ▶ benefits
    - ▷ hypoperfusion of brain or heart mandates immediate volume expansion to maintain SBP between 80 and 90 mm Hg
    - ▷ transfuse isotonic crystalloid and uncrossmatched blood immediately for patients in severe shock to maximize the oxygen-carrying capacity to vital organs
  - ▶ risks
    - ▷ can dislodge hemostatic clots
    - ▷ will dilute necessary clotting factors and can provoke coagulopathy
- ▶ some utilize the PASG with pelvic or femur fractures to control hemorrhage
- ▶ the Trendelenberg position has no proven benefit and can be harmful with head or chest injuries

Disability (Neurologic)

Management

- ▶ determine level of responsiveness
  - ▶ GCS (see Table 7–1, p. 73)
- ▶ for patients with altered sensorium, rapidly rule out or empirically treat the following medical possibilities
  - ▶ hypoglycemia
    - ▷ if low glucose reading on chemstrip testing, administer intravenous dextrose (1 ml/kg of 50% solution up to 50 ml)

- ▶ opioid intoxication
  - ▹ if small pupils and hypoventilation, administer intravenous naloxone (0.01 mg/kg in children or 0.4–2 mg in adults)
- ▶ Wernicke's encephalopathy
  - ▹ in alcoholics and others with poor nutritional state, administer intravenous thiamine (100 mg in adults)
- ▶ if head injury and GCS below 11
  - ▶ obtain emergent neurosurgical consultation
  - ▶ immediately perform orotracheal intubation after rapid sequence induction
    - ▹ provides airway protection
    - ▹ provides supplemental oxygen (start with 50% FiO_2)
    - ▹ provides adequate ventilation
  - ▶ for trans-tentorial herniation
    - ▹ appreciate clinical findings of progressively decreasing responsiveness, unilateral pupillary dilation, and contralateral hemiparesis
    - ▹ hyperventilate to halt progression (induces cerebral vasoconstriction and reduces intracranial pressure)
    - ▹ consider immediate burr holes in the resuscitation area or decompressive craniotomy in the operating room
    - ▹ administer intravenous mannitol (1.5–2 g/kg) to reduce intracranial pressure
  - ▶ arrange for immediate, noninfused head CT
    - ▹ contraindicated if patient is hemodynamically unstable
    - ▹ in some cases the neurosurgeon may elect to perform burr holes, emergent decompressive craniotomy, or place an intracranial pressure (ICP) monitor based on the clinical examination before CT confirmation
  - ▶ load with phenytoin for prophylaxis against seizures

Expose (Undress) and Environment (Temperature Control)

Management

- ▶ patients are often only partially undressed in the prehospital setting
- ▶ rapidly and completely undress every trauma patient to uncover occult signs of trauma
  - ▹ minimize heat loss by then keeping patient covered with a blanket between examinations
- ▶ log roll and inspect the back when the patient requires spinal immobilization
  - ▶ requires a minimum of three individuals to perform safely
  - ▶ one individual maintains the head-neck-shoulder orientation during the entire process

▶ the patient is rolled towards one individual while another inspects and palpates the back (Figure 3–1)

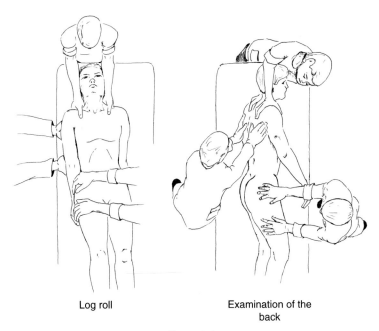

Log roll

Examination of the back

Figure 3–1

Resuscitation Phase

▶ perform any necessary procedures not already completed on the primary survey such as
  ▶ intubation
  ▶ venous central line insertion
  ▶ tube thoracostomy
  ▶ FAST (focused assessment by sonography in trauma) examination or DPL
▶ continue fluid and blood infusion as clinically necessary
▶ when emergent operative intervention is anticipated, inform appropriate consultants and ready the operating room team

Adjuncts to Consider

Monitoring

▶ cardiac rhythm
▶ pulse oximetry
▶ place urinary catheter for urine output measurement

Screening Radiographs

▶ chest (AP)
▶ cervical spine (AP, lateral, and odontoid)
▶ pelvis (AP)

Treatment

▶ gastric catheter to evacuate the stomach
    ▶ prevents aspiration and facilitates ventilation
▶ supplemental oxygen
▶ in non-trauma centers consider initiating the transfer process

Rapid History

▶ take a rapid, "AMPLE" history
    ▶ allergies
    ▶ medications
    ▶ past medical history
    ▶ last meal
    ▶ events preceding the event
▶ determine co-morbid factors that may be responsible for the traumatic event
    ▶ substance abuse is highly associated with all types of trauma
    ▶ a syncopal episode may be the cause of a fall or motor vehicle collision
    ▶ a suicide attempt may be evidenced by a temporal association with depression or a major stressor

Secondary Survey

Approach

Rapid and Complete

▶ ideally performed in 5–10 minutes
▶ every inch of skin should be visually inspected and every major bone palpated

–29–

Examples

▶ head and face
  ▶ palpate through scalp lacerations for a skull step-off
  ▶ inspect for Battle's sign (ecchymosis over the mastoid area)
  ▶ palpate all facial bones, assess facial sensation, mid-face stability, extraoccular muscle function
▶ eyes
  ▶ check gross visual acuity (ability to read a name tag), pupillary size, and reactivity to light
  ▶ inspect for raccoon eyes, anisocoria, ocular palsy, hyphema, ruptured globe, dislocated lens
  ▶ evert the eyelid when there is either eye pain or conjunctival injection in order to uncover foreign bodies
  ▶ use the fundoscope to identify retinal or vitreous hemorrhages, papilledema
  ▶ fluorescein facilitates the diagnosis of corneal abrasion or penetration
  ▶ remove and save contact lenses
▶ ears
  ▶ use otoscope to identify hemotympanum, CSF otorrhea
    ▶ remove and save hearing aids
▶ nose
  ▶ inspect for septal hematoma
▶ oropharynx
  ▶ assess airway patency
  ▶ inspect for tooth injuries, expanding intraoral hematomas
    ▶ remove and save dentures
▶ neck
  ▶ while maintaining immobility, palpate spinous processes for deformity or crepitance
  ▶ inspect for expanding anterior hematoma and tracheal shift
▶ chest
  ▶ inspect for flail chest
  ▶ auscultate for absent or asymmetric breath sounds
  ▶ palpate for subcutaneous emphysema and bony tenderness of sternum/ribs
▶ back
  ▶ if omitted in the primary physical survey, log roll to visualize and palpate the back while the cervical spine is immobilized
▶ abdomen
  ▶ inspect for ecchymoses, distension
  ▶ palpate for tenderness, peritoneal signs
  ▶ in many centers the FAST examination is becoming part of the primary survey for blunt abdominal trauma (see p. 194)
▶ pelvis
  ▶ assess stability by gentle compression of the iliac wings and symphysis pubis

▶ rectum
  ▶ perform a digital rectal examination to assess prostate position, rectal tone, and the presence of gross blood
▶ genitalia
  ▶ in males inspect for scrotal hematoma/ecchymosis, blood at the penile meatus, testicular hematoma
  ▶ in females inspect for vaginal bleeding and perform a gentle bimanual examination
▶ extremities
  ▶ inspect for deformity and swelling
  ▶ palpate for tenderness, crepitus, limited joint movement, and abnormal pulses
▶ neurologic
  ▶ perform careful mental status, cranial nerve, sensorimotor, and reflex examination
    ▹ whenever possible, assess baseline prior to sedation or paralysis

Laboratory Utilization

Hematocrit

▶ obtain as a baseline in all patients with a significant mechanism of injury
▶ patients requiring crystalloid resuscitation for hemorrhagic shock benefit from serial hematocrit measurement in order to determine the degree of hemodilution and the need for blood transfusion
▶ hematocrit determination is a poor "screening test" for occult hemorrhage
  ▶ patients not receiving a rapid crystalloid bolus may have a normal initial hematocrit despite significant hemorrhage
    ▹ the compensatory movement of extravascular fluid into the vascular system after hemorrhage (hemodilution) takes several hours when fluid resuscitation is not initiated
  ▶ conversely, patients without shock who are routinely given a rapid crystalloid bolus "to see if the hematocrit will drop" can have untoward consequences
    ▹ pulmonary edema may develop in the elderly and those with cardiac disease
    ▹ normovolemic patients often experience a hematocrit drop of 2–3 points per liter of fluid infused as a rapid bolus (false positive test)

Creatinine

▶ obtain when contrast study anticipated

Glucose

▶ determine rapidly in patients with altered sensorium to rule out hypoglycemia

Amylase/Lipase

▶ although some obtain amylase and/or lipase levels in abdominal trauma, routine use is not justified because of low specificity
▶ sensitivity for pancreatic injuries
  ▶ elevated in 80% with blunt and 25% with penetrating pancreatic injury
  ▶ lipase is more accurate than amylase, so ordering both tests is unnecessary
  ▶ facial injuries may cause elevation of amylase (salivary), which should not be misinterpreted
  ▶ progressive elevation increases suspicion of pancreatic, liver, or bowel injuries

Cardiac Enzymes

▶ obtain when a cardiac event may have precipitated the trauma

Arterial Blood Gases

▶ obtain in patients with altered sensorium, chest trauma, or hemorrhagic shock to assess ventilation and oxygenation
▶ metabolic acidosis is strongly associated with hypoperfusion and is used to assess efficacy of resuscitation

Coagulation Studies

▶ international normalized ratio (INR), prothrombin time (PT), and partial thromboplastin time (PTT) are indicated when
  ▶ operative intervention is likely
  ▶ transfusion is anticipated
  ▶ there is preexisting coagulopathy (e.g., hemophilia) or the patient is on anticoagulant therapy
  ▶ there is known liver disease or heavy alcohol use
  ▶ there is severe head injury
    ▶ tissue thromboplastin released, causing INR increase

Urinalysis

▶ obtain when there is back, flank, or abdominal trauma
▶ positive urine dipstick for blood corresponds to over 5 red blood cells per high-power field

Blood Type and Crossmatch

▶ order in case of
  ▶ significant traumatic mechanism of injury
  ▶ evidence of hemorrhagic shock
  ▶ operative intervention likely

Toxicology Screening

▶ may aid in explaining altered mental status
▶ can be helpful for public health epidemiology

Radiograph Utilization

Cervical Spine

General Principles

▶ high priority since subsequent procedures may depend on whether injury is present
▶ keep the neck immobilized until cervical spine injury is clinically or radiographically excluded
▶ can clear clinically for injury despite mechanism when all of the following conditions are met
  ▶ no cervical pain or tenderness
  ▶ no paresthesias or neurologic deficits
  ▶ normal mental status
    ▶ no altered sensorium from intoxicants or head injury
  ▶ no distracting pain
  ▶ the patient is at least 5 years old

Three Views (lateral, AP, odontoid)

▶ this series is the mainstay in most institutions to radiographically exclude cervical spine injuries
▶ order on all patients with mechanism for injury that cannot be clinically excluded
▶ the lateral must reveal the C7–T1 interface

Oblique Views

▶ order "trauma oblique" views as neck motion is required with conventional obliques
▶ helpful when the three-view series is suspicious of fracture or dislocation

Flexion–Extension Views

- ▶ order when suspicion of injury remains high despite negative nondynamic radiographs
    - ▶ for instance, pain out of proportion to cervical strain or focal spinous process tenderness
- ▶ helpful when severe degenerative arthritic changes make interpretation of nondynamic views difficult
- ▶ contraindicated when nondynamic radiographs are suspicious for fracture/ subluxation or new neurologic deficit is present
- ▶ cervical movement must be performed by a reliable patient (sober and co-operative), while a physician is in attendance, and halted at the point of pain or neurologic symptoms

Cervical Spine CT

- ▶ order when plain radiographs are suspicious of fracture or when all seven cervical vertebrae and the C7–T1 interface cannot be visualized
    - ▶ order 2–3 mm cuts one body above and below the suspicious area
    - ▶ contrast unnecessary
- ▶ unhelpful for diagnosing ligamentous injuries

Chest

- ▶ the initial radiograph is typically supine and AP when the patient is immobilized, hemodynamically unstable, or uncooperative
- ▶ whenever possible, obtain an upright radiograph to appreciate free intraabdominal air (pneumoperitoneum) and to achieve a more accurate assessment of mediastinal width
- ▶ radiopaque markers for penetrating wounds are often helpful

Abdomen

- ▶ useful to locate missiles or foreign bodies in penetrating trauma
- ▶ not indicated in blunt trauma

Pelvis

- ▶ obtain AP to screen for pelvis fracture when pain, tenderness, or mechanism of injury exists with an altered sensorium
- ▶ if fracture is seen or suspected, the following views may offer more information
    - ▶ inlet views are best for visualizing the posterior components

▶ outlet or tangential views are best for anterior components
▶ Judet views are best for visualizing the acetabulum

Thoracic or Lumbo-Sacral Spine

▶ obtain when pain, tenderness, neurologic findings, or mechanism of injury exist with an altered sensorium
▶ patients with back pain after a low-energy, hyperflexion/extension mechanism (e.g., typical MVC) but no direct trauma can be clinically excluded
▶ T12–L1 is the most common site of subluxation and fractures

Extremity Views

▶ obtain for areas of pain, swelling, or deformity
  ▶ include joints above and below known fractures
▶ portable C-arm fluoroscopy units are being used in place of conventional radiographs in some centers to increase efficiency

Reassessment

Continuous Monitoring

▶ perform frequent reassessments throughout the resuscitation
  ▶ continuous vital signs and pulse oximetry
  ▶ focused physical reexamination
    ▶ serial abdominal examinations are performed in patients with mechanism for intraabdominal injury since a normal initial examination does not exclude intraabdominal injury
    ▶ serial evaluation of neurologic status is necessary for all head and spinal injured patients
    ▶ check restrained extremities for adequate perfusion

Repeat Physical Survey

▶ also called the tertiary survey
▶ many perform another complete head-to-toe examination in severe trauma patients before the final disposition is made
  ▶ this practice helps avoid a missed diagnosis especially in the multiple blunt trauma patient because occult minor fractures are often uncovered after swelling and pain increase and when more attention can be paid to the less severe injuries
  ▶ this is ideally performed by on-coming physicians when change of shift occurs

Disposition

Transfer

General Principles

▶ comply with federal EMTALA (COBRA) regulations, hospital policy, and the wishes of the patient/family
▶ it is common for non-trauma centers to routinely transfer patients to trauma centers
  ▶ transfer should be initiated as soon as the needs of the patient exceed the capability of the center to address them
    ▷ do not delay transfer to perform tests or treatment
    ▷ do not delay tests or treatment while awaiting the transfer team
  ▶ there should be a preexisting understanding between centers and a defined procedure to properly and expeditiously arrange transfer

Procedure

▶ stabilize the patient as well as possible
▶ inform the patient/family of the reasons why transfer is necessary
▶ give physician-to-physician and nurse-to-nurse report to the trauma center
▶ send copies of the physician and nurse evaluation and progress notes, test results, radiographs, and transfer forms with the patient
  ▶ any paper report that becomes available after transfer should be faxed immediately
  ▶ routinely utilize an advanced life-support ambulance staffed by paramedics
  ▶ the nurse or physician may need to accompany an unstable patient
  ▶ some trauma centers dispatch their own transfer team to pick up unstable patients

Refusal of Treatment

General Principles

▶ only competent patients can leave against medical advice
  ▶ the patient must meet the following criteria
    ▷ an adult who is fully oriented and not under the influence of any mind-altering substances
    ▷ fully aware of the clinical impression and optimal management plan
    ▷ able to appreciate the potential consequences of refusing care
  ▶ in general the more life-threatening the medical problem the more confident the physician must be that the patient is fully competent to refuse necessary treatment

▶ carefully document the criteria by which competency was ascertained and that the patient was informed of the clinical impression, optimal management, and risks incurred by noncompliance with the plan

▶ have the patient sign a document attesting to the above

▶ provide good aftercare instructions, necessary medications, and referrals for outpatient care

▶ there is no reason to resent or mistreat a patient who leaves against medical advice

4

Airway Management

Intubation Indications

▶ in general, endotracheal intubation is required to relieve or prevent the following medical problems
  ▶ airway obstruction
  ▶ aspiration
  ▶ hypoventilation
  ▶ hypoxia
▶ the following are the most common indications for endotracheal intubation in the setting of emergency trauma
  ▶ cardiopulmonary arrest
  ▶ advanced hemorrhagic shock
  ▶ severe head injury
  ▶ significant airway burn
  ▶ penetrating face or neck wounds
  ▶ flail chest
  ▶ pulmonary contusion

Orotracheal Intubation

General Principles

▶ primary means of airway management
▶ use in-line stabilization of cervical spine when injury is possible based on mechanism
  ▶ maintain the existing relationship between head, neck, and shoulders
  ▶ do not apply traction
▶ requires rapid sequence induction or deep sedation
▶ anticipate difficult intubation when
  ▶ short muscular neck
  ▶ limited cervical movement
  ▶ distance from mentum to hyoid under 3 fingerbreadths
  ▶ unable to open mouth over 3 cm wide
  ▶ large tongue

Technique

▶ see p. 420

Patient Preparation Options

Rapid Sequence Induction

▶ advantages
  ▶ controlled situation
  ▶ dose and response remain constant
  ▶ technically less difficult intubation since no patient movement
  ▶ aspiration risk decreased using cricoid pressure
  ▶ with adequate preoxygenation, the duration of action of succinyl-choline is usually shorter than the time oxygen desaturation occurs due to apnea
▶ disadvantages
  ▶ paralysis is not immediately reversible
    ▷ with nondepolarizing agents, if unable to intubate or ventilate with a bag-valve-mask, an immediate life-threatening situation is created

Sedation Without Neuromuscular Blockade

▶ advantages
  ▶ spontaneous ventilation and airway reflexes preserved
  ▶ reversible
  ▶ large doses insure patient compliance
▶ disadvantages
  ▶ variable doses required
    ▷ large doses needed in some patients requiring more time for adequate sedation to be achieved
    ▷ must continually re-dose if the patient becomes agitated or combative during the procedure
  ▶ slower onset than paralysis
    ▷ more prolonged course of hypoxia
  ▶ patient motion makes intubation technically more difficult
  ▶ prolonged sedation after intubation with higher doses
  ▶ laryngospasm possible since laryngeal muscles not relaxed

Local Airway Anesthesia

▶ advantages
  ▶ ventilation remains intact
▶ disadvantages
  ▶ technically most difficult due to movement of mandible/closing of mouth/patient motion
  ▶ uncomfortable unless combined with sedation

▶ technique
  ▶ goal—block afferent sensory nerves in oral cavity, larynx, trachea
  ▶ agents
    ▷ Lidocaine—oral spray, viscous transtracheal spray, or aerosolized
    ▷ superior laryngeal nerve block

Rapid Sequence Induction

General Principles

▶ minimizes aspiration risk of administering induction and paralytic agents to the patient with a (presumed) full stomach
▶ the following sequence represents one specific method of inducing general anesthesia before intubation

1. preoxygenate with 100% oxygen
2. lidocaine 1.5 mg/kg (for severe hypertension/increased ICP)
3. defasciculating dose (optional): pancuronium 0.01 mg/kg, vecuronium 0.01 mg/kg, or rocuronium 0.06 mg/kg
4. atropine 0.02 mg/kg (for children <5 years old)
   WAIT 3 MINUTES
5. succinylcholine 1.5 mg/kg
6. sedative agent (optional): etomidate 0.3 mg/kg or thiopental 3–5 mg/kg
7. apply cricoid pressure
   WAIT 30 SECONDS
8. intubate as soon as patient is flaccid

Assemble necessary equipment, medications, and team members

1—Preoxygenation

▶ 100% oxygen for 3–5 min
▶ perform while setting up the intubation equipment
▶ use 100% nonrebreather oxygen mask
▶ allows for 3–5 min of apnea without significant desaturation
▶ do not ventilate patient (if unnecessary) prior to first intubation attempt
  ▶ ventilation with the BVM increases the likelihood of gastric insufflation and subsequent vomiting and aspiration

---

While preoxygenating for 3–5 minutes, consider the following drugs:

2—Lidocaine

▶ attenuates cardiovascular response to intubation and is used by many when increased ICP suspected

▶ reduces bronchospasm and airway reactivity following tracheal intubation
▶ dose is 1.5 mg/kg IVP

3—Fasciculation Prophylaxis (see Table 4–1)

▶ a low, "defasciculation dose" of a nondepolarizing paralytic may be given before succinylcholine
▶ many use in the setting of increased ICP and open globe injuries to temporize the pressure rise during fasciculations
▶ will increase risk of aspiration, so begin applying cricoid pressure earlier (see below)
▶ agents and doses (10% of minimum paralytic doses)
  ▶ rocuronium, 0.06 mg/kg
  ▶ vecuronium, 0.01 mg/kg
  ▶ pancuronium, 0.01 mg/kg

4—Atropine

▶ prevents reflex bradycardia in children under 5 years old caused by succinylcholine
▶ recommended when ketamine is used as induction agent to prevent hypersalivation
▶ dose
  ▶ adults 0.4 mg
  ▶ children 0.02 mg/kg (maximum 0.4 mg, minimum 0.1 mg)

> **Wait 2 minutes before the following induction agents if any of the above optional drugs were given**

5—Paralytic Agents (see Table 4–1)

▶ depolarizing
  ▶ succinylcholine 1.5 mg/kg IVP
    ▹ preferred agent
    ▹ onset in 30–60 s (after fasciculations terminate); duration 5 min
    ▹ contraindicated in patients with burns, crush injuries, or paralysis over 48 h and under 6 months old (since can cause severe hyperkalemia)
    ▹ consider nondepolarizing paralytic in patients with increased intracranial pressure or open globe injuries
▶ nondepolarizing
  ▶ rocuronium 0.6–1.2 mg/kg
    ▹ use when succinylcholine is contraindicated
    ▹ onset 1–2 min; duration 30 min
  ▶ vecuronium
    ▹ use when succinylcholine is contraindicated and rocuronium is unavailable
    ▹ high dose (0.25 mg/kg): onset in 1–2 min and duration 60–90 min
    ▹ low dose (0.1 mg/kg): onset in 3–5 min and duration 25–40 min

Table 4–1 Neuromuscular blocking drugs

Paralytic	Dosage (paralytic)	Dosage (fasciculation, prophylaxis)	Onset	Duration	Advantages	Disadvantages
succinylcholine	RSI: 1–2 mg/kg		<1 min	5 min	rapid onset short duration	increases ICP and intraocular pressure exacerbates existing hyperkalemia avoid in subacute (2–40 days) burn or crush injuries or paralysis
rocuronium	RSI: 0.6–1.2 mg/kg M: 0.6 mg/kg	0.06 mg/kg	2 min	30 min	quick onset	
vecuronium	RSI: 0.1 mg/kg (0.25 mg/kg for high dose) M: 0.1 mg/kg	0.01 mg/kg	3–5 min (1–2 min)	25–40 min (60–90 min)	preferred in renal insufficiency	
pancuronium	M: 0.1 mg/kg	0.01 mg/kg	3–5 min	45–60 min		long duration
atracurium	M: 0.4 mg/kg	0.04 mg/kg	3–5 min	20–35 min	metabolism not renal or hepatic dependent	histamine release—avoid in asthmatics hypotension with dose over 0.04 mg/kg

RSI = Rapid Sequence Induction, M = Maintenance of Paralysis

6—Sedation (see Table 4–2)

▶ since sedative agents are more rapid-acting
  ▶ administer sedative immediately after paralytic agent to achieve onset of the paralysis and sedation simultaneously and reduce aspiration risk
  ▶ alternatively, administer sedative immediately before paralytic agent to ensure there is no chance of event recall
▶ preferred agent
  ▶ etomidate (Amidate) 0.3 mg/kg (range of 0.2–0.6 mg/kg) IVP
    ▹ GABA-like, nonnarcotic, nonbarbiturate hypnotic
    ▹ onset under 60 s; duration 3–5 min
    ▹ minimal hemodynamic effects
    ▹ does not cause histamine release or bronchospasm
    ▹ short-term adrenal suppression
▶ alternative agents
  ▶ midazolam (Versed) 0.1–0.3 mg/kg IVP
    ▹ benzodiazepine
    ▹ onset 1–2 min; duration 1–2 h
    ▹ lower dose in elderly
    ▹ increase dose in alcoholics
  ▶ thiopental sodium (Pentothal) 3–5 mg/kg IVP
    ▹ barbiturate
    ▹ onset 20–40 s; duration 5–10 min
    ▹ best agent with suspected increased intracranial pressure
    ▹ lower dose in elderly and hypotensive patients
    ▹ withhold if severely hypotensive/hypovolemic
  ▶ ketamine (Ketalar) 1–2 mg/kg IVP
    ▹ dissociative anesthetic
    ▹ onset 60 s; duration 15 min
    ▹ minimal respiratory depression and protective airway reflexes maintained
    ▹ may raise blood pressure, so often used in hypotensive patients and contraindicated when increased ICP
    ▹ bronchodilator, so excellent choice in status asthmaticus

7—Cricoid Pressure (Sellick Maneuver)

▶ initiate after sedative or paralytic administered to prevent passive regurgitation and subsequent aspiration since posterior aspect of cricoid occludes the esophagus behind it
▶ facilitates intubation by moving larynx into view
  ▶ used in conjunction with the "BURP" procedure, which means applying backward (posterior), upward, rightward pressure to achieve an ideal view
▶ release after successful intubation and endotracheal (ET) cuff inflated
  ▶ suction immediately if any regurgitation of gastric contents

Table 4-2 Sedative and induction agents

Sedative	Dosage	Onset	Duration	Advantages	Disadvantages
etomidate	0.2–0.6 mg/kg	< 60 s	3–5 min	maintains BP better than thiopental no histamine release short duration, nonnarcotic	myoclonic movements during induction
thiopental	3–5 mg/kg	20–40 s	5–10 min	use when increase ICP rapid onset profound sedation	exacerbates hypotension—lower dose or avoid
ketamine	1–2 mg/kg	30–60 s	15 min	bronchodilator, maintains BP maintains airways reflexes	increases ICP and exacerbates hypertension pretreat with atropine 0.4 mg to prevent hypersalivation
midazolam	induction: 0.1–0.3 mk/kg sedation (titrate): 0.02–0.04 mg/kg	2 min	1–2 h	excellent amnestic properties rapid onset benzodiazepine reverse with flumazenil 0.2 mg IVP (up to 1 mg)	exacerbates hypotension lower dose when used with opiates
fentanyl	induction: 2–10 mcg/kg sedation (titrate): 2–4 mcg/mg	< 60 s	30–60 min	rapid onset reversible with naloxone	exacerbates hypotension skeletal muscle rigidity occurs rarely lower dose when used with benzodiazepine

> **While holding cricoid pressure, wait until the patient becomes flaccid**

8—Intubate

▶ confirm correct position of ETT by auscultation, radiograph, or capnometry
▶ if intubation is unsuccessful after attempting for 60 s, then ventilate with bag-valve-mask and try again
▶ if unable to intubate or ventilate after paralysis, prepare for surgical airway or alternate technique

Sedative-Aided Intubation

General Principles

▶ preferred when anatomically difficult oral intubation is anticipated or when bag-valve-mask ventilation may be technically difficult
▶ rapid-onset, short-duration agents preferred (see Table 4–2)

Opiates

▶ advantages
  ▶ rapid-onset
  ▶ potent analgesia and significant sedation
  ▶ reversible
    ▹ use 0.04–0.4 mg of naloxone in incremental doses
▶ general principles
  ▶ higher dose when used as sole agent for sedation and in opiate users
  ▶ lower dose with concomitant benzodiazepine use
  ▶ cautions include hypoventilation, hypotension, bradycardia, and muscle rigidity
▶ fentanyl (Sublimaze) 2–4 mcg/kg IVP
  ▶ onset 45 s; duration 30–60 min
▶ alfentanil (Alfenta) 20–40 mcg/kg IVP
  ▶ onset 30 s; duration 10 min
  ▶ superior to fentanyl since faster onset and shorter duration

Benzodiazepines

▶ general principles
  ▶ amnestic and sedative properties
  ▶ muscle relaxant

- ▹ higher doses needed in chronic alcohol abusers
- ▹ reversible with flumazenil 0.2 mg IVP (to max. 1 mg)
  - ▹ use with caution—may induce seizures
- ▶ midazolam (Versed) 0.1–0.3 mg/kg IVP is used most commonly
  - ▹ onset 1–2 min; duration 30–120 min
  - ▹ lower dose in elderly
  - ▹ increase dose in alcoholics

Ketamine

- ▶ ketamine (Ketalar) 1–2 mg/kg IVP
  - ▹ dissociative anesthetic
  - ▹ onset 60 s; duration 15 min
  - ▹ less respiratory depression and protective airway reflexes maintained
  - ▹ may raise blood pressure, so often used in hypotensive patients and contraindicated when ICP is increased
  - ▹ bronchodilator, so would be excellent choice in status asthmaticus

Nasotracheal Intubation

Advantages

- ▶ consider in spontaneously breathing patient when technically difficult oro-tracheal intubation is anticipated
  - ▹ with cervical spine injury, cervical spine remains fully immobilized
  - ▹ with mandibular injury, head and jaw motion unnecessary for intubation
  - ▹ avoids paralysis or excessive sedation of patient
- ▶ facilitates surgery to repair intraoral trauma

Technique

- ▶ see p. 425

Contraindications

- ▶ apnea
- ▶ midface trauma
- ▶ basilar skull fracture or increased ICP suspected
- ▶ coagulopathy
  - ▹ coumadin administration
  - ▹ cirrhosis
  - ▹ hemophilia

Alternative Techniques

Fiberoptic Intubation

General Principles

▶ reliable method only with experienced operator
▶ difficult when blood and secretions are present
▶ often impractical when immediate airway is necessary
  ▶ equipment must be set up
  ▶ generally takes more time to secure airway than by conventional means

Indications

▶ restricted cervical spine motion
  ▶ secondary to fracture or subluxation
▶ limited ability to open mouth
▶ severe facial fractures
▶ penetrating neck trauma with airway distortion
▶ history of prior intubation difficulty

Retrograde Guidewire

General Principles

▶ consider as an alternative to cricothyrotomy and translaryngeal jet ventilation
▶ neck motion unnecessary

Indications

▶ failure to rapidly achieve endotracheal intubation
▶ severe maxillofacial trauma where nasotracheal intubation is contraindicated and orotracheal intubation is impeded by intraoral bleeding

Technique

▶ see p. 434

Contraindications

▶ coagulopathy
▶ expanding hematoma over cricothyroid membrane
▶ inability to open mouth for guidewire retrieval

Digital Intubation

General Principles

▶ patient must be deeply sedated or paralyzed

Indications

▶ when more conventional methods have failed
▶ when upper airway is obscured by blood or secretions
▶ short neck
▶ when endotracheal equipment is missing or fails

Technique

▶ see p. 436

Laryngeal Mask Airway

General Principles

▶ special mask sits in the hypopharynx and increases likelihood of BVM ventilation
▶ see p. 427 for technique

Esophageal–Tracheal Combitube

General Principles

▶ dual-lumen tube can pass blindly into the esophagus or the trachea and allow BVM ventilation via ports from one lumen or the other (Figure 4–1)

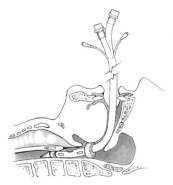

Figure 4–1

Surgical Airways

Cricothyrotomy

General Principles

▶ preferred over tracheostomy for immediate surgical airway because faster, technically less difficult, and fewer complications
▶ does not require cervical spine movement

Indications

▶ unable to obtain an airway by alternate means generally due to
  ▶ anatomical difficulty
  ▶ distortion due to injury
  ▶ foreign body lodged in upper airway
  ▶ intraoral hemorrhage
  ▶ edema from thermal or chemical burn

Technique

▶ see p. 428

Contraindications

▶ age under 5–10 years (depending on child's size)
▶ significant injury to larynx or cricoid cartilage
▶ tracheal transection
▶ preexisting laryngeal pathology
▶ expanding anterior neck hematoma

Tracheostomy

Indications

▶ younger pediatric patients requiring a surgical airway
▶ laryngeal fracture
▶ tracheal transection
▶ expanding hematoma over cricothyroid membrane
▶ laryngeal foreign body

Technique

▶ see p. 430

Contraindication

▶ expanding anterior neck hematoma

Percutaneous Transtracheal Jet Insufflation

General Principles

▶ allows oxygen delivery
▶ temporizing procedure in children under 5 years old who cannot be endotracheally intubated while awaiting tracheostomy
▶ positive-pressure jet of oxygen forced through catheter placed through cricothyroid membrane with an insufflation:exhalation ratio of 1:3

Indications

▶ failure to rapidly achieve endotracheal intubation

Technique

▶ see p. 432

Contraindications

▶ total obstruction of airway above the vocal cords
▶ tracheal transection
▶ damage to cricoid cartilage or larynx

Advantages over Surgical Airway

▶ more rapidly performed (when equipment is immediately available)
▶ less bleeding
▶ smaller scar

Disadvantages

▶ aspiration still possible
▶ typically inadequate ventilation
▶ barotrauma can occur including subcutaneous emphysema, pneumothorax, and pneumomediastinum

Special Situations

Head Injury

General Principles

▶ gagging provoked by laryngoscopy causes increased ICP
▶ succinylcholine does not increase ICP when used in conjunction with
  ▶ adequate sedation
  ▶ pretreatment dose of a nondepolarizing neuromuscular blocking agent

Technique

▶ rapid sequence induction with orotracheal intubation recommended with the following adjuncts
▶ give lidocaine 1.5 mg/kg IVP at 3 min preintubation
▶ give paralytic agent
  ▶ if succinylcholine is used, give defasciculating dose of nondepolarizing agent at 2 min preintubation (see Table 4–1, p. 43)
▶ immediately follow with adequate dose of thiopental sodium (Pentothal)
  ▶ 3–5 mg/kg IVP
  ▶ onset 20–40 s and duration 5–10 min
  ▶ use lower dose in elderly or hypotensive patients(1–2 mg/ks)

Penetrating Neck Injury

General Principles

▶ airway distortion or disruption must be expected and airway control maintained
  ▶ expanding hematoma can compress trachea or hypopharynx
  ▶ distorted anatomy may be delayed while hematoma accumulates, making airway management progressively more difficult
▶ prophylactic airway intervention is advised for asymptomatic patients at high risk to develop airway compromise
  ▶ patients with neck gunshot wounds should be intubated because of propensity for collateral injuries, progressive swelling due to blast effect, and cavitation
  ▶ intubate whenever there is any indication of respiratory distress or evidence of an expanding hematoma
▶ have two suction devices available since bleeding can be brisk
▶ avoid nasotracheal intubation if airway is penetrated
  ▶ may dislodge clot and cause hemorrhage or result in false passage
▶ cervical spine immobilization
  ▶ less of concern than with blunt trauma

- ▶ in penetrating trauma with normal neurologic examination, an unstable cervical spine is unlikely
  - ▷ under emergent conditions it is permissible to manipulate the neck in this setting to facilitate orotracheal intubation
- ▶ the specific airway management technique depends on the mechanism and clinical findings

Techniques

- ▶ *with gunshot wound to neck and no airway compromise*
  - ▶ perform prophylactic orotracheal intubation using rapid sequence induction technique
- ▶ *with penetrating wound to neck and minimal signs of airway compromise when bag-valve-mask ventilation is anticipated without difficulty*
  - ▶ use rapid sequence induction and orotracheal intubation
- ▶ *with penetrating wound to neck and moderate to severe airway distortion, loss of normal muscle tone with paralysis can complicate oral intubation and make bag-valve-mask difficult or impossible*
  - ▶ use topical airway anesthesia in conjunction with reversible sedation
  - ▶ consider awake fiberoptic intubation
  - ▶ induce a reversible state of general anesthesia with high doses of opiates and benzodiazepines
    - ▷ use fentanyl 5–10 mcg/kg or alfentanil 40 mcg/kg
    - ▷ combine with midazolam 0.05 mg/kg
  - ▶ consider ketamine if above methods fail
    - ▷ patient maintains airway protective reflexes
    - ▷ minimal respiratory depression when given slowly
  - ▶ attempt nasotracheal intubation only if wound has not penetrated the airway
  - ▶ prepare for surgical airway if intubation is unsuccessful
- ▶ *with expanding hematoma over anterior neck*
  - ▶ avoid paralytic agents since bag-valve-mask may be difficult
  - ▶ use judicious amounts of topical airway anesthesia, adequate yet reversible sedation, and attempt oral intubation
    - ▷ if oral intubation is unsuccessful, reverse sedative agent(s)
  - ▶ fiberoptic intubation is ideal when equipment and skilled personnel are immediately available
  - ▶ retrograde guidewire intubation is contraindicated since it may exacerbate bleeding
  - ▶ attempt nasotracheal intubation if the wound has not penetrated the airway
  - ▶ percutaneous translaryngeal jet ventilation can temporize the situation
    - ▷ performed by placing cannula in trachea above sternal notch if hematoma precludes placement through cricothyroid membrane
  - ▶ prepare for difficult cricothyrotomy or tracheotomy
    - ▷ surgical airway intervention is difficult because of distorted anatomy and may result in severe hemorrhage

▶ *with suspected (partial or complete) transection of trachea near suprasternal notch*
  ▶ avoid endotracheal intubation attempt since it may complete transection and push proximal segment into chest
  ▶ gentle fiberoptic intubation is permissible when equipment and skilled personnel are immediately available
  ▶ formal tracheostomy is preferred
  ▶ while it may be possible to pass a tracheostomy tube through the wound, this greatly increases risk of completing transection and pushing proximal segment into chest
  ▶ if trachea retracts into chest, prepare for emergency median sternotomy to retrieve proximal segment
▶ *with respiratory arrest*
  ▶ begin bag-valve-mask ventilation
  ▶ attempt orotracheal intubation
  ▶ if unsuccessful, proceed with surgical airway

Potential Cervical Spine Injury

General Principles

▶ assume cervical spine injury until radiographically excluded
▶ lateral radiograph alone misses about 15% of cervical injuries

Techniques

▶ orotracheal intubation with in-line cervical stabilization
  ▶ maintain existing relationship between the head–neck–shoulders
  ▶ axial traction should not be used since may cause disruption of spinal cord
▶ blind nasotracheal intubation with topical anesthesia and intravenous sedation
  ▶ cervical spine immobilization maintained
  ▶ preferred when anatomically difficult orotracheal intubation is anticipated
▶ consider awake fiberoptic intubation when unstable cervical spine injury is likely
▶ perform cricothyrotomy if the aforementioned means are unsuccessful

Hypotensive Patient

General Principles

▶ immediate resuscitation critical
▶ expeditious airway control optimal

Technique

▶ many sedative agents lower blood pressure
  ▶ administer succinylcholine without sedative agent when the patient is significantly hypotensive and already "self-sedated" due to cerebral hypoperfusion
  ▶ etomidate or ketamine are excellent agents for sedation of moderately hypotensive patients since they have minimal hemodynamic effects

Penetrating Globe Injury

General Principles

▶ use nondepolarizing agents over succinylcholine if no difficulty is anticipated with intubation
  ▶ succinylcholine-induced fasciculations may increase in intraocular pressure
  ▶ in emergent situations, reduced risk of aspiration supersedes increased intraocular pressure concerns

Burn Injury

General Principles

▶ aggressive airway management is essential
  ▶ significant upper airway edema or bronchospasm can develop when mucosal burns or carbonaceous sputum are present
  ▶ pneumonitis and noncardiogenic pulmonary edema may cause hypoxia
  ▶ treat concurrent carbon monoxide or cyanide inhalation
▶ indications for endotracheal intubation
  ▶ airway mucous membrane burns
  ▶ significant inhalation injury
  ▶ dyspnea or stridor
  ▶ airway edema

Technique

▶ orotracheal intubation
  ▶ may be technically difficult because of airway swelling/distortion and thick, carbonaceous sputum
  ▶ consider awake fiberoptic intubation
  ▶ succinylcholine
    ▶ associated with mild hyperkalemia in the acutely burned patient but not contraindicated
    ▶ serious potassium elevation occurs when given to patients with significant burns between 2 days and 6 weeks old

▶ nasotracheal intubation
  ▷ avoid if nasopharyngeal burns
▶ cricothyrotomy
  ▷ perform if other methods fail

Pediatric Intubation

Key Differences

▶ head size
  ▷ proportionately larger in children
  ▷ child normally in "sniffing position" when supine
    ▹ no need to elevate the occiput during orotracheal intubation
▶ tongue
  ▷ proportionately larger in children
  ▷ use laryngoscope blade to move tongue aside
▶ epiglottis
  ▷ floppy, shorter, and more "U-shaped" in children
  ▷ use straight blade in children under 8 years old to lift the epiglottis
▶ airway diameter
  ▷ in children, smallest at cricoid ring
  ▷ natural seal occurs with the appropriate size tube
  ▷ use uncuffed ET tubes in children under 10 years old
    ▹ cuffed tubes cause tracheal stenosis

Technique

▶ straight blade recommended in young children
  ▷ size 0—premature infants
  ▷ size 1—under 2 years old
  ▷ size 2—over 2 years old
▶ child is already in "sniffing position" when supine

Tube Size

▶ estimated size
  ▷ tube size = (16 + age)/4
  ▷ same caliber as child's little fingernail width
▶ have available at least one size larger and one smaller than that estimated

5

Shock

General Principles

▶ inadequate tissue perfusion results from decreased or maldistributed cardiac output from a variety of etiologies
▶ clinical symptoms relate to the end organs affected
▶ uncompensated shock causes hypoperfusion of end organs and results in several possible clinical events
  ▶ decreased CNS perfusion causes agitation or altered mental status
  ▶ selective vasoconstriction occurs in kidneys, skin, gut, and muscles
  ▶ myocardial ischemia can occur in individuals with underlying coronary artery disease
  ▶ hypoventilation and hypoxia can occur in individuals with underlying pulmonary disease
  ▶ anaerobic metabolism is initiated
  ▶ disseminated intravascular coagulation (DIC) may develop
▶ "terminal shock" occurs when irreversible damage has occurred to vital organs and leads to death within hours to days

Hemorrhagic

General Principles

▶ this type accounts for the overwhelming majority of trauma patients in shock
▶ once hemorrhagic shock is appreciated it is essential to determine and control the site of hemorrhage
▶ clinical findings in hemorrhagic shock are due to compensatory mechanisms
  ▶ excess sympathetic nervous system stimulation
  ▶ diminished peripheral and renal blood flow
▶ pulses that are palpable correlate with minimum SBP levels
  ▶ carotid, 60 mm Hg
  ▶ femoral, 70 mm Hg
  ▶ radial, 80 mm Hg
  ▶ pedal, 100 mm Hg

▶ the classification system of hemorrhagic shock relates to varying percentages of blood volume lost (Table 5–1)

  ▶ adult blood volume (in liters) is estimated by 7% of ideal body weight (in kg)

    ▷ for instance, a 70 kg person (average-size adult male) has a blood volume of about 5 liters

Table 5–1 Summary of Hemorrhagic Shock Classes

	I	II	III	IV
Blood loss (ml, in a 70 kg adult)	< 15% (< 750)	> 15% (750–1500)	> 30% (1500–2000)	> 40% (> 2000)
HR (bpm)	< 100	> 100	> 120	> 140
SBP (mmHg)	Normal	Normal	< 90	< 70
Capillary refill (s)	< 1	1–2	> 2	Absent
RR (/min)	< 20	20–30	30–40	> 40
Mental status	Appropriate	Anxious or giddy	Confused or inappropriate	Comatose
Urine output (ml/h)	> 30	20–30	5–15	Negligible

Class I

▶ under 15% blood loss (under 750 ml in average adult males)

▶ this degree of blood loss is well compensated by reduced blood flow to the kidneys, skin, gut, and muscles

▶ typical clinical findings include

  ▶ vital signs

    ▷ normal SBP

    ▷ normal HR

    ▷ orthostatic change in SBP or HR may be appreciated

    ▷ normal RR

  ▶ skin

    ▷ normal

  ▶ mental status

    ▷ normal

  ▶ urine output

    ▷ over 30 ml/h

  ▶ objective physical findings are scarce in early hemorrhagic shock due to adaptive mechanisms whereby the heart and brain can receive up to a fourfold increase in blood flow during this phase

▶ when hemorrhage is controlled, resuscitate with isotonic crystalloid using the "3:1" rule whereby volume of crystalloid replacement is triple the estimated blood loss

Class II

▶ over 15% blood loss (over 750 ml in average adult males)
▶ typical clinical findings
  ▶ vital signs
    ▷ normal SBP, increased DBP, decreased pulse pressure
    ▷ HR over 100
    ▷ RR over 20
  ▶ skin
    ▷ slightly delayed capillary refill (1–2 s)
  ▶ mental status
    ▷ anxious appearing
  ▶ urine output
    ▷ 20–30 ml/h
▶ when hemorrhage is controlled, resuscitate with crystalloid using the "3:1 rule"

Class III

▶ over 30% blood loss (over 1500 ml in average adult males)
▶ typical clinical findings
  ▶ vital signs
    ▷ SBP under 90 mm Hg
    ▷ HR over 120
    ▷ RR over 30
  ▶ mental status
    ▷ anxious or confused
  ▶ skin
    ▷ capillary refill delayed over 2 s
  ▶ urine output
    ▷ 5–15 ml/h
▶ start crystalloid bolus and anticipate the need for a blood transfusion
  ▶ if intracavitary bleeding not yet controlled
    ▷ begin blood transfusion immediately
    ▷ consider "permissive hypotension" (see p. 63) by maintaining the SBP between 80 and 90 mm Hg, using a ratio of 1.5 liters crystalloid for each unit of blood

Class IV

▶ over 40% blood loss (2000 ml in average adult males)
▶ typical clinical findings
  ▶ mental status
    ▷ combative or comatose

- ▶ vital signs
  - ▹ SBP under 70 mm Hg
  - ▹ HR over 140
  - ▹ RR over 35
- ▶ skin
  - ▹ cool, diaphoretic
  - ▹ mottled, ashen, gray, pale
  - ▹ capillary refill absent
- ▶ urine output
  - ▹ negligible
- ▶ start rapid crystalloid bolus and blood transfusion
  - ▶ if intracavitary bleeding not yet controlled
    - ▹ consider "permissive hypotension" (see p. 63) by maintaining the SBP between 80 and 90 mm Hg using a ratio of 1.5 liters crystalloid for each unit of blood

Laboratory Findings

Hemodilution

- ▶ passive or compensatory hemodilution
  - ▶ occurs with translocation of interstitial fluid from the intracellular to the intravascular space
  - ▶ takes several hours
    - ▹ two-thirds of circulating plasma volume can be restored in 6 h
    - ▹ fluid mobilization rate varies from 100 to 1000 ml/h
- ▶ active hemodilution due to fluid resuscitation is immediate
  - ▶ expect to drop the hematocrit approximately 3 points for each liter of crystalloid administered to a hypovolemic patient
- ▶ hematocrit (or hemoglobin) measurement
  - ▶ a singular value is important in establishing a baseline but unhelpful in determining occult hemorrhagic shock soon after injury
    - ▹ anemia may be a preexisting condition
  - ▶ serial hematocrit measurement over several hours are very helpful

Base Deficit

- ▶ quantifies the degree of metabolic acidosis due to an elevation in serum lactate from anaerobic cellular metabolism that occurs with shock
  - ▶ amplitude correlates directly with shock severity
- ▶ the presence of a base deficit under −7 mmol/L suggests consideration of fluid resuscitation even if clinical signs of shock are absent

Humoral Compensatory Response

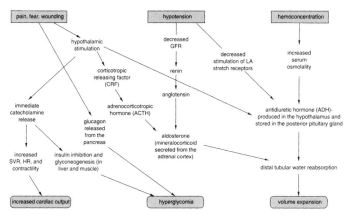

<u>Cardiogenic</u>

General Principles

▶ the key to this diagnosis is appreciating an elevated central venous pressure (over 20 mm Hg) in the setting of hypotension
   ▶ usually evidenced by jugular venous distension while sitting up or the presence of a prominent S3 heart sound

Pathophysiology

Causes

▶ blunt myocardial injury
   ▶ rare cause of cardiogenic shock
▶ preexisting cardiac dysfunction is the most common cause
▶ myocardial infarction
   ▶ may have precipitated a traumatic injury
      ▶ consider syncope or seizure when there is an unclear cause of single motor vehicle collisions and in unexplained falls
▶ myocardial ischemia due to coronary artery hypoperfusion
   ▶ occurs in those with underlying coronary artery disease in hemorrhagic shock or even with the physical/emotional stress of trauma

Mechanics

▶ inadequate pumping (loss of inotropy)
  ▶ causes
    ▹ hemorrhagic shock with preexisting cardiac dysfunction
    ▹ concurrent coronary ischemia
    ▹ contused myocardium with loss of contractility
▶ cardiac inflow obstruction
  ▶ causes
    ▹ tension pneumothorax causing resistance to venous return
    ▹ pericardial tamponade causing resistance to diastole (filling phase)

Treatment

▶ pump failure
  ▶ first ensure adequate volume by measuring central venous pressure or pulmonary artery pressures
  ▶ then consider the following
    ▹ inotropes and vasopressors
    ▹ mechanical ventilation to reduce myocardial workload
    ▹ placement of an intraaortic balloon pump
▶ tension pneumothorax is treated with immediate needle decompression followed by tube thoracostomy
▶ pericardial tamponade is treated with pericardiocentesis/pericardotomy

Neurogenic

General Principles

▶ neurogenic shock should not be confused with spinal shock: the latter refers to neuropraxia associated with incomplete spinal cord injuries
▶ neurogenic shock involves the loss of systemic vascular resistance (sympathetic tone) due to disruption of descending autonomic pathways in cervical and high thoracic spinal cord injuries, which results in significant hypotension
  ▶ skin signs of shock are not evident since loss of vasomotor tone causes peripheral vasodilation
  ▶ loss of sympathetic innervation also causes absence of compensatory tachycardia and provides a diagnostic clue
▶ this state is transient and resolves within a week

Treatment

▶ volume replacement
  ▶ adequacy best judged by central venous pressure measurement
▶ alpha-1 vasopressors
  ▶ high dose dopamine
  ▶ epinephrine
  ▶ ephedrine

6

Fluids

Resuscitation Goals

▶ when there is no intracavitary bleeding or after it has been controlled the goals are
  ▶ normal vital signs
  ▶ adequate urine output
    ▹ over 0.5 ml/kg/h in adults
    ▹ over 1 ml/kg/h in children under 10 years old
    ▹ over 2 ml/kg/h in children under 1 year old
  ▶ no base deficit
  ▶ normal central venous pressure
    ▹ can use large-bore peripheral IV catheter
    ▹ normal is 4–8 cm H_2O and can still be associated with class I or II shock
▶ while the classification for hemorrhagic shock is based on presumed blood loss, fluid resuscitation is primarily by physiologic response and secondarily by presumed or estimated blood loss
▶ when intracavitary bleeding is not yet controlled the goal is "permissive hypotension"
  ▶ aggressive fluid resuscitation in the prehospital and hospital environments has been proven deleterious when hemorrhage remains uncontrolled since
    ▹ elevated pressure dislodges or prevents formation of protective thrombus
    ▹ dilution lowers blood viscosity, which decreases resistance to flow around an incomplete thrombus
    ▹ dilution causes progressive anemia and loss of coagulation factors
  ▶ the goal is to maintain SBP 80–90 mm Hg
  ▶ maintain multiple, large-bore IV catheters so that rapid fluid resuscitation can begin immediately if the patient becomes pulseless
  ▶ "permissive hypotension" is inappropriate in patients with severe head injuries since cerebral perfusion pressure must be optimized

Crystalloid

General Principles

▶ refers to isotonic salt solutions
▶ inexpensive
▶ nonantigenic

Types

▶ normal saline (0.9%)
  ▶ least expensive
  ▶ compatible with blood products
  ▶ risk for hyperchloremic metabolic acidosis with massive infusion
▶ lactated Ringer's (LR) solution
  ▶ more expensive
  ▶ incompatible with blood products

Utilization in Hemorrhagic Shock

▶ use 3 ml crystalloid for every ml of blood loss
  ▶ known as the "3:1 rule"
▶ bolus 1 liter increments in adults
  ▶ reduce to 250–500 ml in the elderly and those with a suspected cardiomyopathy
    ▶ consider early invasive monitoring to prevent fluid overload
▶ bolus 20 ml/kg increments in children
▶ reassess the patient after each fluid bolus
▶ after 3 boluses, if the patient remains hemodynamically unstable
  ▶ begin transfusing blood
  ▶ aggressively identify the source of blood loss
  ▶ consider immediate transfer to the operating room if intraabdominal hemorrhage is suspected
▶ the inability to correct hypotension within 15 minutes requires consideration of immediate operative hemorrhage control

Other Adjuncts

Nonblood Colloids

General Principles

▶ effective volume expanders but no proven benefit over crystalloid

▶ detrimental effects shown with regard to myocardial, renal, and respiratory function

Types

▶ albumin
▶ dextrans
▶ hetastarch

Hypertonic Saline

General Principles

▶ used in trauma research protocols at the present
▶ causes rapid expansion of the intravascular volume far beyond the amount infused
  ▶ free water moves from the intracellular space to the hyperosmolar plasma
▶ adverse effects include
  ▶ pulmonary edema
  ▶ hypernatremia
  ▶ hyperosmolar coma

Blood Products

General Principles

▶ to prolong storage time an acid–citrate–dextrose solution is added to blood
  ▶ citrate is responsible for a decline in 2,3-diphosphoglycerate, which increases hemoglobin oxygen affinity ("left shift"), and impairs oxygen delivery for about 24 h after the transfusion
▶ one unit of packed red blood cells (PRBCs) is about 250 ml with a hematocrit of 70%
▶ whole blood (before plasma and platelets are separated) is ideal
  ▶ generally unavailable for use in trauma

Uncrossmatched Blood

▶ type O, Rh-negative is the "universal donor"
  ▶ does not react with the major antigens, Rh, A, or B
  ▶ 50% of the population is type O
▶ use Rh-negative blood in premenopausal women to prevent Rh sensitization

▶ transfuse immediately when class III or IV shock is evident and intracavitary bleeding not yet controlled
  ▸ do not wait for a type-specific or crossmatched product
▶ each unit raises the hematocrit by 3% if hemorrhage is controlled
  ▸ give children PRBCs in 10 ml/kg increments

Type-Specific Blood

▶ expect availability within 20 min
▶ screens for the major antigens (A, B, O, Rh)

Crossmatched Blood

▶ expect availability within 40 min
▶ screens more specifically to prevent even minor antigenic reactions by in vitro mixing and testing of the patient and donor blood samples

Autologous Blood

General Principles

▶ commonly known as autotransfusion
▶ blood collected from patient's body cavity into collection bag containing citrate solution is later reinfused through a filter into same patient
  ▸ usually from large hemothoraces via a chest tube
▶ recovery of at least 500 ml makes this procedure practical
▶ in most cases autotransfusion represents 25% of the blood the patient will receive and thus the risks of banked blood are reduced but not eliminated

Advantages

▶ immediately available and already warm
▶ no risk of transmitting viral hepatitis or HIV
▶ no risk of transfusion reaction

Disadvantages

▶ rare risk of air embolism
▶ risk of contamination by intestinal contents
  ▸ often when intrathoracic blood used in a patient with a bowel injury and an undetected diaphragm rupture

Indications for Blood Transfusion

Physiologic Criteria

▶ transfuse patients presenting in class III or IV shock immediately
  ▶ when intracavitary bleeding not yet controlled
  ▶ otherwise, after 3 liters of crystalloid

Hematocrit

▶ maintain the hematocrit above 20% in all trauma patients
▶ maintain the hematocrit above 30% to maximize the oxygen-carrying capacity in the following situations
  ▶ elderly patient
  ▶ serious underlying cardiac or pulmonary disease
  ▶ aggressive, on-going, uncontrolled bleeding

Transfusion Risks

Coagulopathy

Pathophysiology

▶ nearly 90% of the coagulation factors (within plasma) and 70% of the platelets are removed from whole blood to make PRBCs
▶ hypothermia causes prolonged clotting times and thrombocytopenia
▶ DIC can complicate trauma though rare in the first hour of treatment
▶ 25% with severe head injury have associated coagulopathy

Prevention

▶ give 1 U fresh frozen plasma (FFP) for every 5 U PRBCs after the first 5 U PRBCs
▶ give 10 U platelets if bleeding (or oozing) and the count is under 50,000/mm^3
▶ warm blood and fluids to prevent hypothermia and DIC

Hypothermia

Pathophysiology

▶ blood is stored at 4°C and multiple transfusions not warmed to body temperature cause hypothermia
▶ hypothermia itself increases coagulopathy

Prevention

▶ measure the core temperature of all patients requiring vigorous resuscitation
▶ use warmed fluids and blood whenever possible
▶ cover the patient with blankets as soon as the secondary survey is complete

Incompatibility Reactions

Acute Intravascular Hemolysis

▶ rare occurrence due to ABO incompatibility
▶ 80% due to clerical errors involving misidentification of the sample or patient
▶ potentially fatal
▶ clinical signs develop within 15 minutes and are proportional to the amount of blood transfused
  ▶ fever, chills, anxiety, shock, flank pain, chest pain and dyspnea
  ▶ progressive anemia, renal failure, jaundice
  ▶ disseminated intravascular coagulation (DIC)
▶ when suspected
  ▶ stop the transfusion immediately
  ▶ infuse crystalloid to maintain urine flow and adequate blood pressure
  ▶ consider diuretics and renal dose dopamine to increase GFR
  ▶ follow coagulation laboratory parameters closely
  ▶ if DIC develops, treat with heparin

Acute Extravascular Hemolysis

▶ due to antibodies other than ABO and also rare
▶ usually benign
▶ clinical signs include
  ▶ fever, progressive anemia, increase in bilirubin
  ▶ positive direct antiglobulin test
  ▶ disseminated intravascular coagulation (DIC)
▶ when suspected
  ▶ stop the transfusion immediately
  ▶ treat with acetaminophen

Nonhemolytic Febrile Reactions

▶ common with an incidence of up to 5% of all transfusions
▶ due to white cell or platelet antibodies
▶ clinical signs include fever, chills, headache, myalgias, nausea, and vomiting
▶ treat with acetaminophen
▶ stop the transfusion immediately
▶ after two such reactions use leukocyte-poor products

Allergic and Anaphylactic-like Reactions

▶ clinical signs include
   ▹ fever
   ▹ urticaria, bronchospasm, and anaphylaxis
   ▹ noncardiogenic pulmonary edema

Treatment

▶ treat like an allergic reaction
   ▹ epinephrine (if bronchospasm or anaphylaxis)
   ▹ antihistamines and steroids
   ▹ stop the transfusion immediately

Citrate Toxicity

▶ hypocalcemia is common due to citrate toxicity
▶ measure ionized calcium serially after multiple-unit blood transfusions
▶ supplement calcium as needed
   ▹ if the ionized calcium cannot be measured, give 1 g calcium gluconate for every 4 U PRBCs transfused

Infections

Viral Hepatitis

▶ Hepatitis B (HBV)
   ▹ risk is currently 1 in 66,000 with donor screening
▶ Hepatitis C (HCV)
   ▹ formerly called "non-A, non-B"
   ▹ accounted for 90% of hepatitis transmitted by transfusion before screen became available in 1992
   ▹ 30% develop chronic active hepatitis and 10% develop cirrhosis
   ▹ risk is currently 1 in 100,000 with donor screening
▶ Hepatitis D (HDV)
   ▹ causes infection only in the presence of HBV and those infected are at a greater risk for hepatic failure
   ▹ testing to detect the presence of hepatitis B should prevent HDV transmission
▶ Hepatitis G (HGV)
   ▹ described in 1996 and present in approximately 2% of U.S. blood donors
   ▹ association with liver disease is unclear as the majority of infected individuals do not have hepatic abnormalities
   ▹ presently blood donors are not routinely tested

HIV

▶ risk is currently about 1 in 700,000 with donor screening

Bacterial Infection

▶ due to improper blood collection, component preparation, and storage procedures
  ▶ very unusual occurrence with adherence to aseptic techniques
  ▶ *Klebsiella* or *Pseudomonas* are the causative agents in two-thirds of cases
▶ clinical signs include erythroderma, fever, chills, septic shock
▶ send blood for gram stain and culture to confirm the diagnosis
▶ treat with circulatory support and antibiotics

Part II

ANATOMIC AREAS OF INJURY

Head Trauma

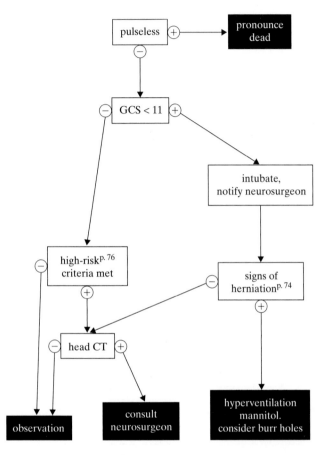

7

Head

Severity Determination

Glasgow Coma Scale (GCS)

▶ add the best score from each of the following categories (Tables 7–1 and 7–2) and use the result as a method to judge injury severity
▶ GCS aids in categorizing degree of blunt head trauma (BHT)
  ▶ mild means GCS over 13
  ▶ moderate means GCS 9–13
  ▶ severe means GCS under 9, which is an accepted definition of "coma"

Other Clinical Findings

▶ focal neurologic findings
▶ symptoms/signs of increased intracranial pressure (ICP)

Table 7–1 GCS: Adults

	6	5	4	3	2	1
Eye opening			Spontaneous	To voice	To pain	None
Verbal		Full oriented	Confused but conversant	Inappropriate	Sounds only	None
Motor	Follows commands	Localizes pain	Withdraws to painful stimuli	Decorticate posturing	Decerebrate posturing	None

Table 7–2 GCS: Infants

	6	5	4	3	2	1
Eye opening			Spontaneous	To voice	To pain	None
Verbal		Smiles or babbles	Irritable and inconsolable	Cries or screams with pain	Moans with pain	None
Motor	Appropriate for age	Withdraws to touch	Withdraws to painful stimuli	Decorticate posturing	Decerebrate posturing	None

Increased ICP

General Principles

Pathophysiology

▶ ICP is a function of the volume of brain parenchyma, blood, CSF, and any space-occupying lesion
  ▶ ICP under 10 mm Hg is normal
  ▶ ICP over 20 mm Hg requires treatment
  ▶ ICP over 40 mm Hg is immediately life-threatening
▶ intracranial bleeding or brain swelling causes a rapid increase in the "volume" of the fixed intracranial space and causes ICP to rise
  ▶ physiologic compensation to a limited degree occurs through a reduction in venous blood and CSF volume
▶ cerebral perfusion pressure (CPP) equals mean arterial pressure (MAP) minus ICP
  ▶ a rise in ICP decreases CPP with resultant brain ischemia
  ▶ maintaining adequate CPP is critical in protecting brain from ischemia
  ▶ the goal is to maintain CPP about 70 mm Hg

Cerebral Blood Flow

▶ ventilatory regulation of cerebral blood flow (CBF) occurs through CO_2-dependent vasoactivity
  ▶ hypoventilation causes vasodilatation and increases ICP
  ▶ normal ventilation prevents vasodilatation and optimizes ICP
  ▶ hyperventilation causes vasoconstriction and decreases CPP acutely
    ▶ $PaCO_2$ below 25 mm Hg associated with CBF under 50% and worse outcome
▶ CBF equals CPP divided by the CVR (cerebral vascular resistance)
  ▶ autoregulation between vasoconstriction and vasodilation maintains CBF
  ▶ autoregulation is lost when CPP is under 50 mm Hg

Herniation Syndrome

▶ when compensatory mechanisms fail, uncontrolled ICP results in rapid brain position shifting
  ▶ fatal if not immediately reversed

Clinical Findings

Symptoms

▶ severe headache
▶ continuous vomiting

Signs

▶ diminishing level of consciousness
▶ Cushing's reflex
  ▶ progressive hypertension and bradycardia
  ▶ late and ominous finding
▶ respiratory depression
▶ change in size, shape, or reactivity of pupil
▶ motor weakness or posturing
▶ triad of typical transtentorial uncal herniation
  ▶ rapidly deteriorating LOC
  ▶ unilateral pupillary dilation
  ▶ contralateral hemiparesis

Management

▶ airway/breathing
  ▶ perform immediate rapid sequence induction and intubation for all patients with GCS below 11 (see p. 41)
  ▶ maintain PCO_2 between 35 and 40 mm Hg
  ▶ avoid hyperventilation below a PCO_2 of 35 mm Hg except to halt the progression of brain herniation
  ▶ administer oxygen to maintain PaO_2 over 80 mm Hg
▶ treat hemorrhagic shock adequately to maintain MAP above 90 mm Hg
▶ avoid severe systemic hypertension
  ▶ increased capillary filtration pressures with transcapillary leakage may increase ICP
▶ drugs
  ▶ mannitol 1.5–2 g/kg IV over 30–60 min
  ▶ steroids (e.g., dexamethasone) are without proven benefit and not recommended
  ▶ maintain adequate sedation
    ▶ use benzodiazepines and opiates
    ▶ consider on-going paralysis
  ▶ prophylactic anticonvulsants (e.g., phenytoin or phenobarbital)
    ▶ used to prevent early posttraumatic seizures in high risk patients
  ▶ barbiturate coma
    ▶ pentobarbital loading dose of 10 mg/kg body weight over 30 minutes, followed by 1–1.5 mg/kg/h dosing
    ▶ slows brain metabolic activity and reduces cerebral oxygen requirements
    ▶ use only for refractory intracranial hypertension in hemodynamically stable, salvageable, severe head injury patients
▶ immediately notify neurosurgeon or transfer to a facility with a neurosurgeon
▶ arrange immediate head CT
  ▶ allows a rapid and accurate diagnosis
  ▶ perform only if hemodynamically stable

- ▸ can start with a central cut which usually shows the surgical lesion in order to minimize the time in CT
- ▸ if progressive herniation, consider immediate burr holes even before CT
- ▶ burr holes/decompressive craniotomy
  - ▸ criteria include clinical evidence of transtentorial herniation after closed head trauma
  - ▸ life-saving in up to 90% if performed without delay
- ▶ criteria for ICP monitor
  - ▸ GCS under 9 and abnormal head CT
  - ▸ GCS under 9 and two of the following regardless of head CT findings
    - ▹ age over 40 years
    - ▹ systemic hypotension (MAP under 90 mm Hg)
    - ▹ clinical signs of increased ICP
  - ▸ patients with potential intracranial injury requiring general anesthesia for a nonneurosurgical procedure and no time for a preoperative head CT
  - ▸ patients with known intracranial injury undergoing general anesthesia for a nonneurosurgical procedure
    - ▹ allows anesthesiologist follow CPP
- ▶ general guidelines for neurosurgical intervention
  - ▸ GCS of 9–15 with midventricular shift of over 5 mm
  - ▸ GCS of 9–15 with ICP over 25 mm Hg or neurologic deterioration
  - ▸ GCS under 9
    - ▹ some do not proceed when criteria for brain death are met or the situation is otherwise deemed futile

Diagnostics

Risk for Intracranial Injury

Low

- ▶ no diagnostic investigation indicated when
  - ▸ asymptomatic
  - ▸ mild headache
  - ▸ "dizziness"
  - ▸ scalp wound or hematoma

High

- ▶ immediate head CT indicated when
  - ▸ GCS under 15 (and changed from baseline)
  - ▸ patient has repetitive questioning of what happened or profound amnesia
  - ▸ focal neurologic signs

- ▶ skull fracture documented on plain radiograph or suspected clinically
- ▶ highly focused blunt trauma
    - ▷ hammer/golf ball strike
    - ▷ tangential gunshot wound
- ▶ penetrating intracranial injury
- ▶ posttraumatic seizures
- ▶ definite loss of consciousness after head trauma
- ▶ posttraumatic vomiting or severe headache
- ▶ head trauma in a patient with a preexisting coagulopathy or taking warfarin (Coumadin)

Skull Radiographs

General Principles

- ▶ do not obtain as a compromise when head CT indicated
    - ▶ accurate for detecting skull fractures
    - ▶ highly inaccurate for detecting intracranial lesions
- ▶ presence of skull fracture greatly increases risk of intracranial injury
    - ▶ order head CT when present

Indications

- ▶ possible skull fracture or penetrating intracranial injury and head CT/MRI unavailable
    - ▶ if positive, transfer patient to trauma center
- ▶ age less than 2 years with significant mechanism for blunt head trauma and criteria for head CT not met
    - ▶ circumstances of injury often unclear
    - ▶ facilitates identification and documentation of child abuse
    - ▶ diastatic fractures associated with leptomeningeal cysts
    - ▶ if positive, obtain head CT

CT

General Principles

- ▶ performed rapidly (within minutes)
- ▶ reliably identifies surgically correctable intracranial injury

Indications

- ▶ high risk criteria for intracranial injury met (see above)

Magnetic Resonance Imaging (MRI)

▶ not recommended for evaluation of acute head trauma unless head CT unavailable
▶ superior to CT in detecting subacute or chronic lesions
▶ specific lesions better visualized on MRI than CT include
   ▶ isodense (subacute) bilateral subdural hematomas that do not cause midline shifting
   ▶ shearing mechanism causing diffuse axonal injury
   ▶ nonhemorrhagic contusions and edema

Skull Fracture

General Principles

▶ obtain head CT if any type of skull fracture clinically suspected or diagnosed by plain radiography

Linear

▶ curvilinear and nondisplaced
▶ no specific treatment if no intracranial injury except head injury observation
▶ obtain head CT since at increased risk for intracranial injury
▶ multiple fractures in children associated with abuse
▶ treatment
   ▶ if no other injuries, discharge with appropriate analgesic and head injury aftercare instructions (see p. 524)

Basilar

▶ fracture through the skull base
   ▶ includes occipital bones, sphenoid, ethmoid, and/or temporal bones
▶ clinical findings
   ▶ mastoid ecchymosis called "Battle's sign"
   ▶ nontender periorbital ecchymoses called "raccoon eyes"
   ▶ hemotympanum
      ▶ can also be caused by direct strike over the tympanic membrane (barotrauma) and not due to a basilar skull fracture
   ▶ CSF rhinorrhea or otorrhea
      ▶ bloody CSF differentiated from tissue bleeding because it is thinner (lower hematocrit) and causes a "target pattern" when a drop is placed on filter paper
   ▶ cranial nerve VII palsy

► treatment
  ► admit for neurologic observation
  ► if there is CSF leak, monitor for meningitis
    ► 80% resolve spontaneously
    ► some cases require a lumbar drain
  ► prophylactic antibiotics are not indicated

Open

► scalp, skin, nasal sinuses, or middle ear violated and contiguous with fracture site
► resultant CSF leak common
► treatment
  ► same as for basilar skull fracture

Depressed

► mechanism
  ► caused by great force over small surface area
► treatment
  ► admit for neurologic observation
  ► surgical elevation for
    ► adults—fragments driven more than 5 mm below inner table of the skull
    ► children—fragments below the inner table by an amount greater than the thickness of the skull

Intracranial Injury

Subdural Hematoma

General Principles

► due to disruption of the bridging veins (between the cerebral cortex and venous sinuses) with subsequent bleeding into the subdural space (between the dura and the arachnoid)
► more common in the elderly
  ► less resilient bridging veins
  ► atrophy results in more tension on the bridging veins when the brain is jarred
► most common in the parietal region

Radiographic Findings

▶ acute phase is under 2 days
  ▶ hyperdense on CT (Figure 7–1)

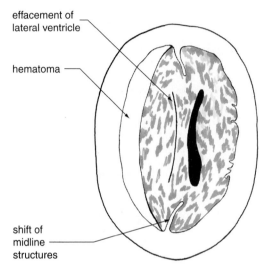

Figure 7–1

  ▶ generally appears as a crescent along inner table of skull conforming to the brain contours
▶ subacute phase is 2 days–2 weeks
  ▶ isodense on CT with respect to the brain parenchyma during this phase and therefore can be very difficult to appreciate (IV contrast helpful)
▶ chronic phase is over 2 weeks
  ▶ hypodense on CT with respect to the brain parenchyma and usually obvious but when bilateral can be confused with severe cortical atrophy (IV contrast helpful)

Treatment

▶ obtain prompt neurosurgical consultation
  ▶ evacuation necessary when
    ▶ associated mass effect (over 5 mm shift)
    ▶ focal neurologic findings
    ▶ posterior fossa location
    ▶ increased ICP
  ▶ evacuation within 4 h improves clinical outcome and decreases mortality

Epidural Hematoma

General Principles

▶ less common than subdural hematoma
▶ due to arterial bleeding within epidural space, usually from temporal bone fracture across the groove of the middle meningeal artery
▶ most common in the temporal region
▶ "classic presentation"
  ▶ lucid interval between trauma and appearance of symptoms
  ▶ occurs in less than one-third

Radiographic Findings

▶ hyperdense lenticular (biconvex) shape due to intimate attachment of dura to inner table which inhibits diffuse spread of blood (Figure 7–2)

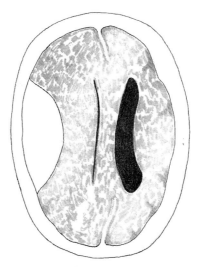

Figure 7–2

Treatment

▶ emergent neurosurgical evacuation

Intraparenchymal Hemorrhage

General Principles

▶ bleeding most common in inferior frontal and anterior temporal lobes
  ▶ areas where brain strikes bone during deceleration
▶ clinical findings include altered level of consciousness, confusion, and focal deficits depending on size and location of hematoma

Radiographic Findings

▶ hyperdense focal area within the brain parenchyma

Treatment

▶ control increased ICP
▶ focal hematoma may be amenable to neurosurgical evacuation

Diffuse Axonal Injury

General Principles

▶ shear force causes microscopic hemorrhages in the following areas
  ▶ gray–white junction
  ▶ white matter tracts
  ▶ periventricular area
  ▶ corpus callosum
▶ clinical findings
  ▶ physical findings range from mild neurologic impairment to coma

Radiographic Findings

▶ generally a paucity of CT findings
  ▶ may see small hyperdense speckles at the gray–white junction
▶ best visualized on MRI

Treatment

▶ control increased ICP if necessary
▶ expectant management

Subarachnoid Hemorrhage

General Principles

▶ clinical findings include severe headache and nuchal rigidity

Radiographic Findings

▶ blood in ventricles, cisterns, or within sulci
  ▹ look for hyperdense "outlining" of the paramesencephalic (quadrigeminal) cistern and in the Sylvian fissure

Treatment

▶ admit for close observation
▶ neurosurgical consultation
▶ when associated with communicating hydrocephalus, requires shunt
  ▹ subarachnoid blood impairs CSF resorption and ICP can increase as a result

Disposition Considerations

Discharge

▶ low risk criteria for intracranial injury
▶ high risk criteria for intracranial injury and the following satisfied
  ▹ GCS of 15 and a normal neurologic examination
  ▹ normal head CT
▶ explain and provide "Head Injury" aftercare instructions (see p. 524)
  ▹ it is reasonable to prescribe effective analgesics for severe headache as long as CT was performed and negative and if the patient understands the need to return if the condition worsens
▶ discharge to care of a responsible adult who will monitor patient

Admission

▶ abnormal GCS or neurologic examination
▶ persistent vomiting
▶ abnormalities found on CT
▶ significant intoxication
▶ no responsible adult to care for patient with significant injury mechanism

8

Eye

Evaluation

History

- mechanism of injury
- pain
  - foreign body sensation
  - photophobia
- visual symptoms
  - floaters
  - decreased visual acuity
  - flashing lights
  - diplopia

Visual Acuity

- mandatory in all patients with eye or facial trauma
- if glasses unavailable
  - use pinhole
  - allow patient to look through ophthalmoscope and dial to best refraction
  - use near-vision scale

Examination

Inspection

- exophthalmos/enophthalmos
- deformity of external eye structures
- conjunctiva for foreign bodies, lacerations, and blood
- evert the upper lids to look for foreign bodies in the upper fornices

Palpation

- tenderness of periorbital bones
- step-off for fractures
- crepitus for medial orbital fractures

Pupils

- size
- shape
- reaction to light
  - direct response
  - consensual response
    - look for afferent pupillary defect

Extraocular Motion

- check in all directions
- test for diplopia
- observe for symmetrical movement of the eyes

Anterior Segment

- cornea
  - foreign body
  - abrasion using fluorescein staining and cobalt blue light
  - laceration/penetration
  - Seidel test
    - gently paint fluorescein on cornea, examine with cobalt blue light using slit lamp, and then search for aqueous humor leaking from wound and changing the color of the fluorescein from brown to green
- hyphema
- iris for irregularities
- lens for dislocation
- depth of anterior chamber can be assessed by the lateral light test

Direct Ophthalmoscopy

- retina for hemorrhages, tears and detachment
- clarity of the vitreous
- search for foreign bodies

Intraocular Pressure

- perform only when no suspicion for globe rupture or corneal laceration
- low pressure associated with
  - globe rupture
  - early iritis since ciliary body shuts down production of aqueous
- elevated pressure associated with
  - late iritis since trebecular meshwork clogs

Test Ordering

Plain Radiographic Studies

▶ see Plain Radiograph Interpretation (p. 484)

Waters' View

▶ best delineates orbital floor
▶ signs of orbital floor fracture include
  ▶ air–fluid level in maxillary sinus
  ▶ opacification of maxillary sinus
  ▶ "teardrop" sign of intraorbital fat protruding from the orbital floor

Caldwell's View

▶ best delineates
  ▶ medial orbital wall
  ▶ lateral and superior orbital rims
▶ check ethmoid and frontal sinuses for
  ▶ air–fluid level

Lateral View

▶ best delineates orbital roof
▶ check maxillary and frontal sinus for
  ▶ fracture
  ▶ air–fluid level

CT

Technique

▶ axial and coronal views (after cervical spine cleared)
▶ 1–2 mm cuts

Indications

▶ acute enophthalmos or proptosis
▶ unexplained decrease in visual acuity
▶ intraorbital emphysema
▶ metallic foreign body location/identification
▶ improved fracture definition necessary
▶ intraorbital hemorrhage

MRI

▶ superior for viewing soft tissues and nonmetallic foreign body identification
▶ contraindicated when metallic foreign body is suspected

Ultrasound

Indications

▶ lens rupture
▶ vitreous hemorrhage
▶ retinal detachment
▶ nonmetallic intraocular foreign body identification

Caution

▶ do not perform if globe rupture is suspected

Specific Injuries

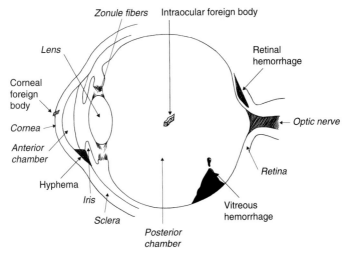

Figure 8–1

Corneal Abrasion

Clinical Findings

▶ sudden and severe eye pain
  ▶ intense foreign body sensation
▶ marked relief with topical anesthetics

- photophobia
- conjunctival injection
- tearing

Diagnosis

- fluorescein staining of cornea reveals epithelial defect under cobalt blue light source

Cautions

- search carefully for foreign body
  - evert the eyelids to evaluate the conjunctival fornices
- always maintain a high suspicion of intraocular foreign body
  - classic history is abrupt onset of eye pain after an explosion or while pounding, drilling, or grinding metal

Treatment

- prophylactic antibiotic (ointment or drops)
  - gentamicin, tobramycin, erythromycin, or ciprofloxacin
- topical nonsteroidal anti-inflammatory agent (NSAID) drops
  - ketorolac or diclofenac
- consider a cycloplegic to reduce ciliary spasm from secondary iritis
  - cyclopentolate 0.5% 1–2 gtt
- patch large abrasions for 24 h to prevent blinking
  - discourage driving or operating machinery while patch in place
- no contact lens wearing for 3 days
- patching raises temperature of the cornea, promotes bacterial growth, and should be avoided when infection risk is high such as in
  - contact lens wearers
  - scratches from organic material
- follow up in 24–48 h, especially important when
  - central or large abrasion
  - contact lens wearer
- tetanus prophylaxis

Corneal Foreign Body

Clinical Findings

- severe pain or foreign body sensation
- conjunctival injection

Diagnosis

- imbedded foreign body easily visualized on slit lamp examination
- evert upper lid to search for retained foreign bodies

▶ obtain orbital radiograph or CT if history is consistent with possible intraocular foreign body

Treatment

▶ removal
  ▶ only attempt in cooperative patients
  ▶ achieve topical ocular anesthesia with tetracaine or proparacaine drops
  ▶ dislodge foreign body
    ▷ use 25-gauge needle or foreign body spud (which looks like a spatula)
    ▷ perform under direct slit lamp visualization with patient's head and operator's hand firmly stabilized
  ▶ residual rust ring removal
    ▷ ferrous oxide particles will diffuse through cornea if not removed
    ▷ most defer to ophthalmologist and removal may be delayed up to 24 h
    ▷ electric-powered corneal burr is used by some emergency physicians
  ▶ deeply embedded foreign bodies or foreign bodies in central visual axis require urgent ophthalmologist referral
▶ further treatment after removal
  ▶ prophylactic antibiotic (ointment or drops)
    ▷ gentamicin, tobramycin, erythromycin, or ciprofloxacin
  ▶ cycloplegic to reduce ciliary spasm and secondary iritis
    ▷ cyclopentolate 0.5% 1–2 gtt
  ▶ ophthalmologic follow-up in 24 h
  ▶ tetanus prophylaxis

Intraocular Foreign Body

General Principles

▶ classic history is onset of eye pain after an explosion or while pounding, drilling, or grinding metal
  ▶ sometimes initially painless and then followed by progressive eye pain

Clinical Findings

▶ decreased visual acuity
▶ small lid or globe defect
  ▶ can be misinterpreted as a corneal abrasion
▶ positive Seidel test

Radiographic Findings

▶ plain orbital radiographs reveal presence of a metallic foreign body
▶ CT necessary for precise localization

▶ MRI or ultrasound useful to diagnose and localize nonmetallic foreign bodies

Treatment

▶ emergent ophthalmologic consultation
▶ avoid eye manipulation and place metal eye shield to prevent inadvertent pressure on globe
▶ antiemetics for nausea/vomiting
▶ keep the patient NPO
▶ prophylactic antibiotics
　▶ use first-generation cephalosporin and aminoglycoside
▶ tetanus prophylaxis

Subconjunctival Hemorrhage

Mechanism

▶ common injury from
　▶ blunt or penetrating trauma
　▶ sneezing, coughing, or valsalva

Clinical Findings

▶ painless, smooth red areas over bulbar conjunctiva
▶ visual acuity normal
▶ bullous subconjunctival hemorrhage
　▶ can be the result of a scleral rupture so rule this out when visual acuity is reduced

Treatment

▶ should heal spontaneously within 4 weeks
▶ when healing is delayed, check coagulation profile and bleed time

Hyphema

Mechanism

▶ traumatic disruption of vessels in iris or ciliary body resulting in anterior chamber bleeding

Clinical Findings

▶ blurred vision
▶ pain
▶ photophobia

▶ presence of blood in anterior chamber
  ▶ blood layers out inferiorly due to gravity and may appear as meniscus at bottom of anterior chamber if given sufficient time to settle (Figure 8–2)
  ▶ complete opacification results in "eight ball" appearance of eye and lack of red reflex

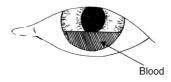

Figure 8–2

Treatment

▶ urgent ophthalmologic consultation
▶ elevate head of bed to 45°
▶ avoid eye manipulation and use metal eye shield to prevent inadvertent pressure on globe
▶ when unable to exclude retinal detachment or lens dislocation due to hyphema, consider an ocular ultrasound
▶ screen patients of African descent for sickle cell disease
▶ measure the intraocular pressure and, when over 30 mm Hg, initiate pressure-lowering agents
  ▶ timolol, brimonidine (Alphagan), dorzolamine (Trusopt), mannitol
  ▶ pilocarpine has fallen out of favor because it increases inflammation
  ▶ parenteral acetazolamide has more complications (e.g. metabolic acidosis) than topical carbonic anhydrase inhibitors, which are equally efficacious
▶ cycloplegia may enhance patient comfort
  ▶ use cyclopentolate or homatropine TID to "freeze" the pupil
    ▶ temporary cycloplegia causes movement of the iris root, which is the usual source of bleeding
▶ topical steroids may minimize discomfort from traumatic iritis
  ▶ prednisolone
▶ aminocaproic acid (Amicar)
  ▶ prevents conversion of plasminogen to plasmin
  ▶ delays clot dissolution
  ▶ decreases rate of rebleeding
▶ analgesia
  ▶ acetaminophen with or without codeine may be used
  ▶ do not use aspirin and other NSAIDS
▶ antiemetics
▶ surgical management
  ▶ uncontrolled intraocular pressure rise
  ▶ total hyphema not resolved within a week
▶ small hyphemas in cooperative patients may be managed as outpatients with quiet activity

Traumatic Iritis

Mechanism

▶ blunt trauma to iris and ciliary body resulting in inflammatory reaction in anterior chamber leading to ciliary muscle spasm

Clinical Findings

▶ pain with direct and consensual photophobia
  ▶ due to iris and ciliary body irritability
▶ decreased visual acuity due to constricted pupil and inflammation of the anterior chamber
▶ perilimbal injection called "ciliary flush" (Figure 8–3)

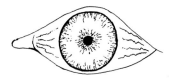

Figure 8–3

▶ check intraocular pressure and, if greater than 30 mm Hg,
  ▶ notify ophthalmologist
  ▶ initiate pressure-lowering agents
    ▶ brimonidine, dorzolamide, timolol, acetazolamide, and/or mannitol
▶ white blood cells and flare (protein) seen in anterior chamber
  ▶ due to leakage of white blood cells and protein from inflamed ciliary body
  ▶ seen using the slit lamp and passing a narrow strip of light across the anterior chamber (Figure 8–4)

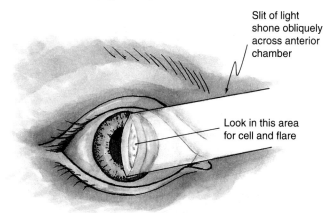

Slit of light shone obliquely across anterior chamber

Look in this area for cell and flare

Figure 8–4

Treatment

- ▶ cycloplegia
    - ▶ cyclopentolate or homatropine
- ▶ steroid ophthalmic drops
    - ▶ prednisolone
- ▶ refer to ophthalmologist for reevaluation in a few days

Traumatic Mydriasis

Mechanism

- ▶ small tear in sphincter muscle fibers

Clinical Findings

- ▶ unilateral dilated pupil
    - ▶ in the comatose patient, traumatic mydriasis cannot be easily differentiated from herniation syndrome (with CN III palsy)

Treatment

- ▶ spontaneous improvement occurs in time

Traumatic Dislocated Lens

Mechanism

- ▶ compression of globe disrupts zonule fibers
- ▶ partial subluxation is more common than complete dislocation
    - ▶ common in Marfan's syndrome

Clinical Findings

- ▶ markedly decreased visual acuity
- ▶ complete dislocation can be backward into vitreous (Figure 8–5) or forward into the anterior chamber

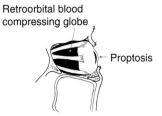

Figure 8–5

▶ pupillary dilation can facilitate visualization of the lens dislocation
▶ lack of red reflex
▶ iridodonesis
  ▶ a trembling or shimmering of the iris after rapid eye movement is an in-
    direct sign of posterior lens dislocation

Treatment

▶ ophthalmologic consultation
▶ surgical removal if lens in anterior chamber
▶ refractive correction or surgery done for posteriorly displaced lens

Vitreous Hemorrhage

Mechanism

▶ tearing of retinal vessels causes bleeding into the vitreous

Clinical Findings

▶ "floaters"
▶ severe loss of vision
▶ inability to visualize fundus due to hazy vitreous
▶ decreased red reflex

Treatment

▶ ophthalmologic consultation
▶ elevation of head
▶ avoid straining
▶ platelet-inhibiting medications are contraindicated
▶ consider vitrectomy for persistent nonabsorbing blood

Chorioretinal Injury

Mechanism

▶ concussive globe injury
▶ can be a complication of "shaken baby syndrome"
▶ results in preretinal and retinal hemorrhage

Clinical Findings

▶ floaters from vitreous hemorrhage
▶ flashing lights from traction and stimulation of retinal neurons

▶ visual field defects
▶ normal to poor visual acuity depending on location of hemorrhage
▶ fundoscopic examination reveals hazy gray membrane of detached retina

Treatment

▶ emergent ophthalmologic consultation for repair

Globe Rupture

Mechanism

▶ penetrating trauma
▶ blunt trauma (rarely) can result in scleral rupture at limbus or site of insertion of intraocular muscles

Clinical Findings

▶ laceration of bulbar or palpebral conjunctiva
▶ extrusion of orbital contents
▶ bloody chemosis
  ▶ hemorrhagic bulging of bulbar conjunctiva overlying scleral rupture
▶ decreased visual acuity
▶ vitreous hemorrhage
▶ positive Seidel test

Treatment

▶ ophthalmologic consultation for emergency surgical repair
▶ avoid eye manipulation and use metal eye shield to prevent inadvertent pressure on globe
▶ antiemetics for nausea/vomiting
▶ keep the patient NPO
▶ prophylactic antibiotics
  ▶ use first-generation cephalosporin and aminoglycoside
▶ tetanus prophylaxis

Globe Lacerations

Bulbar Conjunctival Lacerations

▶ small lacerations (under 1 cm) heal spontaneously
  ▶ prophylactic antibiotic (ointment or drops)
  ▶ ophthalmologic follow-up
▶ large lacerations (over 1 cm) require repair
  ▶ repair by ophthalmologist
  ▶ examine closely for globe rupture

Corneal Laceration

▶ difficult to delineate full from partial thickness tear
▶ positive Seidel test
▶ teardrop-shaped pupil results
▶ treatment
  ▸ rigid metal shield
  ▸ emergent ophthalmologic consultation

Retrobulbar Hemorrhage (Figure 8–6)

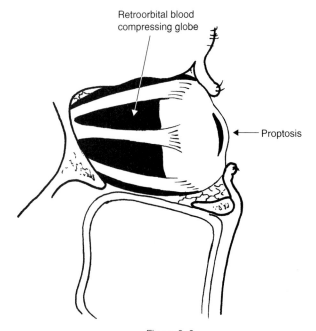

Retroorbital blood
compressing globe

◄─── Proptosis

Figure 8–6

Mechanism

▶ vascular orbital plexus hemorrhage after blunt trauma
  ▸ rare and sight-threatening injury
▶ causes increased intraorbital pressure from posterior force transmitted to globe
  ▸ high pressures will occlude central retinal arterial flow ("orbital compartment syndrome")

Clinical Findings

▶ pain
▶ diplopia
▶ proptosis with resistance to retropulsion
▶ nausea and vomiting
▶ afferent pupillary defect
▶ decreased visual acuity and diplopia
▶ elevated intraocular pressure
▶ circumferential subconjunctival hemorrhage

Diagnosis

▶ orbital CT demonstrates hematoma

Treatment

▶ emergent ophthalmologic consultation
▶ conservative therapy
  ▶ elevate head of bed
  ▶ apply ice pack
  ▶ avoid platelet-inhibiting medications
▶ aggressive therapy if afferent pupil defect or intraocular pressure over 30 mm Hg
  ▶ initiate pressure lowering agents
    ▶ brimonidine, dorzolamide, timolol, acetazolamide, and/or mannitol
  ▶ emergent lateral canthotomy and cantholysis indicated if poor perfusion of central retinal artery
    ▶ expands orbital volume and decreases intraocular pressure
    ▶ apply hemostat to the incision site for one minute (to compress the tissues and reduce bleeding) then make a 1 cm horizontal incision across the lateral canthus, cutting the inferior arm of the lateral canthal tendon

Periorbital Lacerations

General Principles

▶ search for associated ocular injury
▶ repair with 6-0 nylon interrupted suture
▶ remove suture in 3–5 days
▶ closure of complex lacerations usually performed by ophthalmologist

Treatment

- ▶ refer the following complex lacerations to an ophthalmologist
    - ▶ lid margin lacerations
        - ▹ complex three-layer closure needed
    - ▶ canalicular system laceration
        - ▹ medial one-third of lid may injure canalicular ducts with resultant persistent tearing
        - ▹ operative repair with stinting of duct required
    - ▶ canthal tendon laceration
        - ▹ penetrating wound of medial or lateral canthus may interrupt canthal tendons
    - ▶ levator muscle laceration
        - ▹ deep laceration of upper lid
        - ▹ multilayer closure needed to prevent posttraumatic ptosis
    - ▶ orbital septum laceration
        - ▹ deep wound of upper lid
        - ▹ septum runs between the tarsus and superior orbital rim
        - ▹ orbital fat protrudes from wound
        - ▹ high incidence of globe perforation
        - ▹ meticulous multilayered closure needed

Chemical Injury

Mechanism

- ▶ alkaline substances cause liquefactive necrosis
    - ▶ continues to penetrate and dissolve tissues until removed
    - ▶ causes extensive damage to deeper ocular structures
- ▶ acid substances produce coagulation necrosis
    - ▶ precipitation of tissue limits penetration
- ▶ irritants (e.g., mace or pepper spray) cause severe pain, redness, and flow of tears for a limited period

Substances

- ▶ alkaline
    - ▶ lye and other drain or oven cleaners
    - ▶ detergents and bleach
    - ▶ lime in plaster and concrete
    - ▶ cements and mortar
    - ▶ chemical detergents

▶ acid
  ▶ toilet cleaners
  ▶ battery acid
▶ irritants
  ▶ pepper spray
  ▶ mace

Clinical Findings

▶ pain
▶ burning
▶ conjunctival and scleral injection
▶ corneal epithelial defects or clouding

Treatment

▶ begin irrigation immediately after the exposure and continue en route to hospital with water or normal saline
▶ evert the lids quickly and wipe away all debris in the fornices
  ▶ this may be facilitated by using a topical anesthetic
  ▶ defer a detailed physical examination until adequate irrigation has completed
▶ continue irrigation for at least 30 minutes in the emergency department
  ▶ several liters may be needed with alkaline exposures
  ▶ use Morgan lens to facilitate the process
▶ test pH of tears with litmus paper a few minutes after each liter of irrigant
  ▶ the goal is to return the pH of eye to the 7–8 range
▶ topical antibiotic ointment
  ▶ gentamicin, tobramycin, erythromycin, or ciprofloxacin
▶ cycloplegia and mydriasis for patient comfort
  ▶ cyclopentolate or homatropine
▶ some believe topical steroids in acute stage decrease inflammation and promote epithelial regeneration
▶ apply pressure patch between applications of drops/ointment
▶ tetanus prophylaxis

Thermal Burn

Clinical Findings

▶ pain
▶ conjunctival injection
▶ fluorescein uptake in affected areas with cobalt blue lamp examination

Treatment

▶ superficial
  ▶ irrigation and topical antibiotics
▶ partial and full thickness
  ▶ antibiotic ointment and tetanus prophylaxis
  ▶ transfer to burn center

9

Face

General Principles

Associated Injuries

▶ associated intracranial injuries are common and take precedence
▶ cervical spine injuries occur in 10% of patients with severe maxillofacial trauma

Airway Problems

▶ common due to
  ▶ oral hemorrhage or edema
  ▶ Le Fort fractures, which can cause retroposition of palate
  ▶ aspiration of teeth
  ▶ mandibular fractures, which can cause loss of anterior tongue support
▶ immediate cricothyroidotomy is necessary when orotracheal intubation fails
▶ nasotracheal intubation and nasogastric tubes are contraindicated when there is severe midface trauma
  ▶ the tube can pass through a cribriform plate fracture into the cranium
▶ consider allowing the patient to hold the suction catheter and use as needed

Facial Hemorrhage

▶ keep the head of the bed elevated where possible
▶ apply pressure
▶ infiltrate using lidocaine with epinephrine to induce vasoconstriction
  ▶ except at tip of nose
▶ identify bleeding source and ligate bleeding vessels that are isolated
  ▶ do not blindly clamp or ligate

Nasal Fracture

Types

▶ nondisplaced

▶ depressed
▶ laterally displaced

Clinical Findings

▶ nasal pain and deformity
▶ edema and tenderness
▶ epistaxis
▶ crepitus and hypermobility

Diagnosis

▶ clinical diagnosis without radiographs is reasonable for uncomplicated nasal fractures
▶ obtaining radiographs is controversial
  ▸ do not change the treatment and thus is an unnecessary cost
  ▸ often desired by patients who "just want to know for sure if it is broken"

Complications

▶ a septal hematoma can lead to necrosis of the septum if not appreciated and evacuated through a nasal mucosal incision
▶ severe epistaxis

Management

▶ control epistaxis by performing the following maneuvers (listed in recommended sequence)
  ▸ apply a topical alpha-agonist for vasoconstriction
    ▸ phenylephrine or cocaine
  ▸ attempt chemical cauterization with a silver nitrate application stick
  ▸ nasal packing
    ▸ place anterior pack, bilaterally if necessary to increase pressure
    ▸ if unsuccessful, place posterior pack or balloon tamponade device
  ▸ intubate the patient and apply pressure with transoral gauze pack
    ▸ nasal intubation will worsen the bleeding
    ▸ oral intubation will be difficult due to the bleeding
    ▸ surgical airway may be necessary
  ▸ consider angiographic embolization
  ▸ attempt selective internal or external carotid ligation as a last-ditch effort
▶ consider closed reduction of gross nasal bone deformities after topical anesthesia and inferior orbital nerve block
▶ minor fractures require referral and closed reduction within 5–7 days
  ▸ pediatric nasal fractures have potential for severe deformity due to continued growth and must be followed carefully

▶ patients receiving anterior nasal packing must be seen within 48 h for removal and reassessment
▶ patients receiving posterior packs require admission

Maxillary Fracture

Le Fort I (Figure 9–1)

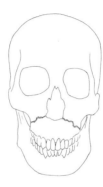

Figure 9–1

Definition

▶ transverse or "horizontal" fracture across the inferior maxilla that separates the entire maxillary dental arch away from the mid-face
▶ fracture may be unilateral or bilateral

Clinical Findings

▶ can elicit motion of maxilla while the nasal bridge remains stable
▶ all the Le Fort fractures commonly have malocclusion of the teeth

Radiographic Findings

▶ CT demonstrates the following sequence of fractures
  ▶ nasal aperture
  ▶ inferior maxilla
  ▶ lateral wall of maxilla
  ▶ pterygoid plate
▶ Waters' view shows bilateral maxillary clouding in all Le Fort fractures though fracture lines are often not evident

Management

▶ consult maxillofacial surgeon since fixation is required
  ▶ intermaxillary fixation
  ▶ direct wiring
  ▶ mandibular arch bar
▶ nasal packing usually controls associated epistaxis
▶ apply ice and offer analgesia
▶ administer prophylactic antibiotics

Le Fort II (Figure 9–2)

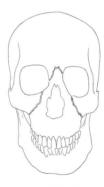

Figure 9–2

Definition

▶ "pyramidal" fracture of the maxilla that extends obliquely upward from the pterygoid plates, through the upper portion of the maxillary sinus and across the bridge of the nose
▶ inferior orbital rim is often involved with the upper portion of the fracture line

Clinical Findings

▶ can elicit motion of maxilla along with the nasal bones
▶ nasal flattening (unless masked by the swelling)
▶ traumatic telecanthus is common (eyes move apart due to disruption of the medial canthal ligaments)
▶ CSF rhinorrhea occurs if the cribriform plate is injured

Radiographic Findings

▶ CT demonstrates the following sequence of fractures
  ▶ frontal process of the maxilla
  ▶ nasal bones
  ▶ medial orbital wall
  ▶ maxillary sinuses
  ▶ pterygoid plate

Management

▶ consult maxillofacial surgeon since operative fixation is required
  ▶ intermaxillary fixation
  ▶ direct wiring
▶ nasal packing usually controls associated epistaxis
▶ apply ice and offer analgesia
▶ administer prophylactic antibiotics

Le Fort III (Figure 9–3)

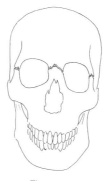

Figure 9–3

General Principles

▶ "craniofacial disjunction" that separates the entire facial skeleton from the cranial vault
▶ fracture line extends upward from the pterygoid plates through the lateral orbit and orbital rim and then separates transversely across the frontozygomatic suture line and the nasal ethmoidal region

Clinical Findings

▶ severe airway obstruction is the rule
▶ can elicit motion of maxilla, nasal bones, zygoma
▶ causes "beachball" or "dish" face (facial flattening and elongation with eyes markedly swollen shut)
▶ CSF rhinorrhea more common

Radiographic Findings

▶ CT demonstrates separation of the entire midface from the cranium
▶ midface becomes retropositioned at about 45°
  ▶ separation or fracture of the zygomaticofrontal sutures
▶ opacification of the maxillary and ethmoid sinuses
▶ vertical elongation of the orbits

Management

▶ immediate airway attention may be necessary
▶ consult maxillofacial surgeon since operative fixation is required
  ▶ direct wiring
▶ nasal packing usually controls associated epistaxis
▶ apply ice and offer analgesia
▶ administer prophylactic antibiotics

Zygomatic Fracture

Zygomatic Arch Fracture

Clinical Findings

▶ preauricular depression and point tenderness
▶ trismus
  ▶ due to impingement of the coronoid process of the mandible on the arch during mouth opening

Diagnosis

▶ fracture best seen on submental–vertex radiographic view

Management

▶ consult maxillofacial surgeon
▶ apply ice and analgesia
▶ possible open elevation when
  ▶ cosmetic correction desired
  ▶ entrapment of the mandible persists

Tripod Fracture

Three Parts

▶ diastasis (widening) of the zygomaticotemporal suture
▶ diastasis of the zygomaticofrontal suture
▶ fracture of the infraorbital foramen (across the anterolateral wall of the maxillary sinus)

Clinical Findings

▶ cheek edema and facial flattening
▶ circumorbital ecchymosis
▶ infraorbital nerve anesthesia common
▶ concomitant globe injuries common

Diagnosis

▶ CT best defines extent of fractures
▶ Waters' view (Figure 9–4)
  ▸ opacification of the maxillary sinus
  ▸ widening of the zygomaticofrontal suture
  ▸ disruption of the inferior orbital rim

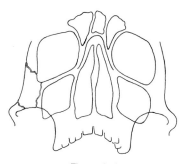

Figure 9–4

▶ submental–vertex radiographic
  ▸ for zygomatic arch evaluation

Management

▶ consult maxillofacial surgeon
▶ apply ice and analgesia
▶ requires surgical fixation if displaced
▶ refer for elective repair if not displaced

Orbital Floor Fracture

Mechanism (Figure 9–5)

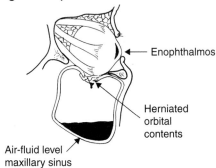

Enophthalmos

Herniated
orbital
contents

Air-fluid level
maxillary sinus

Figure 9–5

▶ blunt object with a radius of curve of under 5 cm strikes orbit
  ▶ often a fist or ball smaller than a 16 inch softball
▶ rapid increase in intraorbital pressure causes fracture along the weakest parts of orbital wall
  ▶ usually inferior
  ▶ sometimes medial
▶ herniation of contents through the fracture into the inferior portion of orbital wall and potential entrapment of the inferior rectus muscle in the fracture

Clinical Findings

▶ pain
  ▶ greatest with vertical eye movement
▶ periorbital tenderness, swelling, ecchymosis
▶ impaired ocular motility (especially with upward gaze) or diplopia
  ▶ due to inferior rectus entrapment (Figure 9–6)

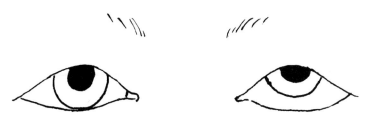

Figure 9–6

▶ infraorbital hypoesthesia
  ▶ due to compression/contusion of the infraorbital nerve
▶ enophthalmos
  ▶ due to herniation of orbital fat through the fracture
  ▶ may be masked by orbital edema
▶ periorbital emphysema
  ▶ due to fracture into a sinus
▶ normal visual acuity
  ▶ unless associated ocular injury

Radiographic Findings

▶ CT
  ▶ coronal views optimal (after cervical spine cleared)
  ▶ provides detail of orbital wall and floor fracture
  ▶ excludes retrobulbar hemorrhage
▶ Waters' view (Figure 9–7)

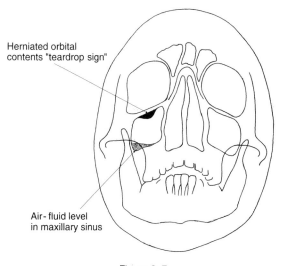

Herniated orbital
contents "teardrop sign"

Air- fluid level
in maxillary sinus

Figure 9–7

  ▶ see p. 484 for method of interpretation
  ▶ fractures of inferior or medial orbit are difficult to visualize
  ▶ "teardrop sign" of herniated orbital fat and muscle in the roof of the
    maxillary sinus
  ▶ depressed bony fragments into maxillary sinus
  ▶ maxillary sinus clouding or air–fluid level due to bleeding
  ▶ orbital emphysema

Management

▶ perform a complete ophthalmologic examination to assess for potential eye injuries
▶ spontaneous resolution of entrapment or diplopia occurs with reduction of edema over several days in the majority
　▶ persistent entrapment or cosmetically unacceptable enophthalmos requires orbital reconstruction
▶ refer to maxillofacial surgeon or ophthalmologist
　▶ significant orbital floor fractures may result in late enophthalmos
▶ medications
　▶ tetanus immunization
　▶ decongestant for 3 days
　　▷ oxymetazoline (Afrin) nasal spray
　　▷ pseudoephedrine orally
　▶ prophylactic antibiotics
　　▷ first generation cephalosporin or erythromycin for 5 days
▶ avoid straining or nose blowing

Mandibular Fracture

Anatomy (Figure 9–8)

General Principles

▶ multiple fractures occur in the majority

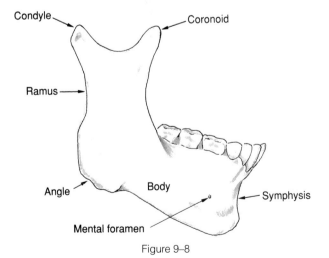

Figure 9–8

► most frequent fracture sites
  ► angle (30%)—bilateral displaced angle fractures cause a "bucket handle defect" causing loss of anterior tongue support and are at risk of airway obstruction
  ► condyle (30%)—bilateral condylar fractures cause anterior bite
  ► body (30%)—often cause mental nerve anesthesia when at mental foramen
► least frequent fracture sites (10%)
  ► ramus—often overriding
  ► coronoid—rare
  ► symphysis—diastasis or fracture unlikely since bone is thick anteriorly

Clinical Findings

► pain and decreased range of motion
► malocclusion or pain with teeth clenching (cannot bite tongue blade)
► inability to fully open the mouth
► separation of teeth interspaces with intraoral bleeding
► preauricular pain with biting occurs with condylar fractures

Radiographic Evaluation

► panoramic view (panorex) is best
► mandible series acceptable
  ► PA and lateral
  ► right and left lateral oblique views to include the condyles
  ► Townes' view to include the condyles

Management

► closed reduction with occlusion fixation (interdental wiring and elastics) for 4–6 weeks appropriate in 90%
► open reduction required for severe or unstable fractures
► external fixation required when mandible is edentulous or dentition is poor
► most are open fractures to the oral cavity and require antibiotics
  ► penicillin or clindamycin is recommended

Temporomandibular Dislocation

Etiology

► blow to the chin with an open mouth
► wide opening of mouth in susceptible individuals
► condyles lock anteriorly to the temporal articular eminence and muscle spasm prevents it from sliding back

Clinical Findings

▶ when bilateral, anterior bite with inability to close the mouth
▶ when unilateral, jaw displaced to unaffected side

Management

▶ sedation
▶ reduce by applying downward pressure on posterior molars with operator's thumbs wrapped in gauze
▶ discharge with analgesic, soft diet, and ENT or oral surgeon referral

Parotid Duct/Facial Nerve Injuries

Landmarks (Figure 9–9)

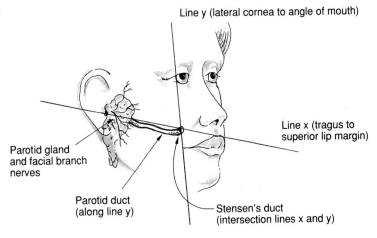

Line y (lateral cornea to angle of mouth)

Line x (tragus to superior lip margin)

Parotid gland and facial branch nerves

Parotid duct (along line y)

Stensen's duct (intersection lines x and y)

Figure 9–9

Clinical Findings

▶ facial nerve injury
  ▶ peripheral cranial nerve VII palsy
▶ parotid duct injury
  ▶ leak of methylene blue instilled via a cannula through Stensen's duct

Management

▶ maxillofacial surgery consultation
  ▶ repair soft tissues in multiple layers
  ▶ parotid duct lacerations repaired over a stent with a drain in place
  ▶ consider microsurgical repair of facial nerve lacerations

Tooth Injury

Ellis Fracture Classification (Figure 9–10)

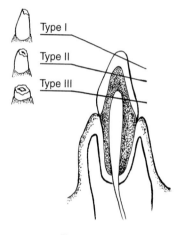

Figure 9–10

Type I

▶ involves enamel only
  ▶ white, chalky appearance
▶ treatment
  ▶ file sharp edges
  ▶ dental referral
    ▶ cosmetic deformity can be corrected using bonding material

Type II

▶ extends into the dentin
  ▶ dentin is identified by its pinkish or yellow appearance, as opposed to the white enamel

- ▶ patients with exposed dentin often complain of hot/cold sensitivity
- ▶ more serious in children under 12 years old
  - ▶ less dentin to protect the pulp against infection once exposed to the oral flora
- ▶ treatment
  - ▶ if a large area of dentin is exposed and the patient is over 12 years old, place calcium hydroxide paste and cover with foil
  - ▶ refer to dentist within 24 h
  - ▶ avoid hot/cold foods or fluids to minimize discomfort

Type III

- ▶ extends into the pulp
  - ▶ after wiping tooth with a cotton applicator, blood indicates exposed pulp
- ▶ severe pain expected due to exposed nerve
  - ▶ sometimes can be asensate when neurovascular supply is disrupted
- ▶ risk for abscess formation
- ▶ treatment
  - ▶ urgent dental consultation
  - ▶ place moistened cotton over the exposed pulp and cover with a piece of dry foil
  - ▶ consider a dental nerve block to control pain

Subluxation

Definition

- ▶ teeth loosened but not avulsed

Clinical Findings

- ▶ mobility evident by pushing tooth with a finger or tongue blade
- ▶ may see blood around the gingival crevice

Treatment

- ▶ minimally mobile
  - ▶ soft diet for several days
- ▶ markedly mobile
  - ▶ stabilization of tooth for 1–2 weeks
    - ▶ arch bars or dental wires
    - ▶ enamel bonding material
- ▶ dental referral

Avulsion

Clinical Findings

▶ tooth obviously malpositioned or completely avulsed from socket
▶ consider CXR to make sure tooth not aspirated

Treatment

▶ if tooth is recovered
  ▶ rinse gently to remove all dirt/debris
    ▹ scrubbing damages remaining periodontal ligament fibers and adversely affects reattachment
  ▶ place back into socket
    ▹ contraindicated for primary teeth since reimplanted primary teeth have a high tendency to ankylose, or fuse to the bone itself
    ▹ must be done promptly since after periodontal fibers are torn there is 1% less chance of regeneration with every passing minute
    ▹ if unable to replace, store in a balanced pH cell culture medium (marketed commercially) or milk
  ▶ splint to adjacent teeth
▶ if tooth is not recovered and there is bleeding from socket
  ▶ patient should bite on gauze soaked for 20 min
  ▶ if still bleeding, pack with absorbable gelatin sponge or oxidized regenerated cellulose and secure with a silk suture
▶ urgent dental referral

Prognosis

▶ most avulsions result in hypoxia and ultimate necrosis of the pulp
▶ object of immediate reimplantation is to keep the periodontal ligament alive, ensuring a retained functional tooth
▶ almost all reimplanted teeth require subsequent root canal therapy in order to
  ▶ debride the pulp
  ▶ render the tooth insensitive to pain
  ▶ fill and seal the pulp chamber with an inert material to prevent infection or chronic inflammation

10

Spine

General Principles

Mechanism

► motor vehicle collisions, 48%
► falls, 21%
► assault, 15%
► sports related, 14%
   ► shallow water diving accounts for most

Anatomic Distribution

► cervical—55%
► thoracic—15%
► thoraco-lumbar junction—15%
► lumbosacral—15%

Stability

► while certain fracture types are considered skeletally stable, it is best to assume instability until consultation with an orthopedic or neurosurgeon
   ► since at least 10% of cervical fractures are associated with another spinal column fracture, maintain full immobilization until absolutely certain an injury is solitary and stable (see Figure 1–4, p. 12)

Hyperflexion Injury

Subluxation

► potentially unstable
► rupture of ligamentous structures without bony fracture
► anterior longitudinal ligament usually remains intact to provide stability

▶ radiographic appearance
  ▶ widening of interspinous space
  ▶ flexion–extension views best demonstrate column displacement

Anterior Wedge Fracture (Figure 10–1)

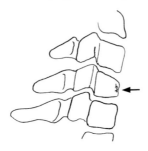

Figure 10–1

▶ stable
▶ anterior compressive forces sufficient to cause impaction of one vertebra by adjacent vertebrae
▶ radiographic appearance
  ▶ compressed anterior vertebral body

Flexion "Teardrop" Fracture (Figure 10–2)

▶ extremely unstable
▶ severe hyperflexion resulting in disruption of all ligaments
▶ disruption of facet joints
▶ common after diving accident
▶ anterior cord syndrome common
▶ radiographic appearance
  ▶ triangular fracture of anterior–inferior corner of vertebral body
  ▶ involved vertebra may be displaced and rotated

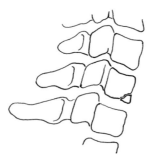

Figure 10–2

Spinous Process "Clay Shoveler's" Fracture (Figure 10–3)

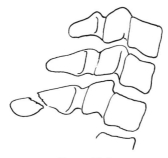

Figure 10–3

▶ stable
▶ in order of likelihood from most to least: C7, C6, T1
▶ no neurologic involvement
▶ mechanisms
 ▶ head and upper cervical spine flexed against pull of ligaments
  ▹ interspinous ligament avulses piece of the spinous process
  ▹ often called "Clay shoveler's" fracture because it often occurred when clay stuck to a shovel while a laborer attempted to throw it, thus provoking cervical hyperflexion
 ▶ direct trauma to spinous process
▶ radiographic appearance
 ▶ avulsion fracture of spinous process

Bilateral Facet Dislocation (Figure 10–4)

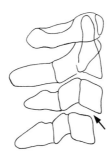

Figure 10–4

▶ unstable
▶ spinal cord injury occurs in most
  ▶ 85% are complete
  ▶ 15% are incomplete
▶ disruption of posterior ligaments with superior facets passing forward and upward, locking over inferior facets
▶ radiographic appearance
  ▶ anterior displacement by 50% of vertebral body AP diameter
  ▶ facets of involved vertebra lie anterior to inferior vertebra
  ▶ most obvious on oblique views

"Chance" Fracture (Figure 10–5)

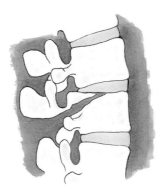

Figure 10–5

▶ flexion–distraction injury involving both fracture and posterior ligament disruption
▶ occurs secondary to distraction of the posterior, middle, and anterior columns
  ▶ anterior column acts as the center of rotation and the body bends around the fulcrum of a lap seat belt
  ▶ horizontal "splitting" occurs from posterior to anterior aspect of body
▶ typical mechanism
  ▶ head-on motor vehicle collision while wearing only a lap seat belt for restraint
▶ seldom associated with neurologic compromise unless a significant amount of translation or dislocation occurs
▶ radiographic appearance
  ▶ increased interspinous process distance on the anteroposterior view.
  ▶ increased posterior height of the vertebral body on the lateral view

Hyperextension Injury

Posterior Arch C1 Fracture (Figure 10–6)

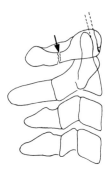

Figure 10–6

▶ stable, though can be confused with a Jefferson fracture (p. 126), which is unstable
▶ compression of posterior arch of C1 between occiput and spinous process of C2
▶ anterior arch and transverse ligament remain intact
▶ radiographic appearance
 ▶ minimally displaced vertical fracture of posterior arch of C1 on lateral view
 ▶ predental space normal
 ▶ no prevertebral swelling
 ▶ lateral masses not displaced on odontoid view

"Hangman's" Fracture (Figure 10–7)

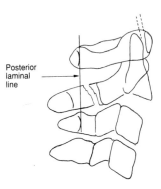

Posterior laminal line

Figure 10–7

▶ unstable
▶ traumatic spondylolysis of C2 caused by abrupt hyperextension
  ▶ fracture of the posterior elements
  ▶ gets its name because it is the goal in judicial hangings
▶ usually results in a high-level complete spinal cord injury which is almost invariably fatal
▶ radiographic appearance
  ▶ vertical pedicle fractures of C2
  ▶ displacement of C1–C2 complex
  ▶ marked prevertebral swelling

Extension "Teardrop" Fracture (Figure 10–8)

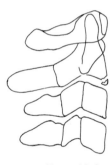

Figure 10–8

▶ unstable
▶ anterior longitudinal ligament pulls anterior–inferior corner of vertebral body away
▶ locations
  ▶ C2 most commonly involved
  ▶ C5–C7
▶ common in older patients falling onto the chin
  ▶ associated with central cord syndrome
▶ radiographic appearance
  ▶ triangular fragment avulsed from the anterior–inferior vertebral body (usually C2) on lateral radiograph

Body Fracture/Dislocation

▶ unstable
▶ force transmitted through lateral masses and posterior elements
▶ comminuted fracture of articular mass with extension to pedicles and lamina
▶ neurologic injury common
▶ radiographic appearance
    ▶ severely comminuted fracture of articular mass
    ▶ anterior displacement of vertebral body

Hyperflexion–Rotation Injury

Unilateral Facet Dislocation

▶ usually stable
    ▶ degree of ligamentous injury determines stability but generally stable since "locked" in place
▶ during flexion and rotation one facet acts as a pivot and the other dislocates with the superior facet riding forward over the tip of the inferior facet and resting in the neural foramen
▶ some present with neurological findings
    ▶ 40% with incomplete cord syndrome
    ▶ 30% with root neuropathy due to narrowing of the neural foramen
    ▶ 10% with complete cord syndrome
▶ radiographic appearance
    ▶ lateral view demonstrates involved vertebral body anteriorly displaced
    ▶ oblique views best show anterior displacement with "shingles" disrupted
    ▶ AP view demonstrates spinous processes above lesion deviated toward side of dislocation

Vertical Compression Injury

Burst Fracture of Body

▶ potentially unstable
▶ explosive comminuted fracture of vertebral body caused by axial load
    ▶ anterior fragments may resemble teardrop fracture
    ▶ posterior fragments may be displaced into spinal canal
▶ neurologic deficits common
    ▶ anterior cord syndrome
▶ radiographic appearance
    ▶ comminution of vertebral body
    ▶ decreased disk space

Jefferson Fracture (Figure 10–9)

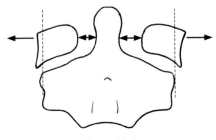

Figure 10–9

- ▶ unstable
- ▶ four-part burst fracture of C1 caused by axial load
  - ▶ two fractures in anterior arch
  - ▶ two fractures in posterior arch
- ▶ often no spinal cord injury since spinal canal is wide at C1
- ▶ commonly caused by diving
- ▶ radiographic appearance
  - ▶ lateral masses shifted laterally on open-mouth radiograph
  - ▶ prevertebral swelling on lateral radiograph

Extension-Rotation Injury

Articular Pillar Fracture

- ▶ stable
- ▶ hyperextension and rotation bring force on to a single pillar resulting in fracture
- ▶ associated anterior longitudinal ligament tear
- ▶ radiographic appearance
  - ▶ fracture in articular pillar
  - ▶ prevertebral swelling on lateral radiograph

Flexion–Rotation Injury

Odontoid Fractures (Figure 10–10)

- ▶ three types (Figure 10–10)
  - ▶ Type I—avulsion at tip of dens at site of alar ligament attachment
    - ▶ stable
    - ▶ uncommon

> ► Type II—transverse fracture at base of odontoid
>> ▸ unstable
>> ▸ most common type
>> ▸ in children under 6 years old, the open epiphysis may appear like a type II odontoid fracture
> ► Type III—fracture through body of C2 involving one or both superior articulating facets
>> ▸ potentially unstable

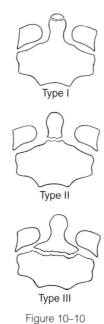

Type I

Type II

Type III

Figure 10–10

► radiographic appearance
>> ► open-mouth view best demonstrates fracture
>> ► conventional tomography best demonstrates fracture
>> ► axial CT may miss transverse fracture

Direct Force Injury

Transverse Process Fracture

► stable
► lumbar most common
► radiographic appearance
>> ► vertical fracture through transverse process seen on AP

Dislocation

Atlanto-Occipital Dislocation (Cranial–Cervical Disruption)

▶ unstable
▶ tearing of all ligamentous connections between C1 and occiput
▶ almost always an immediately fatal injury
▶ radiographic appearance
  ▶ displacement of occipital condyles from superior articulating facets of C1
  ▶ prevertebral swelling
▶ never apply traction or tongs

C1-Rotatory Subluxation

▶ occurs more often in children than adults
▶ open mouth view reveals asymmetry of the odontoid between the lateral masses of C1

Atlanto-Axial Dislocation

▶ unstable
▶ uncommon injury
▶ most seen in children
▶ adults with rheumatoid arthritis also at risk
  ▶ transverse ligament is weakened by chronic inflammation of the synovial joint between the odontoid (axis) and the anterior aspect of C1 (atlas)
▶ neurologic deficit common since rupture of the transverse ligament generally drives the odontoid into the medulla
▶ radiographic appearance
  ▶ increased predental space
    ▶ over 3 mm in adults
    ▶ over 5 mm in children
  ▶ abnormal C1–C2 position
  ▶ open-mouth view shows rotary subluxation and odontoid fracture

Radiography

Plain Radiographs

General

▶ when the spine is protected from further injury by immobilization, radiographs can be deferred until other evaluation and management priorities are met

▶ at least 10% of cervical fractures are associated with another spinal column fracture, mandating a careful search

Thoracic/Lumbar Spine

▶ order AP and lateral views
▶ indications
  ▶ bony tenderness
  ▶ neurologic findings
  ▶ significant mechanism and altered mental status
  ▶ axial load injury pattern such as associated with calcaneal fracture
  ▶ maintain lower threshold in the elderly

Cervical Spine

▶ see Chapter 40, p. 473, for interpretation guidelines
▶ in general, obtain nondynamic cervical radiographic series on every patient with serious traumatic injury above the clavicles
▶ can clinically exclude without radiographs when all of the following conditions are met
  ▶ no cervical pain or tenderness
  ▶ no paresthesias or neurologic deficits
  ▶ normal mental status
    ▶ sensorium not altered by intoxicants or brain injury
  ▶ no distracting pain
  ▶ over 4 years old (accurately communicates)
  ▶ after all the above conditions are met, release the collar straps and confirm there is no pain with slow and independent head movement
  ▶ to clinically exclude thoracic and lumbar spine injuries, gently log roll the patient (see p. 28) and ensure no thoracic or lumbar spinous process tenderness
▶ lateral view alone misses 15% of injuries
▶ three-view is 95% sensitive in radiographically excluding cervical spine injuries
  ▶ lateral (to the C7–T1 interface)
  ▶ AP
  ▶ odontoid (open mouth)
▶ submental view (closed-mouth odontoid) demonstrates odontoid when the patient cannot or refuses to cooperate with the open-mouth odontoid view
▶ oblique radiographs
  ▶ order "trauma obliques" which, unlike conventional obliques, do not require neck motion
  ▶ helpful when three-view suspicious of injury
  ▶ some institutions routinely obtain a five-view series (three-view and bilateral obliques)

▶ flexion–extension radiographs
  ▶ consist of lateral cervical views in both maximal flexion and extension
  ▶ performed only when the following requirements are met
    ▹ patient must be cooperative and sober, and move without assistance, just to the point of discomfort
    ▹ stop if neurologic symptoms develop
    ▹ physician should be present during this procedure
  ▶ obtain when high clinical suspicion of injury despite absence of neurological signs and normal nondynamic radiographs
    ▹ pain out of proportion to that of a cervical strain
    ▹ focal spinous process tenderness
    ▹ interpretation of nondynamic series difficult because of extensive degenerative arthritic changes
  ▶ detects ligamentous instability
  ▶ contraindicated when
    ▹ nondynamic view is suspicious of a fracture or subluxation
    ▹ clinical signs of an acute spinal cord lesion
    ▹ movement provokes neurologic symptoms

CT

General Principles

▶ order 2–3 mm cuts above and below the area of interest
▶ contrast is unnecessary

Indications

▶ fractures seen or suspected on plain radiographs should be followed by CT for better definition
▶ cannot visualize all cervical vertebrae or the C7–T1 articulation on the lateral radiograph
▶ subluxation on flexion–extension views

Advantages

▶ excellent images of complex bony anatomy
▶ spinal cord and canal evaluated
▶ patient can remain in spinal immobilization

Disadvantages

▶ limited utility for ligamentous disruptions
▶ poor visibility of horizontally oriented fractures on axial reconstruction

MRI

General Principles

▶ patient should be stable

Indications

▶ consider whenever neurological signs are present
▶ helpful for patients that require but cannot tolerate flexion–extension views

Advantages

▶ detects bone, ligament and cord injuries

Disadvantages

▶ may not be possible when life-support equipment is required (unless special set-up in place)
▶ lacks high resolution for bony anatomy
▶ often not immediately available

Contraindications

▶ metallic foreign bodies
▶ pacemaker
▶ cerebral aneurysm clips

Spinal Cord Injury

Pathophysiology

▶ from direct trauma or spinal artery interruption
▶ results in cord hemorrhage, edema, and/or neuron disruption

Neurologic Examination

Sensory Function

▶ see Figure 10–11

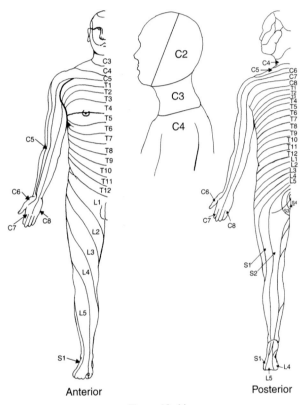

Anterior   Posterior

Figure 10–11

Motor Function

▶ see Table 10–1
▶ American Spinal Injury Association (ASIA) grading system
  ▶ 0 = paralysis
  ▶ 1 = visible flicker or palpable contraction
  ▶ 2 = movement with gravity eliminated
  ▶ 3 = barely able to overcome gravity
  ▶ 4 = less than normal when tested against resistance
  ▶ 5 = normal

Table 10–1 Nerve Function

Nerve Root	Motor/Function	Sensory	Reflex
C4	Diaphragm/ventilation	Suprasternal notch	
C5	Deltoid/shoulder shrug	Below clavicle	Biceps
C6	Biceps/elbow flexion, wrist extension	Thumb	Biceps
C7	Triceps/elbow extension	Middle finger	Triceps
C8	Flexor digitorum/finger flexion	Little finger	
T1	Interossei/spread fingers	Medial forearm	
T4	Intercostal/ventilation	Nipples	
T8		Xiphoid	
T10	Abdominal musculature	Umbilicus	
T12		Pubic symphysis	
L1/L2	Iliopsoas/hip flexion	Upper thigh	
L3	Quadriceps/knee extension	Medial thigh	Patellar
L4	Quadraceps/knee extension	Big toe	Patellar
L5	Extensor hallucis longus/great toe dorsiflexion	Middle toe	
S1	Gastrocnemius and soleus/ankle plantarflexion	Little toe	Achilles
S2/S3/S4	Anal sphincter/bowel and bladder	Perianal area	Bulbocavernosus

Ventilatory Function

▶ vital capacity (VC) reduced
  ▶ 95% in high cervical cord injuries
  ▶ 75% in low cervical cord injuries
  ▶ 50% in high thoracic cord injuries
  ▶ 0% in cord injuries below T10

Clinical Presentation

Neurogenic Shock

▶ must first exclude
  ▶ hemorrhagic shock
  ▶ cardiogenic shock
▶ results from disruption of descending autonomic pathways due to spinal cord injury above T6

▶ loss of sympathetic vascular tone below level of injury causes "neurologic hypotension"
▶ heart rate normal or slow due to unopposed vagal tone
   ▶ bradycardia responds to atropine
▶ skin signs normal despite hypotension because of vasodilation
▶ treat with Trendelenburg position, crystalloid infusion and alpha-agonist
   ▶ high-dose dopamine
   ▶ epinephrine
   ▶ ephedrine
▶ treating with crystalloid alone can precipitate pulmonary edema
▶ consider central venous or pulmonary artery pressure monitoring
▶ resolves usually within 24 h but may last up to a week

Complete Cord Syndrome

▶ pathophysiology
   ▶ complete loss of sensorimotor function below the level of injury
▶ clinical examination
   ▶ neurologic examination clinically determines level of injury (Table 10–1)
      ▶ the sensory level refers to the highest level of normal sensation on both sides
      ▶ the motor level refers to the highest level of motor function (ASIA grade at least 3/5) on both sides
   ▶ "sacral sparing" generally absent
▶ prognosis
   ▶ at onset of injury, 5% with complete cord syndrome may recover
   ▶ when sensorimotor deficit persists
      ▶ after 24 h only 1% recover
      ▶ after 72 h none recover
   ▶ neurogenic shock common

Incomplete Cord Syndrome

▶ pathophysiology
   ▶ incomplete loss of sensorimotor function below the level of injury
   ▶ "spinal shock" refers to neuropraxia associated with incomplete cord syndromes and should not be confused with neurogenic shock
▶ clinical examination
   ▶ may be able to be further subcategorized by the syndromes listed below
   ▶ neurologic examination clinically determines level of injury (Table 10–1)
   ▶ the presence of "sacral sparing" shows potential for recovery and is much more common in incomplete than complete cord syndromes
   ▶ evidence of "sacral sparing" includes
      ▶ perianal sensation
      ▶ rectal sphincter tone
      ▶ slight toe flexion

▶ prognosis
    ▶ in incomplete syndromes over half the patients will eventually walk

Central Cord Syndrome (Figure 10–12)

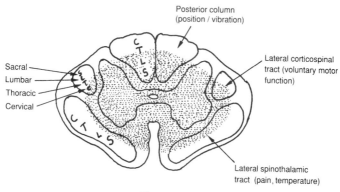

Figure 10–12

(figure labels) Posterior column (position / vibration); Lateral corticospinal tract (voluntary motor function); Lateral spinothalamic tract (pain, temperature); Sacral, Lumbar, Thoracic, Cervical

▶ history
    ▶ typically a forward fall onto the face in an elderly person
▶ pathophysiology
    ▶ during forced hyperextension the ligamentum flavum buckles into the cord, causing contusion of the central part of cord
    ▶ more common in those with cervical osteoarthritis and vertebral canal stenosis
    ▶ central gray matter (motor) and pyramidal/spinothalamic (sensory) tracts affected with greater deficit in upper extremities than lower extremities
▶ clinical examination
    ▶ sensorimotor deficit greater in the upper than lower extremities and distal muscles more involved than proximal
    ▶ fibers controlling voluntary bowel/bladder function are centrally located and often affected, though "sacral sparing" is usually present
    ▶ dysesthesias (painful burning sensation) occur primarily in the upper extremities
▶ prognosis
    ▶ nonoperative therapy
    ▶ 50% regain some function
        ▶ recovery pattern is usually lower extremity strength first, followed by bowel/bladder function, and then upper extremity strength

Brown–Sequard Syndrome (Figure 10–13)

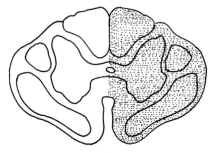

Figure 10–13

- ▶ pathophysiology
  - ▶ hemisection of spinal cord, which is a rare result of penetrating injuries or lateral mass fractures of cervical spine
- ▶ clinical examination
  - ▶ ipsilateral loss of motor strength, vibratory sensation, and proprioception (joint position)
  - ▶ contralateral loss of pain and temperature sensation
- ▶ prognosis
  - ▶ most patients improve

Anterior Cord Syndrome (Figure 10–14)

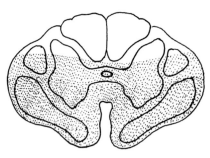

Figure 10–14

- ▶ pathophysiology
  - ▶ interruption of the anterior spinal arteries
    - ▹ as a complication of descending aorta injury or repair
  - ▶ flexion injuries with posterior protrusion of bony fragments or disk herniation causing direct injury to the anterior cord
    - ▹ as with a burst fracture of the vertebral body

▶ clinical examination
  ▶ variable degrees of motor paralysis and absent pain sensation below the lesion
  ▶ preservation of vibratory sensation and proprioception (posterior column intact)
▶ prognosis
  ▶ some improvement may follow but most patients do not regain motor function
    ▷ this injury has the poorest prognosis of all the incomplete cord syndromes
  ▶ surgery required if ventral compression is demonstrated

Conus Medularis

▶ pathophysiology
  ▶ sacral cord injury which may involve lumbar roots
▶ clinical examination
  ▶ areflexic bowel/bladder
  ▶ variable motor/sensory loss in lower extremities

Cauda Equina

▶ pathophysiology
  ▶ usually due to large central lumbar disk herniation with injury to bilateral lumbosacral nerve roots
  ▶ can occur from subluxation at the thoracolumbar junction
▶ clinical examination
  ▶ areflexic bowel/bladder
  ▶ variable motor/sensory loss in lower extremities
  ▶ areflexia in lower extremities

Spinal Cord Injury Without Radiographic Abnormality (SCIWORA)

▶ seen in children because the spinal cord is less elastic than the bony spine and ligaments
▶ associated with paresthesias and generalized weakness
▶ symptoms may be delayed in 25% of cases
▶ consider MRI, which can confirm the diagnosis

Management

General Principles

▶ intubation necessary for those with decreased vital capacity (under 10 ml/kg), tachypnea, or elevated A-a gradient (over 40) since impending ventilatory insufficiency is likely

▶ for all patients with clinical evidence of a spinal cord syndrome
  ▶ obtain immediate neurosurgical consultation for unstable injuries or neurologic findings
  ▶ presume the spine is unstable and maintain immobilization with collar and backboard
    ▷ try to minimize the time a patient with a confirmed unstable spine lies on a backboard by facilitating the consultant in setting up a halo vest or Stryker frame
    ▷ when the spine is determined to be stable, take the patient off the backboard
  ▶ consider transfer to a specialized spinal cord unit after stabilization if necessary
  ▶ assess for other injuries
    ▷ lack of sensation complicates the clinical evaluation and the abdominal examination becomes unhelpful for the determination of intraabdominal injuries

Methylprednisolone (Solumedrol)

▶ consider when subjective symptoms or objective neurologic findings are consistent with a spinal cord injury
  ▶ the National Association of Spinal Cord Injury Studies (NASCIS) showed improvement in ASIA motor scores when initiated as soon as possible and most follow the dosing protocol below if within 8 h of injury
  ▶ many believe these studies were flawed and that the aggregate risk does not outweigh potential benefit
▶ dose
  ▶ bolus = 30 mg/kg over 15 min
  ▶ maintenance = 5.4 mg/kg per h for next 23 h

Penetrating Neck Trauma

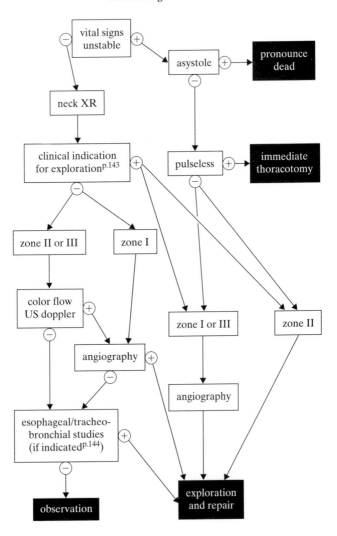

11

Neck

General Principles

► lack of bony protection makes the neck vulnerable to injury
► there are a large number of exposed vital structures
  ► concurrent injury to multiple structures is common
► early protection of airway is of paramount importance
► rapid but thorough diagnostic investigation is indicated

Penetrating Trauma

Anatomic Zones (Figure 11–1)

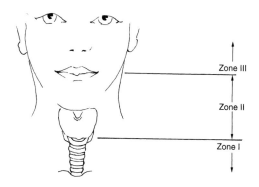

Figure 11–1

Zone I

► below cricoid cartilage
► may cause injury to structures near the thoracic outlet
► may require sternotomy for proximal control

Zone II

▶ above cricoid cartilage and below the angle of the mandible
▶ easiest area to operatively expose, evaluate, and repair injured structures

Zone III

▶ above the angle of the mandible
▶ most difficult area to expose surgically
▶ distal control is difficult or impossible to obtain

Management

Initial Intervention

▶ with significant injuries, immediate airway control is essential
  ▶ an expanding hematoma and laryngeal injury will cause airway compromise and make intubation difficult
    ▹ perform early prophylactic intubation as patients may worsen during diagnostic testing outside the resuscitation area
  ▶ the cervical spine may be considered stable after penetrating trauma as spinal cord injuries do not progress
    ▹ unlike in blunt trauma, cervical spine immobilization in patients with penetrating neck wounds should not hinder endotracheal intubation, especially when the initial neurologic examination is normal
▶ control bleeding with pressure and not clamps
▶ it is permissible to gently separate the wound edges and inspect the wound
▶ never blindly probe penetrating wounds to assess depth or direction as there is a great risk of interrupting hemostasis or worsening injury
▶ patients with clear indications for surgery (i.e., shock, expanding hematoma or uncontrolled bleeding) should be taken emergently to the operating room

Zone I Injuries

▶ operative intervention is indicated for significant injuries identified either on physical examination or on ancillary diagnostic testing

Zone II Injuries

▶ selective exploration approach (recommended by the authors)
  ▶ explore whenever there are significant findings on clinical examination (see Table 11–1)
  ▶ ancillary diagnostic testing is used to exclude occult injury and to identify candidates for exploration and injury repair
    ▹ includes angiography, esophagoscopy, and laryngoscopy

- ▶ advantages
  - ▹ sensitive for injury identification
  - ▹ reduces incidence of negative neck exploration by 30–50%
- ▶ mandatory exploration approach
  - ▶ all wounds that penetrate the platysma undergo operative exploration
  - ▶ advantages
    - ▹ prevents complications related to delayed diagnosis
    - ▹ low surgical morbidity
    - ▹ exploration is technically straightforward (though injury repair may not be)

Table 11–1 Clinical indications for neck exploration—no need for ancillary diagnostic testing

Vascular	History of substantial blood loss
	Active bleeding
	Expanding hematoma
	Decreased carotid pulse
Airway	Hemoptysis
	Crepitus
	Dysphonia
GI	Hematemesis
	Dysphagia
	Crepitus
CNS	Sensory deficit
	Horner's syndrome
	Facial droop
Complicating factors	Lack of cooperation
	Associated injury

Zone III Injuries

- ▶ perform a careful oropharyngeal examination with zone III wounds
- ▶ operative intervention is indicated for significant injuries identified clinically or after diagnostic testing

Vascular Injuries

Clinical Findings

- ▶ airway compromise due to neck swelling or distortion
- ▶ active bleeding
- ▶ shock
- ▶ expanding hematoma
- ▶ decreased pulse (carotid, temporal, facial, and upper extremity arteries)

▶ carotid bruit or thrill
▶ hemothorax
▶ air embolism
▶ neurologic deficit

Imaging (see algorithm, p. 140)

▶ zone I injuries
  ▶ perform angiography on all stable patients
  ▶ assesses the integrity of thoracic outlet vessels whose repair mandates thoracotomy prior to neck exploration
▶ zone II injuries
  ▶ using selective management approach
    ▻ with experienced operator, color flow doppler can be used as screening tool and, if positive, followed by angiography
    ▻ close (inpatient) observation and no imaging modality for those with very low-velocity injuries (i.e., stab or pellet wound)
    ▻ no imaging when clinical criteria for surgery are met
  ▶ using mandatory surgical approach
    ▻ imaging unnecessary as any injuries will be defined at surgery
▶ zone III injuries
  ▶ perform angiography or color-flow doppler on all stable patients
  ▶ an injury amenable to angiographic embolization avoids a technically difficult operation

Esophageal Injuries

General Principles

▶ recognition is sometimes difficult since initial clinical signs may be subtle and generally nonspecific
▶ aggressive diagnostic evaluation is indicated
▶ delayed repair results in high morbidity due to contamination of para-esophageal space

Clinical Signs

▶ neck pain or tenderness
▶ dysphagia
▶ dyspnea
▶ hematemesis
▶ subcutaneous emphysema
▶ resistance of neck to passive motion
▶ crepitation

Diagnosis

▶ general principles
  ▶ no one study should be relied on to exclude esophageal injury
    ▹ use a combination of physical signs, radiographs (plain and with oral contrast), and esophagoscopy to make diagnosis
▶ neck radiography
  ▶ order AP and lateral "soft tissue" views
  ▶ locate missile position
  ▶ findings suggestive of esophageal injury
    ▹ subcutaneous air
    ▹ pneumomediastinum
    ▹ increased prevertebral soft tissue space
▶ chest radiography (CXR)
  ▶ findings suggestive of esophageal injury
    ▹ pleural effusion
    ▹ pneumothorax
    ▹ pneumomediastinum
    ▹ mediastinal widening
▶ esophageal contrast studies
  ▶ general principles
    ▹ up to 40% false negative rate
    ▹ use in conjunction with esophagoscopy to increase sensitivity
  ▶ indications
    ▹ strong clinical signs
    ▹ projectile path proximate to the esophagus
    ▹ presence of subcutaneous air on plain radiographs
  ▶ use gastrografin initially and, if negative, follow by barium
    ▹ barium study is more sensitive, but causes a chemical mediastinitis
▶ esophagoscopy
  ▶ indications
    ▹ clinical suspicion despite a negative contrast study in order to increase diagnostic sensitivity
    ▹ some perform in lieu of contrast studies
  ▶ scope type
    ▹ can be done with flexible type outside the operating room and without neck extension
    ▹ rigid scope is preferred in suspected upper cervical esophageal injuries since blind passage of a flexible scope through the cricopharyngeus may miss a proximate injury

Management

▶ surgical repair and adequate drainage of deep neck spaces required for cervical esophageal and lower hypopharyngeal injuries
  ▶ earlier repair decreases complications

▶ nonsurgical management acceptable for some injuries to upper portion of
   hypopharynx
▶ administer broad-spectrum antibiotics

Laryngeal Injuries

Clinical Findings

▶ voice alteration (dysphonia)
▶ airway compromise
▶ dysphagia
▶ swelling or deformity
   ▸ gently palpate the area to prevent a worsening of the injury
▶ subcutaneous emphysema or crepitus
▶ hemoptysis
▶ bubbling wound

Diagnosis

▶ "soft tissue" neck radiograph
   ▸ may reveal
      ▹ subcutaneous emphysema or prevertebral air
      ▹ laryngeal fracture (when calcified larynx visible)
▶ visualization of endolarynx via indirect or direct laryngoscopy
   ▸ procedure of choice to identify injuries
   ▸ indications
      ▹ positive clinical findings otherwise suspicious for laryngeal injury
   ▸ may reveal mucosal disruptions, bleeding, and displacement
▶ CT
   ▸ accurately identifies the location and extent of laryngeal fractures
   ▸ indications
      ▹ inability to perform laryngoscopy
      ▹ fracture suspected even with negative laryngoscopy

Treatment

▶ early airway management for significant fractures
   ▸ with minimal airway compromise, use rapid sequence induction and
     orotracheal intubation
   ▸ with moderate–severe airway compromise, use awake orotracheal in-
     tubation techniques
   ▸ if a severely fractured larynx is present, tracheostomy is the preferred
     method for airway management
▶ prompt operative repair for displaced fractures
▶ nonoperative management for nondisplaced fractures

Blunt Trauma

General Principles

▶ clinical findings are often more subtle than with penetrating neck trauma
▶ concurrent cervical spine injuries are frequent
▶ mandatory airway management at first sign of airway compromise

Vascular Injury

Clinical Signs

▶ neurologic findings incongruent with head CT
▶ delay between trauma and symptoms typical
▶ carotid artery injury
  ▶ hematoma over lateral neck
  ▶ bruit over carotid circulation
  ▶ Horner's syndrome
    ▹ ptosis, miosis, and anhydrosis
  ▶ stroke syndrome
    ▹ hemiparesis, hemiplegia, and/or aphasia
▶ vertebral artery injury
  ▶ ataxia
  ▶ vertigo and nystagmus
  ▶ hemiparesis
  ▶ dysarthria and diplopia

Diagnosis

▶ clinical diagnosis is challenging since
  ▶ up to 50% without external signs of trauma
  ▶ delayed neurologic deficits are typical
    ▹ 10% present within 1 h
    ▹ 75% present between 1 and 24 h
    ▹ 15% present after 24 h, sometimes weeks later
▶ four-vessel angiography
  ▶ indications
    ▹ strong clinical findings
    ▹ significant mechanism of injury and weak clinical findings
  ▶ includes both carotid and both vertebral arteries since multiple injuries occur in 40%
▶ color-flow doppler ultrasound
  ▶ provides rapid identification and quantification of arterial dissection
  ▶ unable to assess distal upper extracranial and intracranial internal carotid artery
  ▶ operator dependent
  ▶ use as screening role in lower-risk patients

▶ helical CT angiography
  ▶ used as a screening modality for patients at risk for blunt carotid injury
  ▶ decreases time to diagnose cervical arterial injury
  ▶ increases detection rate of cervical arterial injury
▶ MR angiography (MRA)
  ▶ accurately detects carotid and vertebral artery injuries
  ▶ best for follow-up or for stable patients since it is difficult to utilize in acutely injured, unstable patients

Management

▶ depends on size of lesions and clinical picture
▶ options
  ▶ observation
  ▶ anticoagulation
  ▶ antiplatelet agents
  ▶ arterial reconstruction
  ▶ ligation
▶ revascularization is without benefit after extensive intracerebral embolization

Laryngeal Injuries

Mechanism

▶ compression of thyroid and cricoid cartilage against cervical spine
▶ "padded dash syndrome" occurs when the larynx strikes the dashboard in vehicular collisions

Clinical Findings

▶ airway compromise
▶ stridor
▶ pain and tenderness
▶ dysphonia (voice alteration)
▶ dysphagia
▶ subcutaneous emphysema or crepitus
▶ hemoptysis
▶ recurrent laryngeal nerve injury
▶ anterior neck hematoma
▶ intralaryngeal hematoma and edema
  ▶ may not reach maximum until several hours after injury

Diagnosis

▶ "soft tissue" neck radiographs
  ▶ indications
    ▶ positive clinical findings
    ▶ significant mechanism for injury

▹ radiographic findings suggestive of injury
  ▹ subcutaneous emphysema or prevertebral air
  ▹ laryngeal fracture (when calcified larynx visible)
▶ CT
  ▶ accurately identifies the location and extent of laryngeal fractures
  ▶ indications
    ▹ positive clinical or radiographic findings
    ▹ high clinical suspicion for injury
    ▹ aids in preoperative planning in significantly displaced fractures
    ▹ useful when laryngoscopy cannot be performed (e.g., intubated patient)
▶ direct laryngoscopy
  ▶ most accurate test
  ▶ determines function and status of internal soft tissue defects
  ▶ positive findings include edema, hematoma, and mucosal disruptions

Management

▶ protect airway from potential compromise
▶ endotracheal intubation is controversial with severely displaced fractures
▶ tracheotomy is advocated when surgical airway is indicated
  ▶ cricothyrotomy contraindicated
▶ prompt operative repair for displaced fractures or dislocated cartilage
▶ nonoperative management for nondisplaced fractures

Esophageal Injury

General Principles

▶ an exceedingly rare blunt injury
▶ often masked by laryngeal trauma

Clinical Signs

▶ neck pain
▶ dyspnea
▶ hematemesis
▶ subcutaneous emphysema

Diagnosis

▶ "soft tissue" neck radiographs
  ▶ suggestive findings
    ▹ subcutaneous air
    ▹ pneumomediastinum
    ▹ increased prevertebral soft tissue space

▶ esophageal contrast studies
  ▶ general principles
    ▸ significant false negative rate
    ▸ perform in conjunction with esophagoscopy to increase diagnostic yield
▶ indications
    ▸ positive physical findings/high clinical suspicion
    ▸ presence of subcutaneous air on plain radiographs
  ▶ use gastrografin initially and, if negative, follow by barium
    ▸ barium causes a chemical mediastinitis
▶ esophagoscopy
  ▶ indicated when there is clinical suspicion despite a negative contrast study
  ▶ can worsen the injury with the scope, so perform contrast studies beforehand

Management

▶ early surgical therapy for esophageal or large (over 2 cm) pharyngeal perforations
▶ medical therapy for small (under 2 cm) pharyngeal perforations
▶ broad-spectrum antibiotics

Blunt Chest Trauma

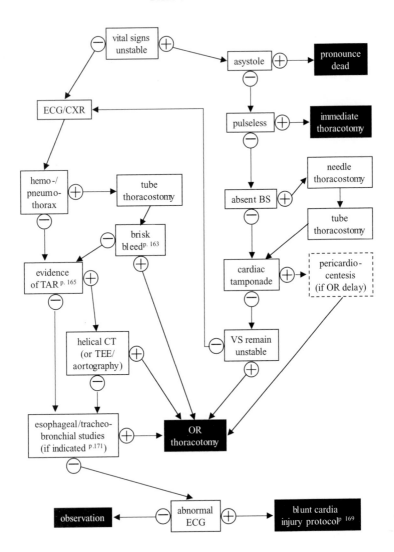

12

Chest: Blunt

General Principles

Testing

- ▶ perform immediate chest radiograph (CXR) after significant blunt mechanism
  - ▶ to define associated injuries
- ▶ when available, FAST examination with thoracic views rapidly detects
  - ▶ significant hemothorax
  - ▶ pericardial effusion

Treatment

- ▶ hemodynamically unstable patients require the following sequential interventions until stability is restored
  - ▶ needle decompression if suspected tension pneumothorax
  - ▶ immediate intubation
  - ▶ fluid resuscitation
  - ▶ thoracotomy in the resuscitation area

Rib Fracture

Pathophysiology

Definitions

- ▶ the term "upper ribs" refers to the first three
- ▶ the term "middle ribs" refers to the middle six
- ▶ the term "lower ribs" refers to the last three

Mechanism

- ▶ AP force causes "outward" fractures usually at the postero-lateral angle, the thinnest portion of the rib

▶ direct blow causes "inward" fractures at the point of impact that can puncture the lung parenchyma

Associated Injuries

▶ upper rib fractures
  ▶ indicates a powerful mechanism of injury since the ribs are well protected by the clavicles, scapulae, and shoulder musculature
  ▶ 36% mortality due to associated intrathoracic injuries
  ▶ 6% have major vascular injuries and aortography/angiography must be considered
  ▶ brachial plexopathy can occur
▶ middle rib fractures
  ▶ lung injuries are common
▶ lower ribs fractures
  ▶ 10% of patients with right-sided fractures have liver injuries
  ▶ 20% of patients with left-sided fractures have spleen injuries

Clinical Findings

Symptoms

▶ localized pleuritic chest pain
▶ pain aggravated by position changes
▶ dyspnea

Signs (Diagnostic)

▶ tenderness
  ▶ point tenderness over a rib, when severe, is strongly associated with the presence of a fracture
  ▶ rib cage compression distant from the fracture will cause focal pain at the fracture
▶ bony crepitance

Chest Radiograph

▶ obtained to exclude associated hemo- or pneumothorax
▶ 50% of rib fractures are missed though upper rib fractures are usually seen

Rib Radiographs

▶ consist of oblique views and increase sensitivity for fractures
▶ generally unnecessary since management decisions can be made based on the clinical diagnosis of rib fractures

Management

Analgesia

▶ adequate pain relief improves compliance with deep breathing exercises
  ▶ prevents development of atelectasis or pneumonia associated with splinting
▶ consider an epidural catheter
▶ intercostal blocks provide temporary pain management (see p. 463)
▶ rib belts, binders, and chest wall taping are not recommended
  ▶ they restrict chest wall movement
  ▶ they are associated with atelectasis and ventilatory insufficiency

Thoracostomy

▶ for any patient who must emergently undergo general anesthesia, perform a prophylactic thoracostomy when there is clinical or radiographic evidence of rib fractures
  ▶ positive pressure ventilation can create a tension pneumothorax if the lung parenchyma was injured

Special Groups

▶ children
  ▶ rib fractures require significant force since the child's chest is more flexible
  ▶ evaluate carefully for intrathoracic injuries
  ▶ associated with child abuse
▶ term pregnant women or elderly patients
  ▶ there is less functional reserve and hypoxia or hypoventilation is more likely
  ▶ presence of multiple rib fractures mandates admission

Flail Chest

Pathophysiology (Figure 12–1)

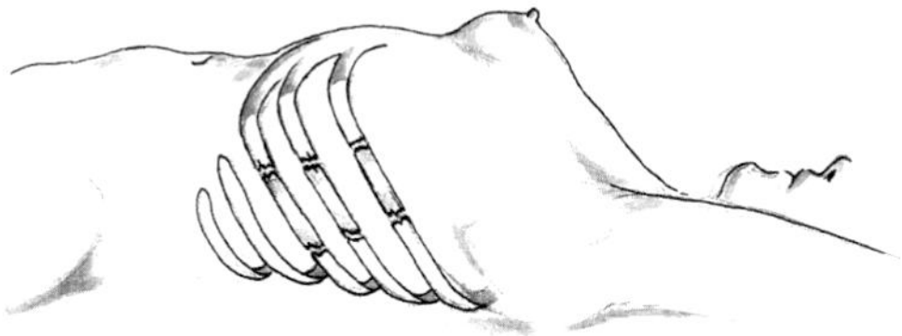

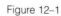

Figure 12–1

- three or more adjacent rib fractures each in two places creates a flail chest
  - segment paradoxically moves in with inspiration and out with expiration
- rarely caused by sternocostal disruption ("sternal flail chest")
- ventilatory failure due to
  - decreased vital capacity
  - *pendaluft*—gas moving from lung to lung with ventilatory effort rather than exchanged with outside air
  - pulmonary contusion
  - mediastinum may shift with respiratory effort causing a decrease in venous return
  - physiologic splinting to reduce pain
- 10% mortality

Clinical Findings/Diagnosis

- careful inspection and palpation reveal the paradoxically moving flail segment
- 20% have a delay in diagnosis of more than 24 h after initial assessment

Management

- in the prehospital setting, to stabilize the flail segment
  - use manual pressure
  - position the patient with the flail segment down
- provide adequate analgesia
  - epidural catheter recommended
- serial ABGs to determine degree of ventilatory insufficiency
- intubate at the first sign of ventilatory failure or hypoxia

Sternal Fracture

Pathophysiology

- mechanism of injury
  - anterior blunt force
  - most commonly from chest impact on steering wheel during MVC
- most often occurs at sternomanubrial joint or the mid-body

Clinical Findings

Symptoms

- anterior chest pain
- dyspnea

Signs

▶ focal tenderness
▶ ecchymosis and hematoma over sternum

Diagnosis

▶ most visualized on a lateral CXR

Management

▶ up to 50% have serious associated injuries including
  ▶ blunt cardiac injury
  ▶ pulmonary contusion
  ▶ traumatic aortic rupture
  ▶ ventricular rupture
▶ normal CXR (except for the sternal fracture) and normal ECG suggests low likelihood for associated serious injury
▶ displaced fractures require reduction
  ▶ attempt closed reduction by depressing the anterior segment
▶ open reduction for unstable fractures or those displaced by over 1 cm overlap
▶ admit patients for
  ▶ observation
  ▶ pain control
  ▶ pulmonary toilet
  ▶ diagnosis and management of other injuries

Scapular Fracture

Pathophysiology

▶ the scapula is a sturdy, mobile, well-protected structure that resists injury
▶ up to 80% of cases harbor serious associated injuries including
  ▶ 50%—pulmonary contusion or hemo-/pneumothorax
  ▶ 50%—ipsilateral upper rib fractures
  ▶ 10%—arterial injury in the ipsilateral extremity
  ▶ 10%—brachial plexus injury

▶ fracture site prevalence (see Figure 12–2)
- ▶ body—50%
- ▶ neck—20%
- ▶ glenoid—15%
- ▶ acromion—10%
- ▶ coracoid—5%

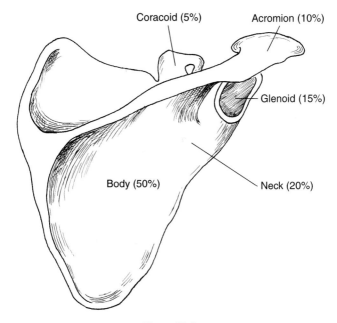

Figure 12–2

Clinical Findings

▶ pain or tenderness
▶ bony crepitus
▶ decreased shoulder motion

Management

▶ shoulder immobilizer and sling is adequate for most
▶ consult orthopedic surgeon
  - ▶ operative repair is necessary for severely displaced fractures
▶ exclude associated injuries

Pulmonary Contusion

Pathophysiology

▶ blunt traumatic force to the chest causes lung parenchymal injury
  ▶ results in interstitial leak of blood and protein
  ▶ severity generally peaks at 48–72 h

Clinical Findings

Symptoms

▶ progressively worsening dyspnea

Signs

▶ tachypnea
▶ decreasing oxygen saturation and increasing A-a gradient

Diagnosis

Chest Radiograph

▶ dense pulmonary infiltrate over the injured area becomes evident 12–24 h after injury so it is a poor *early* clinical predictor
▶ rate of progression of clinical and radiographic findings correlates with severity
▶ CT can confirm diagnosis earlier than plain radiographs

Management

▶ supplemental oxygen
▶ selective intubation
  ▶ hypoventilation
  ▶ hypoxia
▶ avoid overhydration
▶ consider central venous pressure or pulmonary artery monitoring with major contusions

Pneumothorax

Pathophysiology

▶ penetration of pulmonary parenchyma causes air to enter and become trapped in the potential space between the parietal and visceral pleura

▶ an air leak can occur from rupture of a pulmonary bleb during a valsalva or crush mechanism
▶ air in the hemithorax collapses the lung and interferes with ventilation and oxygenation

Clinical Findings

Symptoms

▶ dyspnea
▶ pain in the back, shoulders, or chest (pleuritic)

Signs

▶ tachypnea
▶ subcutaneous emphysema
▶ decreased or absent breath sounds
▶ hyperresonance (tympany) to percussion

Diagnosis

▶ usually evident on the AP CXR
  ▶ size can be roughly estimated by measuring the air space in the periphery of the hemithorax (Figure 12–3)
    ▶ 1 cm = 10%
    ▶ 2 cm = 20%
    ▶ 3 cm = 30%

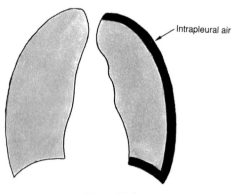

Figure 12–3

▶ upright, expiratory CXRs have increased sensitivity

Management

▶ tube thoracostomy required when
- ▶ medium–large pneumothorax (over 20%)
  - ▹ use small-bore chest tube (22–24 Fr)
- ▶ associated with hemothorax
  - ▹ use large-bore chest tube (36–40 Fr)
- ▶ attach to underwater seal with suction
▶ small pneumothoraces (under 20%) can be managed without thoracostomy if
- ▶ the patient is reliable and otherwise healthy
- ▶ no mechanical ventilation is anticipated
  - ▹ patients who will undergo emergent general anesthesia for any reason require a prophylactic tube thoracostomy
  - ▹ positive pressure ventilation can convert a simple pneumothorax into a tension pneumothorax
- ▶ a repeat CXR in 6–12 h does not show an increase in its size
- ▶ pulmonary symptoms do not worsen

Tension Pneumothorax

Pathophysiology (Figure 12–4)

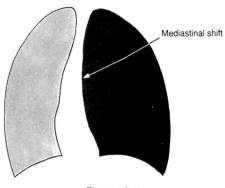

Figure 12–4

▶ air leak acts as a one-way valve with air entering the pleural cavity on inspiration and being unable to escape on expiration
- ▶ causes progressive mediastinal shift that impedes venous blood return to the heart
▶ a simple pneumothorax can be converted to a tension pneumothorax during positive pressure ventilation

Clinical Findings

Symptoms

▶ extreme dyspnea
▶ altered level of consciousness

Signs

▶ hypotension
▶ tachycardia
▶ cyanosis
▶ absent breath sounds
▶ hyperresonance to percussion (tympany)
▶ tracheal deviation away from the affected hemithorax
▶ jugular venous distension
  ▶ absent when there is severe hypovolemia

Diagnosis

▶ must be based entirely on clinical findings
  ▶ while CXR shows mediastinal shift, obtaining one should not precede management when the diagnosis is clinically evident

Management

▶ perform immediate needle decompression
  ▶ insert a large bore (10–16 gauge) angiocath into the second anterior or the fifth lateral intercostal space
▶ perform a tube thoracostomy after decompression

Hemothorax

Pathophysiology (Figure 12–5)

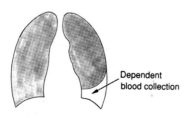

Dependent
blood collection

Figure 12–5

▶ penetration of pulmonary parenchyma or injury to intercostal or internal mammary vessels causes intrathoracic bleeding
▶ massive, continuous bleeding generally results from pulmonary hilar injuries, traumatic aortic rupture, or myocardial rupture

Clinical Findings

Symptoms

▶ dyspnea
▶ pleuritic chest, shoulder, or back pain

Signs

▶ tachypnea
▶ absent breath sounds
▶ dullness to percussion

Chest Radiographs

▶ upright films demonstrate effusions over 300 ml
▶ supine films may show only hemithoracic haziness
▶ very small hemothoraces may remain undiagnosed by chest radiography and often resolve uneventfully

Chest CT Scan

▶ extremely sensitive for even very small hemothoraces

Management

▶ treat hemorrhagic shock
▶ thoracostomy using a large-bore chest tube (i.e., 36–40 Fr) with auto-transfusion setup is mandatory for acute hemothoraces (see p. 449)
▶ utilize autologous blood when over 500 ml collected
▶ the decision to perform an urgent thoracotomy must be correlated with the patient's hemodynamic status, fluid requirements, and associated injuries
▶ guidelines for thoracotomy include the following
  ▶ over 20 ml/kg blood drained initially
  ▶ over 3 ml/kg h continuous bleeding over several hours
  ▶ chest remains more than half full of blood on radiography in spite of chest tube drainage
  ▶ refractory shock

Traumatic Aortic Rupture (TAR)

Pathophysiology (Figure 12–6)

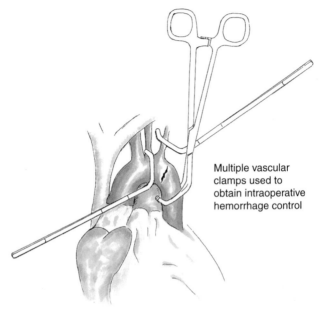

Multiple vascular
clamps used to
obtain intraoperative
hemorrhage control

Figure 12–6

▶ rapid deceleration causes a shear force and tear between the mobile aortic arch and the fixed descending aorta
  ▶ complete rupture is most common and usually results in death at the scene from rapid exsanguination via a proximal tear
  ▶ survivors have incomplete lacerations with the hemorrhage controlled by an intact adventia
  ▶ rarely, survivors have a complete laceration with bleeding tamponaded by a contained mediastinal hematoma
  ▶ tears occur just distal to the left subclavian artery in 85% of survivors
▶ rapid deceleration also causes avulsion at the base of the aortic root and usually results in death at the scene from cardiac tamponade
▶ osseous pinch
  ▶ great vessels "pinched" between compressed sternum and vertebral column
▶ mechanisms of injury
  ▶ falls over 30 feet
  ▶ sudden impact from vehicles traveling over 35 mph

- ► steering wheel or column damaged from chest impact during sudden deceleration
    - ► newer steering columns are designed to collapse as a safety mechanism
- ► pedestrian struck by a vehicle

Clinical Findings

Symptoms

- ► chest pain radiating to back
- ► dyspnea
- ► stridor due to airway compression
- ► hoarseness due to laryngeal compression
- ► dysphagia due to esophageal compression
- ► extremity pain due to ischemia

Signs

- ► physical examination neither sensitive nor specific for TAR
- ► blood pressure
    - ► up to 50% are hypotensive on presentation
    - ► reflex hypertension occurs in some due to stretch of aortic sympathetic fibers
- ► pseudocoarctation syndrome
    - ► upper extremity hypertension with decreased femoral pulses
- ► up to 30% have a harsh systolic murmur often heard in the interscapular area
- ► associated with upper rib, sternal, or scapular fractures although 50% are without external evidence of chest trauma

Chest Radiographic Findings (Figure 12–7)

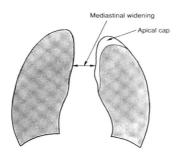

Figure 12–7

- good screening modality
- method
  - supine AP film is often falsely positive due to magnification of the mediastinum
  - upright PA film is more accurate and should be obtained whenever possible
    - 90% sensitive
    - 10% specific
    - compare to a premorbid CXR when available
    - 10% with TAR have normal initial film
- concerning findings in decreasing order of frequency
  - a widened mediastinum is the most sensitive finding though only 8% specific
    - supine CXR: over 8 cm or over 25% of width at that level
    - erect PA CXR: over 6 cm
  - rightward deviation of the trachea, endotracheal tube, or nasogastric tube is the most specific finding
  - downward deviation of left mainstem bronchus
  - obscuration of the aortic knob contour
  - left "apical cap" of extrapleural hematoma
    - appears as a density in the left apex
  - abnormal aortic contour
  - massive hemothorax (usually left)
  - obscured descending aorta
  - wide left paraspinal line
  - thick paratracheal line

Diagnostic Tests

- indications
  - suggestive findings on CXR
  - high-speed deceleration mechanism with suggestive clinical findings
    - falls over 30 feet
    - sudden impact from vehicles traveling over 35 mph
    - steering wheel or column damaged from chest impact during sudden deceleration
    - pedestrian struck by an automobile
- confirmatory test ordering strategy
  - helical CT
    - recommended in stable patients
  - aortography
    - recommended in stable patients with suspicious but nondiagnostic chest CT

▶ transesophageal echocardiography (TEE)
  ▹ recommended in unstable patients with any clinical suspicion for TAR
  ▹ recommended whenever it is not possible to perform CT or aortography
  ▹ results dependent upon operator skill

Helical CT

▶ advantages
  ▶ reduces need for aortography by 50%
  ▶ easily performed if undergoing head or abdominal CT
  ▶ helpful when CXR is equivocal or normal and aortic injury is suspected by clinical findings
  ▶ more cost effective than angiography in ruling out TAR
▶ disadvantages
  ▶ can delay aortography and causes double contrast load when aortography also necessary
  ▶ differentiation of mediastinal hematoma from normal structures requires experienced interpreter
    ▹ due to artifacts, motion, residual thymus, and minimal density of fat pad
  ▶ does not always delineate the arterial laceration
▶ indications
  ▶ stable patients with clinical suspicion for TAR
▶ findings
  ▶ mediastinal hematoma
    ▹ 25% have aortic injury
  ▶ intimal flap
  ▶ pseudoaneurysm
  ▶ abnormal aorta contour
▶ helical CT is superior to conventional CT
  ▶ sensitivity approaches 100%
  ▶ quicker
    ▹ scan time under 1 min allows scanning during one breath hold, reducing motion artifact
  ▶ lower contrast load necessary
  ▶ allows for CT angiography
    ▹ similar information and sensitivity as conventional angiography

Aortography

▶ considered the "gold standard" for diagnosis
▶ defines anatomy preoperatively
▶ helps determine need for cardiopulmonary bypass for ascending aortic injuries
▶ identifies multiple tears, which occur in up to 20%

▶ indications
  ▶ high clinical suspicion of TAR after significant blunt chest trauma
  ▶ abnormal CT scan of chest
  ▶ equivocal TEE results

Transesophageal Echocardiography (TEE)

▶ advantages
  ▶ portable
  ▶ noninvasive
  ▶ rapid (under 30 min with experienced operator)
  ▶ less expensive than aortography
  ▶ demonstrates myocardial and valvular injuries
▶ disadvantages
  ▶ dependent on operator skill
  ▶ probe passage
    ▶ requires stable cervical spine
    ▶ is contraindicated when esophageal or severe maxillofacial injury is suspected
  ▶ preoperative aortogram is desirable after a positive echocardiogram
▶ indications
  ▶ clinical or radiographic suspicion of TAR
  ▶ unable to perform CT or aortography
▶ accuracy in experienced operators
  ▶ sensitivity is 90–100%
  ▶ specificity is 98–100%
▶ findings
  ▶ aortic wall flap
  ▶ periaortic hematoma

Management

▶ hemodynamically deteriorating patients require immediate thoracotomy
▶ hypertensive patients require blood pressure control
  ▶ goal is maintaining systolic pressure at 100–120 mm Hg
  ▶ esmolol followed by nitroprusside is an optimal regime
    ▶ esmolol is rapidly titratable and has a short half-life
    ▶ must initiate beta blockade before afterload reduction since using nitroprusside alone will increase the shear force at the tear
  ▶ some use labetalol as a single agent

Prognosis

▶ 85% sustain complete rupture and die at the scene
▶ 15% survive to the emergency department and if undiagnosed/treated
  ▶ 30% die within a day
  ▶ 60% die within a week
  ▶ 90% die within a month

Blunt Cardiac Injury (BCI)

Pathophysiology

▶ anterior force transmitted to the atria or right ventricle causes contusion to the myocardium and cardiac dysfunction analogous to a myocardial infarction
  ▶ classic mechanism is an unrestrained driver in a head-on collision resulting in a bent steering wheel or broken steering column
  ▶ newer cars have collapsible steering columns to reduce the force transmitted to the chest
▶ unlike a myocardial infarction, the contused area more often heals completely and the clinical course is generally benign
▶ over 50% have clinically significant decrease in cardiac output

Clinical Findings

Symptoms

▶ substernal chest pain
▶ angina-like chest pain

Signs

▶ sternal or parasternal tenderness
▶ tachycardia
▶ dysrhythmia
▶ anterior chest ecchymosis
  ▶ one-quarter have no external evidence of trauma
▶ congestive heart failure and cardiogenic shock are uncommon complications

Diagnosis

General Principles

▶ histologic confirmation at autopsy is the only diagnostic "gold standard"
▶ presumptive diagnosis made by combining the results of the following tests

Electrocardiogram (ECG)

▶ better predictor than clinical findings
▶ best screening modality
▶ clinically significant complications negligible with normal ECG

▶ findings
  ▶ sinus tachycardia is the most common finding
  ▶ premature ventricular complexer (PVCs)
  ▶ right bundle branch block (RBBB)
  ▶ dysrhythmias
▶ acute injury patterns are the most specific findings but infrequent since most injuries are of the atria or right ventricle, areas with little influence on the ECG
▶ any new abnormality on ECG that cannot be explained must be construed as possible evidence of myocardial contusion
  ▶ 50% with abnormalities do not have myocardial contusions but all must be ruled out

Echocardiogram

▶ indicated if patient demonstrates hemodynamical instability
  ▶ transesophageal is better than transthoracic
▶ best used to exclude pericardial effusion
▶ focal areas of hypokinesis offer a presumptive diagnosis

Serum Markers

▶ not recommended since unreliable and do not predict complications
▶ creatine kinase-myocardial band (CK-MB)
  ▶ suggests injury when over 5% total CK
  ▶ 40% false negatives since the typical areas of injury have the least cardiac muscle mass
▶ troponin
  ▶ more specific than CK-MB for myocardial injury
  ▶ not predictive of need for monitoring or further diagnostic testing

Cardiac Radionucleide Testing

▶ nonspecific and does not predict complications
▶ may demonstrate areas of myocardial damage

Management

▶ hemodynamically stable and under 55 years old with a normal ECG and no cardiac history
  ▶ do not require cardiac monitoring for BCI after blunt chest trauma
  ▶ may be discharged if no associated injuries
▶ if either older patient or mild ECG abnormalities (e.g., persistent sinus tachycardia)
  ▶ require 12–24 h of non-ICU telemetry monitoring
▶ obtain echocardiogram if patient develops hemodynamical instability

▶ if hemodynamically unstable patient or concerning ECG abnormality
  ▶ admit to intensive care unit
  ▶ provide close hemodynamic monitoring
    ▷ utilize a central venous pressure or pulmonary artery catheter when necessary
    ▷ obtain cardiology consultation
  ▶ treat dysrhythmias or cardiac arrest using standard ACLS guidelines
  ▶ treat cardiogenic shock with pressors and an intraaortic balloon pump

Myocardial Rupture

Pathophysiology

▶ directly caused by sternal compression or impingement between the sternum and spinal column
▶ indirectly caused when chambers rupture after sudden overdistension associated with lower-body crush injuries

Prognosis

▶ immediate death in the overwhelming majority
▶ 50% mortality in those surviving to the emergency department

Clinical Findings

▶ hemorrhagic shock
▶ pericardial tamponade if the pericardium remains intact
▶ massive hemothorax if the pericardium ruptures

Management

▶ immediate operative repair

Tracheobronchial Disruption

Pathophysiology

▶ traumatic disruption of the tracheobronchial tree can occur with a deceleration mechanism because the trachea is relatively fixed with respect to the bronchi
▶ 80% occur within 2.5 cm of carina, the most vulnerable point
▶ 15% mortality within the first hour
▶ 30% mortality overall

Clinical Findings

Symptoms

▶ dyspnea
▶ chest pain

Signs

▶ subcutaneous emphysema
▶ hemoptysis in up to 50%
▶ massive persistent air leak after thoracostomy
▶ evidence of hypoventilation or hypoxia

Radiographic Findings

▶ pneumomediastinum and air in the cervical soft tissues
▶ large pneumothorax

Diagnosis

▶ assume large air leak through chest tube, mediastinal air, and/or persistent pneumothorax due to tracheobronchial tear until proven otherwise
▶ bronchoscopy will confirm suspicion

Management

▶ endotracheal intubation as necessary
  ▸ with proximal injuries, consider intubating over a fiberoptic broncho-scope to prevent passage of the endotracheal tube into a false space
▶ thoracostomy if pneumothorax present
▶ urgent surgical repair

Esophageal Rupture

General Principles

▶ rare with blunt trauma but can occur with direct force to the lower sternum or epigastrium
▶ the diagnosis is difficult to make
  ▸ one-third are diagnosed within 1 h
  ▸ another third are diagnosed within 24 h
  ▸ last third have diagnosis delayed over 24 h

▶ missed diagnosis results in late mediastinitis and increases morbidity to 50%

Clinical Findings

Symptoms

▶ pain may be out of proportion to physical findings
▶ dyspnea
▶ hematemesis

Signs

▶ neck tenderness
▶ subcutaneous emphysema
▶ pneumomediastinum
▶ pneumopericardium
  ▶ auscultate for "Hamman's crunch," a crunching sound over the heart heard with each systole

Radiographic Findings

Chest Radiograph

▶ increased prevertebral soft tissue space
▶ pneumomediastinum
▶ pneumopericardium
▶ left pleural effusion
▶ pneumothorax without rib fractures

Esophagram

▶ indications
  ▶ clinical suspicion
  ▶ unexplained pneumomediastinum or subcutaneous emphysema
▶ use water-soluble contrast (e.g., gastrografin) first
▶ if the above study is negative or indeterminate, use dilute barium to increase sensitivity
  ▶ unfortunately, barium may worsen mediastinitis

Esophagoscopy

▶ increases the diagnostic yield when used in combination with esophagram
  ▶ perform whenever suspicious of injury even if the esophagram is negative
  ▶ performed after esophagram since scope can worsen undiagnosed injuries

▶ either rigid or flexible scope is acceptable
  ▶ can be done with flexible scope outside the operating room and without neck extension
  ▶ rigid scope is preferred in suspected upper cervical esophageal injuries since blind passage of flexible scope through cricopharyngeus may result in missing a proximate injury

Management

▶ allow nothing by mouth
▶ arrange for immediate surgical repair and mediastinal drainage
▶ naso/orogastric tube and transesophageal echocardiogram are contraindicated
▶ perform thoracostomy if there is effusion or pneumothorax
▶ administer broad-spectrum antibiotics

Diaphragm Rupture

Pathophysiology

▶ 90% on left side since the liver prevents herniation of abdominal organs through right-sided defects
▶ 50% present in shock
▶ 20% mortality due to associated injuries
▶ missed diagnosis results in significant future morbidity
  ▶ incarcerated or strangulated hollow viscus

Diagnosis

▶ CXR
  ▶ stomach, bowel air, and/or tip of a correctly placed nasogastric tube may be seen above diaphragm
  ▶ elevated hemidiaphragm
  ▶ 25% normal
▶ oral contrast upper gastrointestinal study and CT scan may facilitate diagnosis
▶ peritoneal lavage
  ▶ high false negative rate
▶ laparoscopy or thoracoscopy confirms the diagnosis

Management

▶ immediate operative repair
▶ pneumatic anti-shock garment is contraindicated

Traumatic Asphyxia

Pathophysiology

▶ crush mechanism to thorax results in a sudden rise in venous pressure, briefly reversing venous flow in the valveless veins of head and face
▶ generally benign process if normal mentation and no associated injuries

Clinical Findings

Symptoms

▶ perioral cyanosis
▶ facial edema
▶ petechiae of face and neck

Management

▶ supportive care
▶ elevate the head of the bed

Penetrating Chest Trauma

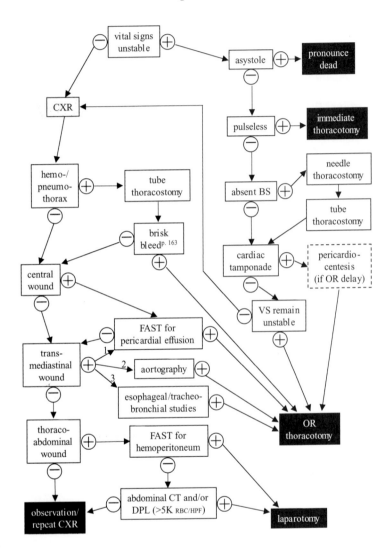

13

Chest: Penetrating

General Principles

Anatomic Considerations

▶ management is best guided by classifying by anatomic area(s) of injury
▶ when injuries are multiple or overlap between anatomic areas, prioritize management in the following order
  ▶ transmediastinal
  ▶ central
  ▶ thoracoabdominal
  ▶ peripheral

Testing

▶ perform immediate chest radiograph (CXR)
  ▶ to define associated injuries
  ▶ to determine missile tract
▶ patients with normal initial CXR require a repeat radiograph immediately if any progression of chest symptoms occurs and after 6 hours otherwise
▶ when available, FAST examination with thoracic views rapidly detects
  ▶ significant hemothorax
  ▶ pericardial effusion
▶ never probe wounds or remove impaled objects
  ▶ this practice can inadvertently worsen injury and/or disrupt hemostasis by dislodging a clot

Treatment

▶ hemodynamically unstable patients require the following sequential interventions until stability is restored
  ▶ needle decompression if suspected tension pneumothorax
  ▶ immediate intubation
  ▶ fluid resuscitation
  ▶ thoracotomy in the resuscitation area

▶ tube thoracostomy is indicated when the path of a bullet is clearly through the thoracic cavity and either:
  ▶ clinical or radiographic confirmation of hemothorax or pneumothorax
  ▶ plan to institute positive pressure ventilation even when the CXR is normal in order to eliminate the possibility of tension pneumothorax

Transmediastinal

General Principles

▶ applies to wounds that traverse the mediastinum
  ▶ the mediastinum contains all the structures sandwiched between the lungs and is approximated by the 3-dimensional space created by connecting the anterior and posterior "boxes" (Figure 13–1)
  ▶ envision the axial chest anatomy and trace the presumed missile tract when considering organs at risk for injury
▶ two-thirds are lethal injuries
▶ consider the following possibilities and rapidly exclude or diagnose
  ▶ pericardial tamponade
  ▶ heart or great vessel injury
  ▶ esophageal or tracheobronchial injury

Management

▶ be prepared to perform immediate thoracotomy should the patient become pulseless
  ▶ clamshell may be necessary to control right chest bleeding
▶ echocardiography reveals cardiac injuries and/or pericardial tamponade
▶ aortography reveals aortic and other great vessel injuries
▶ esophagram followed by esophagoscopy reveals esophageal injuries
▶ bronchoscopy reveals tracheobronchial injuries

Central

Location (Figure 13–1)

▶ this anatomic area is often called "the box"
▶ superior border
  ▶ suprasternal notch and clavicles anteriorly
  ▶ superior aspect of the scapulae posteriorly
▶ inferior border
  ▶ subxiphoid area anteriorly
  ▶ costal margin posteriorly
▶ lateral borders
  ▶ medial to the nipples anteriorly
  ▶ medial to the medial scapular borders posteriorly

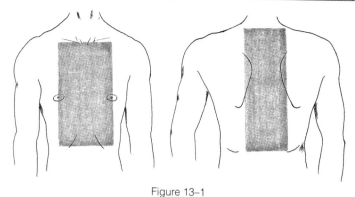

Figure 13–1

Management

▶ anterior central wounds
  ▶ transthoracic or transesophageal echocardiography to exclude an occult hemopericardium
    ▷ repeating after 6 h maximizes accuracy
    ▷ transesophageal study is contraindicated if there is suspicion of an esophageal injury
  ▶ if echocardiogram is unavailable, obtain chest CT
  ▶ if echocardiogram and CT are unavailable, place central venous pressure line to monitor for cardiac tamponade
    ▷ central venous pressure over 15 cm H_2O is suggestive of tamponade
    ▷ falsely low readings occur with hypovolemia or a kinked catheter
    ▷ there may be short time period between initial elevation of central venous pressure and severe clinical deterioration
    ▷ perform immediate pericardial window when hemopericardium is confirmed or suspected physiologically
▶ posterior central wounds
  ▶ obtain echocardiography when
    ▷ missile tracts approach the mediastinum
    ▷ wounds are deep stab
  ▶ obtain arch aortogram when
    ▷ the wound tract is proximate to the aorta
    ▷ there is any clinical or radiographic sign of aortic injury
  ▶ obtain esophagram/esophagoscopy when
    ▷ the wound tract is proximate to esophagus
    ▷ there is any clinical or radiographic sign of esophageal injury

Thoracoabdominal

Location (Figure 13–2)

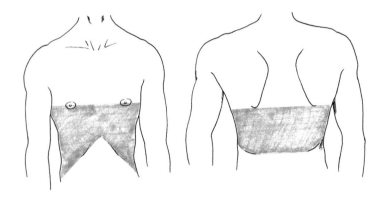

Figure 13–2

▶ below nipples and above the costal margin anteriorly
▶ below scapulae and above the costal margin posteriorly

Management

General Principles

▶ the diaphragm has a great range of excursion rising up to the 4th thoracic vertebra during expiration
▶ diaphragmatic penetration occurs in
  ▶ 45% of thoracoabdominal gunshot wounds
  ▶ 15% of thoracoabdominal stab wounds
▶ missed diaphragmatic injuries can result in significant morbidity
  ▶ herniation and potential strangulation of bowel or stomach into a hemithorax
    ▷ occur more commonly on the left since the liver is protective

Diagnostic Options

▶ diagnostic peritoneal lavage (DPL) (see p. 453)
  ▶ low sensitivity for diaphragmatic injuries, although better than CT
  ▶ use a threshold of 5,000 RBC/mm^3 for increased sensitivity in defining a positive study
    ▷ 25% false negative rate expected using threshold of 100,000 RBC/mm^3

▶ CT
  ▶ defines solid organ, renal, and retroperitoneal injuries accurately
  ▶ low sensitivity (60%) for diaphragmatic injuries
    ▹ helical CT has improved sensitivity over conventional CT
    ▹ use "triple contrast" CT to increase sensitivity for retroperitoneal injuries
  ▶ perform before DPL in stable patients to increase the diagnostic accuracy
    ▹ when performed after DPL, expect intraabdominal lavage fluid and sometimes air that cannot be differentiated from the same findings associated with intraabdominal hemorrhage and ruptured viscus
    ▹ minor right-sided diaphragmatic injuries rarely associated with herniation
  ▶ indicated for posterior thoracoabdominal wounds
▶ ultrasound
  ▶ delineates the subcutaneous and fascial layers, when expert interprets
  ▶ negative examination for fascial penetration excludes injury
▶ laparoscopy
  ▶ 95% accurate so results in few nontherapeutic laparotomies
  ▶ requires general anesthesia
▶ thoracoscopy
  ▶ accurately diagnoses diaphragmatic injuries
  ▶ requires general anesthesia
▶ posterior thoracoabdominal wounds (posterior to the mid-axillary line)
  ▶ additionally require "triple contrast" CT (if stable) to evaluate for retroperitoneal injuries

Disposition

▶ observe patients with an initial negative diagnostic workup and repeat the CXR after 6 h

Peripheral

Location (Figure 13–3)

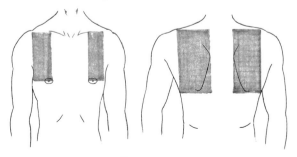

Figure 13–3

- anteriorly
  - lateral to the nipples
  - above the nipple line
- posteriorly
  - lateral to the medial scapular borders
  - above the tips of the scapulae

Management

General Principles

- patients with peripheral stab wounds and a normal initial CXR can be safely discharged when
  - repeat CXR after 6 h remains unchanged
  - repeat clinical examination is unrevealing

Angiography Indications

- enlarging supraclavicular or axillary hematoma
- on-going bleeding (externally or from thoracostomy)
- apical hematoma on CXR
  - need to exclude a brachiocephalic or subclavian artery injury
- upper-extremity pulse deficit or asymmetry
- proximate to major artery or brachial plexus

Cardiac Tamponade

General Principles

- characterized as an inflow obstruction of blood flow to the heart
- occurs in 2% with anterior penetrating chest trauma
- 50% survive when a pulse is present on arrival
- must be rapidly diagnosed or excluded in cases of central chest or trans-mediastinal penetration

Clinical Findings

- cardiogenic shock without pulmonary edema

- ▶ Beck's triad
  - ▶ hypotension
  - ▶ jugular venous distension
    - ▹ although seen in most supine patients without tamponade and not seen in hypovolemic patients with tamponade
  - ▶ muffled heart sounds
    - ▹ although difficult to appreciate in a noisy resuscitation area
- ▶ tachycardia
- ▶ elevated central venous pressure
  - ▶ place central line and measure whenever the diagnosis is entertained
  - ▶ normal pressure is under 10 mm H_2O
    - ▹ central venous pressure over 15 cm H_2O suggestive of tamponade
  - ▶ elevation may not be present in severely hypotensive patients before volume replacement
  - ▶ may be short time period between initial elevation of central venous pressure and severe clinical deterioration
- ▶ pulsus paradoxus
  - ▶ defined as over 10 mm Hg drop in SBP with spontaneous (nonforced) inspiration
  - ▶ neither sensitive nor specific
  - ▶ this is an expected finding in patients with chronic pulmonary disease
- ▶ electrical alternans
  - ▶ changing amplitude or morphology of the QRS complex in a single lead every other beat (Figure 13–4)
  - ▶ pathognomonic
  - ▶ rarely seen

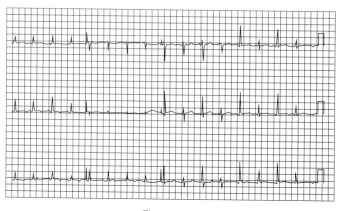

Figure 13–4

Diagnostic Studies

▶ CXR
  ▶ unhelpful
▶ echocardiography
  ▶ diastolic collapse of right ventricle with coexistent pericardial effusion
  ▶ serial transthoracic studies 96% accurate
  ▶ single transesophageal study nearly 100% accurate

Management

▶ if patient becomes profoundly hypotensive or pulseless, intubate, ventilate, and perform an immediate thoracotomy to open the pericardial sac
▶ if unable to perform immediate thoracotomy, consider pericardiocentesis
  ▶ high false negative rate due to clotted blood in pericardial sac
▶ operative pericardiotomy is the definitive treatment

Communicating Pneumothorax

Pathophysiology

▶ often caused by high-energy shotgun blast or large-caliber/high-velocity missile
▶ when the diameter of the chest wall defect exceeds that of the trachea, spontaneous ventilation is impossible since intrathoracic pressure equilibrates with atmospheric pressure
  ▶ the involved lung collapses on inspiration and expands on expiration

Clinical Findings

▶ large defect in the chest wall
▶ called "sucking chest wound" because sonorous air flows through the wound
▶ severe respiratory distress

Management

▶ tape a sterile dressing on three sides to create a one-way (flutter) valve which corrects the defect, allowing air to escape and preventing conversion to a tension pneumothorax (Figure 13–5)
▶ perform tube thoracostomy at site away from the wound and then close the flutter valve dressing

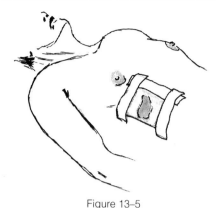

Figure 13–5

▶ consider early endotracheal intubation with positive pressure ventilation
▶ operative repair required for large defects

Air Embolism

Pathophysiology

▶ alveolar–venous communication due to penetrating chest trauma results in air bubbles in the pulmonary veins which, when transmitted to the coronary arteries, can cause myocardial ischemia/infarction

Clinical Findings

▶ consider when cardiac arrest occurs immediately after intubation
▶ CXR may reveal the "box cars" sign of intracoronary arterial air bubbles
▶ maintain a high clinical suspicion since the diagnosis is frequently overlooked

Management

▶ maintain the patient in the left lateral decubitus or Trendelenburg position to sequester the air in the apex of the left ventricle
▶ if cardiac arrest occurs
 ▶ perform immediate thoracotomy
 ▶ cross-clamp the pulmonary hilum on the side of the injury
 ▶ aspirate air from the apex of the atrium, ventricle, pulmonary artery, and aortic root

Esophageal Penetration

General Principles

▶ making the diagnosis is difficult since clinical signs may be subtle
▶ missed diagnosis results in late mediastinitis and increases morbidity to 50%

Clinical Findings

Symptoms

▶ pain may be out of proportion to physical findings
▶ dyspnea
▶ hematemesis

Signs

▶ neck tenderness
▶ subcutaneous emphysema
▶ pneumomediastinum
▶ pneumopericardium
    ▶ auscultate for "Hamman's crunch"—a crunching sound over the heart heard with each systole

Radiographic Findings

Chest Radiograph

▶ increased prevertebral soft tissue space
▶ pneumomediastinum
▶ pneumopericardium
▶ left pleural effusion
▶ pneumothorax without rib fractures

Esophagram

▶ indications
    ▶ clinical suspicion
    ▶ transmediastinal wounds
    ▶ projectile tract proximate to the esophagus
    ▶ unexplained pneumomediastinum or subcutaneous emphysema
▶ use water-soluble contrast (e.g., Gastrografin) first
▶ if the above study is negative or indeterminate, use dilute barium to increase sensitivity
    ▶ unfortunately barium may worsen mediastinitis

Esophagoscopy

▶ increases the diagnostic yield when used in combination with esophagram
  ▶ perform whenever suspicious of injury even if the esophagram is negative
  ▶ performed after esophagram since scope can worsen undiagnosed injuries
▶ should follow negative contrast studies to further increase sensitivity
▶ either rigid or flexible acceptable
  ▶ can be done with flexible probe outside the operating room and without neck extension
  ▶ rigid probe preferred in suspected upper cervical esophageal injuries since blind passage of flexible scope through cricopharyngeus may result in missing a proximate injury

Management

▶ allow nothing by mouth
▶ arrange for immediate surgical repair and mediastinal drainage
▶ naso/orogastric tube and transesophageal echocardiogram are contraindicated
▶ perform thoracostomy if there is effusion or pneumothorax
▶ administer broad-spectrum antibiotics

Thoracotomy

Purpose

Resuscitation Area Thoracotomy

▶ when the patient is potentially salvageable, an immediate thoracotomy allows the following potentially stabilizing maneuvers
  ▶ the limited circulating blood volume is selectively directed to the brain and heart by cross-clamping the descending aorta
  ▶ cardiac tamponade is relieved when pericardial blood is evacuated
  ▶ cardiac, great vessel, or pulmonary parenchymal wounds can be repaired or temporized
  ▶ open cardiac massage may improve perfusion
▶ the highest survival rates are in patients with cardiac stab wounds who suddenly arrest from pericardial tamponade
  ▶ up to 50% will recover if the thoracotomy is performed immediately
▶ thoracotomy is futile when
  ▶ penetrating trauma without pulse/blood pressure and no other sign of life (e.g., reactive pupils, agonal breathing, spontaneous movement, or electrical cardiac activity)
  ▶ blunt trauma without pulse/blood pressure

Operating Room Thoracotomy

▶ each case must be individualized as there are no absolute criteria
▶ the following are generally appreciated guidelines but must be correlated with hemodynamic status and fluid requirements
  ▶ hemodynamic instability despite vigorous resuscitation in the setting of chest trauma
  ▶ aggressive hemorrhage
    ▹ over 20 ml/kg initially via thoracostomy
    ▹ over 3 ml/kg/h continuous bleeding for several hours
  ▶ radiographic evidence of great vessel injury
  ▶ severe tracheobronchial injury suspected
    ▹ continuous, severe hemoptysis
    ▹ massive air leak from the chest tube
    ▹ radiographic or endoscopic evidence
  ▶ evidence of esophageal injury or diaphragmatic rupture
  ▶ suspected or confirmed hemopericardium or cardiac injury
    ▹ foreign body embolus within the heart or pulmonary artery
  ▶ impaled or retained intrathoracic objects

Procedure

▶ see p. 451 for technique of performing a thoracotomy in the resuscitation area

Blunt Abdominal Trauma

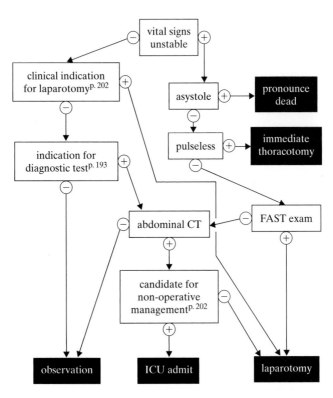

14

Abdomen: Blunt

General Principles

Mechanism

- ▶ sudden direct force can cause laceration of solid organs
- ▶ sudden rise in intraabdominal pressure can cause rupture of hollow organs
- ▶ sudden deceleration (or acceleration) can cause shearing of structures at points of attachment

Organs Injured

- ▶ solid organs most commonly injured in blunt trauma
  - ▶ intraabdominal bleeding causes minimal peritoneal signs in first few hours injury
- ▶ the following are listed in decreasing incidence of injury
  - ▶ spleen
  - ▶ liver
  - ▶ kidney
  - ▶ intraperitoneal small bowel
  - ▶ bladder
  - ▶ colon
  - ▶ diaphragm
  - ▶ pancreas
  - ▶ retroperitoneal duodenum

Physical Examination

General Principles

- ▶ serial examinations by the same examiner improve sensitivity
- ▶ tenderness blunted by intoxicants
- ▶ spinal cord injury masks clinical findings
- ▶ Kehr's sign is left shoulder pain associated with hemoperitoneum and spleen injuries

Abdominal Findings

▶ inspect for skin evidence of blunt trauma
  ▶ contusions or abrasions
  ▶ lap belt ecchymosis
    ▷ associated with mesenteric, bowel, and lumbar spine injuries in 20%
    ▷ occur mostly in children with lap belt and no shoulder restraint
  ▶ periumbilical and flank ecchymosis are late findings in retroperitoneal hematoma
▶ palpate for tenderness, guarding, and/or rigidity
  ▶ 40% with hemoperitoneum are initially without clinical findings
▶ appreciate distension
  ▶ hemoperitoneum of several liters may not visibly increase abdominal girth

Rectal Findings

▶ check for gross blood
▶ determine prostate position
▶ assess sphincter tone

Distal Pulses

▶ assess for absence or asymmetry

Diagnostic Strategy

Basic Data

▶ measure baseline hematocrit
▶ obtain creatinine in case contrast study is necessary
▶ urinalysis
  ▶ absence of hematuria does not rule out genitourinary injury
  ▶ presence of hematuria mandates consideration of a genitourinary injury
▶ elevated amylase/lipase or liver enzymes increase suspicion of intraabdominal injury though specificity is low
▶ obtain pregnancy test in women capable of child bearing
▶ plain radiography
  ▶ plain abdominal radiographs are generally unhelpful
    ▷ upright chest radiograph (CXR) is unlikely to detect pneumoperitoneum despite ruptured viscus
  ▶ pelvic studies may uncover associated fractures

Indications for Further Testing

▶ mechanism for injury with
  ▶ unexplained hemorrhagic shock
  ▶ major chest or pelvic injuries
  ▶ abdominal tenderness
  ▶ diminished pain response due to the following conditions
    ▹ intoxication
    ▹ depressed level of consciousness
    ▹ distracting pain
    ▹ paralysis
  ▶ inability to perform serial examinations
    ▹ patient to undergo general anesthesia

Strategy for Unstable Patients

▶ FAST examination
  ▶ if positive (for intraabdominal fluid)
    ▹ when patient remains unstable, proceed with laparotomy
    ▹ when patient becomes stable, consider CT to evaluate renal system and to determine if patient is a candidate for nonoperative management of a solid organ injury
  ▶ if negative
    ▹ consider DPL to increase sensitivity for intraabdominal source
    ▹ consider other sources of intracavitary hemorrhage
  ▶ if negative and severe pelvic fracture present
    ▹ consider urgent pelvic angiography
▶ diagnostic peritoneal lavage (DPL)
  ▶ if aspiration is positive
    ▹ proceed with laparotomy
  ▶ if lavage is positive and patient remains unstable
    ▹ when no other hemorrhage source or other cause for hypotension is apparent, proceed with laparotomy
  ▶ if lavage is positive and patient becomes stable
    ▹ consider CT to evaluate renal system and to determine if patient is a candidate for nonoperative management of a solid organ injury
  ▶ if aspiration and lavage are negative
    ▹ assume other hemorrhage source or other cause for hypotension

Strategy for Stable Patients

▶ abdominal CT
  ▶ if patient becomes hemodynamically unstable while awaiting CT, perform FAST examination or DPL

> ► consider DPL after CT when
>> ▹ free fluid may not be blood (e.g., ascites)
>> ▹ CT is negative while high clinical suspicion of bowel injury remains (e.g., transaminasemia or lap belt sign present)
► serial abdominal physical and FAST examinations

FAST Examination

Definition

► FAST refers to "focused assessment with sonography for trauma"
► performed by emergency physicians and surgeons
► becoming a mainstay in trauma centers

Advantages

► excellent results reported by emergency physicians and surgeons trained in performing the FAST examination
► inexpensive, noninvasive, and portable
► avoids risks associated with contrast media
► can assess the thorax and retroperitoneum in addition to the peritoneal cavity
► confirms presence of hemoperitoneum in minutes
>> ► decreases time to laparotomy
>> ► great adjunct during multiple casualty disasters
► serial examinations can detect ongoing hemorrhage and increase the diagnostic yield
► confirms placement of DPL fluid
► decreases utilization of DPL and CT
► differentiates pulseless electrical activity from extreme hypotension
► with pregnant trauma patients, determines gestational age and fetal viability

Disadvantages

► requires a minimum of 70 ml of intraperitoneal fluid for positive study
>> ► DPL only requires 20 ml
► accuracy is dependent on operator/interpreter skill and is decreased with prior abdominal surgery
► technically difficult with obese patients and when ileus or subcutaneous emphysema is present
► does not define the exact cause of hemoperitoneum
► sensitivity is low for small-bowel and pancreatic injury
► although clotted blood has a characteristic appearance, one cannot be sure of the exact type of free intraabdominal fluid

Statistical Considerations

▶ overall
▶ sensitivity ranges from 69% to 99%
▶ specificity ranges from 86% to 98%
▶ identification of intraperitoneal fluid differs by view
  ▶ Morrison's pouch
    ▷ 36–82% sensitivity
    ▷ 94–100% specificity
  ▶ perisplenic space
    ▷ 58% sensitivity
  ▶ Douglas' pouch
    ▷ 56% sensitivity

Technique

▶ four basic transducer positions used to search for abnormal fluid (Figure 14–1)
  ▶ hemopericardium
    ▷ epigastric view
  ▶ hemoperitoneum
    ▷ right upper abdominal quadrant for fluid in Morrison's pouch (the space between the right kidney and the liver) (Figure 14–2 on page 196, top)
    ▷ left upper abdominal quadrant for fluid in perisplenic space (Figure 14–3 on page 196, middle)
    ▷ suprapubic transverse and longitudinal view for fluid in Douglas' pouch, optimized by a full bladder (Figure 14–4 on page 196, bottom)

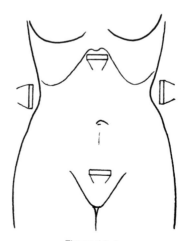

Figure 14–1

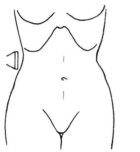
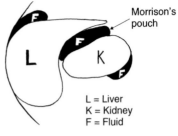

Morrison's pouch

L = Liver
K = Kidney
F = Fluid

Figure 14–2

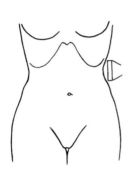
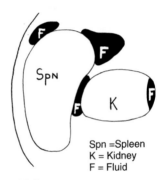

Spn = Spleen
K = Kidney
F = Fluid

Figure 14–3

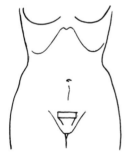
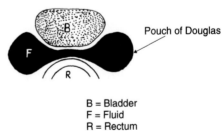

Pouch of Douglas

B = Bladder
F = Fluid
R = Rectum

Figure 14–4

▶ single right intercostal or subcostal longitudinal view of the patient in the Trendelenburg position
  ▶ completed within 1 min
  ▶ increases sensitivity by maximizing the amount of blood in Morrison's pouch

Abdominal CT Scan

General Principles

▶ for blunt trauma, IV and oral contrast are ideal but not essential
  ▶ 400 ml orally at least 20 min prior to and another 250 ml immediately prior to CT
  ▶ 100 ml 60% iodinated IV contrast immediately prior to CT

Advantages

▶ noninvasive
▶ quantifies hemoperitoneum
▶ affords specificity unlike DPL or FAST examination
▶ demonstrates specific organ injuries
▶ allows classification of solid organ injuries
  ▶ aids in identification of nonoperative injuries
▶ identifies retroperitoneal hematoma or injuries
▶ reveals hemo/pneumothorax too small to be seen on CXR
▶ permits a one-position study for patients with pelvic fractures
▶ normal CT in minor trauma patient allows for safe discharge from the emergency department

Disadvantages

▶ requires an experienced interpreter
▶ patients may become hemodynamically unstable while in the radiology department
▶ more time required than for DPL
▶ delays time to laparotomy compared with DPL or FAST examination, which can be done in the operating room when necessary
▶ contrast administration has potential for adverse effects
  ▶ allergic reactions
  ▶ renal dysfunction

Statistical Considerations

▶ 97% sensitivity depending on quality of scanner and experience of interpreter
▶ 95–100% specificity

Potential Findings

► hemoperitoneum
  ► accurately identified
  ► free collections of blood seen in
    ▹ Morrison's pouch (between the liver and right kidney), the most dependent peritoneal recess in the upper abdomen
    ▹ perihepatic space
    ▹ paracolic gutters
    ▹ pelvis
  ► a localized collection of clotted blood adjacent to an organ, often referred to as a "sentinel clot," is an accurate sign of injury
    ▹ clotted blood has higher attenuation than does free blood
► spleen or liver injury
  ► extremely sensitive and specific
    ▹ accuracy for splenic injury exceeds 95%
  ► essential in the nonoperative management of solid organ injuries
► kidney injury and function
  ► depicts the type and extent of renal injury more accurately than IVP or formal ultrasound
  ► best displays perirenal hematomas and extravasation of urine
  ► best distinguishes between the categories of renal trauma
  ► essential in nonoperative management of renal injuries
► pancreatic injury
  ► often difficult to appreciate
  ► may see retrogastric fluid or overt transection
  ► follow-up scans in 12–24 h may be helpful since radiographic signs may be delayed
► bowel and mesenteric injury
  ► signs
    ▹ thickened bowel wall
    ▹ fluid between bowel loops (rather than in dependent regions)
    ▹ mesenteric streaking
    ▹ extravasation of oral contrast material
    ▹ high-density clot adjacent to the involved bowel ("sentinel clot")
    ▹ intraperitoneal air (absent in 50% with bowel injury)
► diaphragm
  ► approximately 60% sensitive in diagnosing injury
    ▹ improved with helical scanner and experienced interpreter
► urinary bladder
  ► CT can distinguish type of bladder rupture
    ▹ intraperitoneal rupture requires operative repair
    ▹ extraperitoneal rupture treated with drainage catheter
  ► technique
    ▹ instill contrast into the bladder and scan with a clamped Foley catheter
    ▹ follow with plain drainage radiographs to help detect extravasation
    ▹ delayed images may be required to detect extravasation

Contraindications

▶ any degree of hemodynamic instability or high potential for the patient to become unstable in the radiology department
▶ need for laparotomy already established

Diagnostic Peritoneal Lavage (DPL)

Advantages

▶ accurate detection of hemoperitoneum
▶ rapid, technically easy, and inexpensive
▶ low incidence of complications

Disadvantages

▶ insensitive for diaphragmatic, bowel, and subcapsular injuries
▶ misses all retroperitoneal injuries
▶ lack of specificity
  ▶ results in some unnecessary laparotomies
  ▶ exact nature of injury not defined
  ▶ false positive results with pelvic fractures

Statistical Considerations

▶ for blunt abdominal trauma and using 100,000 RBC/mm3 to define a positive study
  ▶ accuracy is 98% in blunt trauma
  ▶ 1% false positives
  ▶ 1% false negatives
▶ false negative rate increases with prior abdominal surgery since adhesions may prohibit sampling of entire cavity
▶ about 15% of positive DPLs result from minor intraabdominal injuries that do not require operative repair
  ▶ result in nontherapeutic laparotomies

Contraindications

▶ absolute
  ▶ need for laparotomy already established
▶ relative
  ▶ morbid obesity
  ▶ previous abdominal surgery
  ▶ pregnancy (use open, supraumbilical technique)

Techniques (see p. 453)

▶ consider open or semi-open technique when
  ▶ prior abdominal surgery
  ▶ coagulopathy
  ▶ morbid obesity
  ▶ pregnancy
  ▶ pelvic fracture
▶ closed
  ▶ transcutaneous approach using Seldinger technique
  ▶ minimal risk with appropriate patient selection
  ▶ aspiration typically completed within 5 min
  ▶ lavage typically completed within 20 min
▶ semi-open
  ▶ dissect to the linea alba and then place catheter using Seldinger technique or trocar
▶ open
  ▶ dissect to and open the peritoneum and place catheter in intraperitoneal cavity under direct visualization
  ▶ thought to be the safest technique in general
  ▶ supraumbilical approach is mandatory in patients with pelvic fractures in order to avoid a preperitoneal hematoma associated with retroperitoneal bleeding
  ▶ recommended in patients with prior abdominal surgery to decrease the chance of injury to adhesed bowel with closed techniques
  ▶ suprafundal approach necessary in term pregnant patients to reduce the risk to the uterus
  ▶ aspiration typically completed within 15 min
  ▶ lavage typically completed within 30 min

Interpretation

▶ aspiration
  ▶ positive when 10 ml of gross blood is aspirated via either the intraperitoneal needle or catheter and obviates the need to lavage
    ▶ if under 10 ml aspirated, return blood to the abdomen prior to lavage in order to get an accurate count
▶ lavage red blood cell (RBC) count
  ▶ subjectively positive when too turbid to read newsprint through a test tube of lavage fluid
  ▶ objectively positive when over 100,000 RBC/mm^3
  ▶ only 20 ml of intraabdominal blood is necessary to achieve count of 100,000 RBC/mm^3
  ▶ indeterminate when 20,000–100,000 RBC/mm^3
  ▶ when indeterminate, consider repeat lavage a few hours later or follow with an abdominal CT to increase diagnostic accuracy
  ▶ negative when under 20,000 RBC/mm^3

- lavage white blood cell (WBC) count
  - positive when over 500 WBC/mm^3
  - frequently falsely elevated when DPL delayed more than 7 h after injury
  - positive predictive value of only 23%
  - not used at some centers due to low sensitivity and specificity
- lavage enzyme assays
  - amylase positive when over 20 IU/L
  - alkaline phosphatase positive when over 3 IU/L
  - associated with small-bowel or pancreatic injury
  - high false negative rate
- the presence of bacteria, bile, or vegetable matter in lavage fluid indicates a hollow viscus injury

Complications

- overall rate is under 1%
- more common with closed, Seldinger technique
- types
  - development of abdominal wall hematoma
  - injury to bowel, bladder, mesentery, or blood vessel
  - wound infections and peritonitis
- a patient with a negative DPL should be admitted and observed for the development of complications

Laparoscopy

Advantages

- accurately characterizes the extent of organ injuries and determines the need for laparotomy
  - defines which intraabdominal injuries may be safely managed nonsurgically
- more sensitive than DPL or CT in uncovering
  - diaphragmatic injuries
  - hollow viscus injuries

Disadvantages

- pneumoperitoneum may elevate ICP and increase work of ventilation
- general anesthesia usually necessary
  - some centers will perform with local anesthesia and intravenous sedation/analgesia
- difficult to visualize the spleen
- patient must be hemodynamically stable

Complications

- ▶ insertion can cause bleeding or injury
- ▶ gas embolism possible with solid organ venous disruption and pneumoperitoneum

Laparotomy Indications

Absolute Criteria

- ▶ peritonitis
- ▶ pneumoperitoneum or pneumoretroperitoneum
- ▶ evidence of diaphragmatic defect
- ▶ gross blood from stomach or rectum
- ▶ abdominal distension with hypotension
- ▶ evisceration
- ▶ positive diagnostic test for an injury requiring operative repair

Nonoperative Injury Management

General Considerations

- ▶ criteria for nonoperative management
  - ▸ patient hemodynamically stable after initial resuscitation
  - ▸ continuous patient monitoring for 48 h
  - ▸ surgical team immediately available
  - ▸ adequate ICU support and transfusion services available
  - ▸ absence of peritonitis
  - ▸ normal sensorium
- ▶ patient selection is based primarily on hemodynamic status and secondarily on injury grade (see Table 14–1)
- ▶ angioembolization may be alternative to surgical intervention
- ▶ all patients with solid organ injury managed nonoperatively require admission for observation, serial hematocrit measurement, and repeat imaging

Liver Injury

- ▶ 90% success rate for nonoperative therapy in properly selected patients
- ▶ ideal candidates for nonoperative therapy
  - ▸ hemodynamically stable
  - ▸ low-grade hepatic injury
  - ▸ minimal free peritoneal fluid on CT
  - ▸ no evidence of other abdominal injury
  - ▸ normal coagulation studies

Table 14–1 Solid Organ Injury Grading

Grade	Description
Spleen	
I	▶ subcapsular hematoma under 10% of surface ▶ laceration under 1 cm deep
II	▶ subcapsular hematoma 10–15% of surface ▶ laceration 1–3 cm deep
III	▶ subcapsular hematoma over 50% or expanding ▶ intraparenchymal hematoma over 5 cm or expanding
IV	▶ laceration involving segmental or hilar vessels
V	▶ Shattered spleen ▶ hilar devascularization injury
Liver	
I	▶ Subcapsular hematoma under 10% of surface ▶ laceration under 1 cm deep
II	▶ subcapsular hematoma 10–50% of surface ▶ laceration 1–3 cm deep and under 10 cm in length
III	▶ subcapsular hematoma over 50% or expanding ▶ laceration over 3 cm deep or over 10 cm in length
IV	▶ parenchymal disruption involving 25–75% of a lobe
V	▶ parenchymal disruption involving over 75% of a lobe ▶ retrohepatic vena cava or hepatic vein injury

Spleen Injury

▶ over 90% success rate for nonoperative therapy in properly selected adult and pediatric patients
▶ candidates
  ▶ hemodynamically stable
  ▶ minimal free peritoneal fluid on CT
  ▶ normal coagulation status
▶ advantages
  ▶ reduced risk of sepsis since spleen remains functional
▶ disadvantages
  ▶ transfusion more likely and carries inherent risks

Penetrating Abdominal Trauma

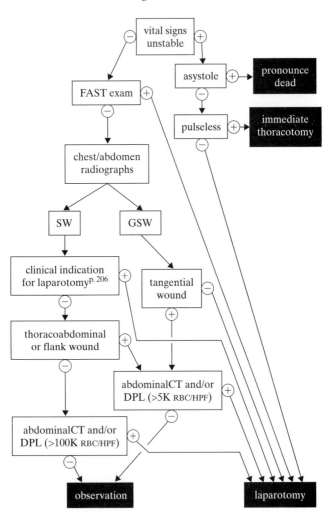

15

Abdomen: Penetrating

General Principles

Clinical Findings

▶ inspect location of wound sites
▶ palpate abdomen for tenderness, distension, and peritoneal signs
  ▶ physical examination insensitive for peritoneal penetration
▶ check distal pulses for symmetry and quality
▶ perform digital rectal examination and check for gross blood
▶ never probe wounds
  ▶ may worsen injuries and disrupt hemostasis, resulting in uncontrolled hemorrhage
  ▶ instead, gently separate skin edges to see if base of wound can be visualized

Basic Management

▶ establish at least two large-bore intravenous catheters
▶ type and crossmatch for at least 4 units PRBC
▶ administer tetanus toxoid and prophylactic antibiotics as necessary
▶ with thoracoabdominal penetration
  ▶ when tube thoracostomy is not otherwise indicated, place prophylactically for those who will undergo positive pressure ventilation
    ▶ eliminates possibility of delayed tension pneumothorax
▶ when there is profound, worsening hypovolemic shock unresponsive to aggressive resuscitative measures, prepare for immediate thoracotomy

Data

Laboratory

▶ measure baseline hematocrit and creatinine
▶ obtain urinalysis
  ▶ absence of hematuria does not rule out genitourinary injury
  ▶ presence of hematuria mandates consideration of a genitourinary injury

▶ obtain pregnancy test in women capable of bearing children

Radiography

▶ mark wound sites with radiopaque objects such as taped-on paper clips or ECG electrodes
▶ obtain AP upright chest and supine abdomen/pelvis radiographs (at a minimum)
▶ when a foreign body is seen radiographically, obtain views in two planes to localize it

Stab

General Principles

▶ left upper quadrant injury is most common in stab wounds
  ▶ since instrument is usually held in perpetrator's right hand
▶ 60% of anterior stab wounds violate the peritoneum
  ▶ half require repair of an intraabdominal injury
▶ risk of intraabdominal injury requiring repair varies by stab wound entry site
  ▶ anterior or flank, 30%
  ▶ thoracoabdominal, 15%
  ▶ back, 10%
▶ in those without a clinical indication for laparotomy, 50% will require laparotomy after diagnostic testing

Radiography

Upright CXR

▶ pneumothorax
▶ pneumoperitoneum indicates peritoneal penetration

Abdomen

▶ exclude retained foreign body
▶ clues to injuries
  ▶ separation of loops of bowel by intestinal fluid
  ▶ loss of the psoas shadow
  ▶ air around the right kidney or along the right psoas margins

Laparotomy

Indications

▶ hemodynamic instability

▶ gross blood from the nasogastric tube or rectum
▶ evisceration
▶ clinical or radiographic evidence of diaphragm injury
▶ peritoneal findings on the abdominal examination
▶ retained stabbing implement
▶ positive diagnostic test for an injury requiring operative repair

Local Wound Exploration (LWE)

General Principles

▶ dissection of wound tract under local anesthesia through an extended incision
▶ goal is to identify base of the wound or that peritoneal penetration has occurred

Indication

▶ single anterior abdominal wound
  ▶ defined as the area below the costal margins, above the inguinal creases, and between the anterior axillary lines

Contraindications

▶ need for laparotomy already established
▶ thoracoabdominal wounds since high potential for iatrogenic complications
▶ multiple stab wounds
▶ technically difficult
  ▶ obesity
  ▶ uncooperative patient

Findings

▶ if wound base clearly demonstrated and peritoneum not violated, can discharge patient after appropriate wound care
▶ if inconclusive or positive, further diagnostic workup (e.g., DPL or CT) recommended
  ▶ some perform serial abdominal examinations in the stable patient without further diagnostic testing

FAST Examination

General Principles

▶ see p. 194
▶ poor diagnostic accuracy for diaphragmatic or hollow viscus injuries

Indications

▶ hemodynamically unstable patient
  ▸ fluid in peritoneum is an indication for laparotomy
▶ thoracoabdominal wounds
  ▸ experienced ultrasonographer can delineate subcutaneous and fascial layers
  ▸ negative examination for fascial penetration excludes injury

Abdominal CT

General Principles

▶ use IV and oral contrast for all
▶ "triple contrast" includes rectal contrast (Gastrografin enema) to increase the detection of retroperitoneal injuries

Indications

▶ helpful in flank and back stab wounds to evaluate for renal and retroperitoneal injuries
▶ determines location and extent of solid organ injury for anterior and thoracoabdominal wounds

Disposition

▶ positive CT mandates emergent surgical exploration
▶ if negative, admit for observation and serial abdominal examinations

Diagnostic Peritoneal Lavage

Indications

▶ abdominal, thoracoabdominal, back, or flank stab wound

Contraindications

▶ need for laparotomy already established

Red Blood Cell (RBC) Count Criteria

▶ differing interpretation based on anatomic location
▶ anterior abdominal stab wound
  ▸ 100,000 RBC/mm^3 positive study to predict intraabdominal injury
    ▹ false negative rate 5%
    ▹ false positive rate 7%
    ▹ accuracy 90%

▶ back and flank stab wounds
  ▶ back defined as the area between the lower tip of scapulae and upper iliac crest with the posterior axillary lines as the lateral borders
  ▶ flank defined as the area between the anterior and posterior axillary lines and from the 6th intercostal space to the iliac crests
  ▶ 5,000 RBC/mm^3 defines peritoneal penetration and is considered a positive study
  ▶ if negative, perform triple-contrast CT which also evaluates retroperitoneal injury
▶ thoracoabdominal stab wounds
  ▶ defined as the area below nipples and above the costal margin anteriorly and below scapulae and above the costal margin posteriorly
  ▶ 5,000 RBC/mm^3 defines peritoneal or diaphragmatic penetration and is considered a positive study

White Blood Cell (WBC) Count Criteria

▶ unreliable marker of injury
▶ "positive" when over 500 WBC/mm^3
▶ frequently falsely elevated when DPL delayed more than 7 h after injury
▶ not used at many centers due to low sensitivity and specificity

Enzymes

▶ amylase positive when over 20 IU/L
▶ alkaline phosphatase positive when over 3 IU/L
▶ each associated with small bowel injury
  ▶ combined elevation increases suspicion of small bowel injury
▶ high false negative rate

Other

▶ bacteria, bile, or vegetable matter indicate a hollow viscus injury

Disposition

▶ positive DPL mandates emergent surgical exploration
▶ if negative, admit for observation and serial abdominal examinations

Comparing DPL and CT

CT

▶ better detects retroperitoneal injury than DPL
  ▶ essential in flank and back wounds

DPL

▶ better detects small bowel injury than CT
▶ preferred in anterior abdominal wounds
▶ better detects diaphragmatic injury than CT
  ▶ preferred in thoracoabdominal wounds

CT Followed by DPL

▶ increases diagnostic yield

Laparoscopy

▶ excellent modality with experienced operator
▶ readily identifies diaphragmatic injuries in thoracoabdominal stab wounds
▶ major role with stab wounds in avoiding unnecessary laparotomy

Gunshot

General Principles

▶ in low-velocity injury, damage is confined to missile tract
▶ in high-velocity injury, blast effect and cavitation occur in addition to damage by the missile tract
▶ 85% of anterior gunshot wounds violate the peritoneum
  ▶ of these, 95% require repair of an intraabdominal injury
▶ organs occupying the most space are more often injured
  ▶ the following ordered by decreasing incidence of injury
    ▹ liver
    ▹ small bowel
    ▹ stomach
    ▹ colon
    ▹ spleen
    ▹ kidney
    ▹ pancreas

Radiography

Abdomen

▶ AP required
▶ lateral view added when retained missile is seen on AP to determine precise location

Laparotomy

Indications

▶ missile tract clearly enters abdominal cavity
▶ clinical evidence of peritoneal penetration
▶ positive diagnostic study in tangential wounds or pellet wounds

Local Wound Exploration (LWE)

Indications

▶ tangential abdominal gunshot wounds and peritoneal penetration uncertain
▶ very low-velocity, superficial wound from pellet gun

Contraindications

▶ need for laparotomy already established
▶ thoracoabdominal wounds, since there is high potential for iatrogenic complications
▶ technical difficulty, such as in obese or uncooperative patients

Findings

▶ if base of wound is clearly demonstrated and peritoneum not violated
  ▶ perform FAST, DPL, or CT to exclude solid organ injury from the blast effect
▶ if penetration of peritoneum is demonstrated, laparotomy indicated
▶ if inconclusive, consider CT, DPL, or laparoscopy

DPL

Indications

▶ suspected tangential abdominal gunshot wounds

Contraindications

▶ need for laparotomy already established

Red Blood Cell Count Criteria

▶ tangential gunshot or BB/pellet wounds
  ▶ over 5,000 RBC/mm^3 defines a positive study
    ▹ suggests peritoneal penetration
    ▹ 100,000 RBC/mm^3 is too high and results in 20% false negative rate for tangential wounds

Disposition

▶ positive DPL mandates emergent surgical exploration
▶ if negative, admit for observation and serial abdominal examinations

Abdominal CT

Indications

▶ suspected tangential gunshot wounds to the flank and back following a negative DPL
  ▶ use "triple contrast" (e.g., oral, intravenous, and rectal contrast)
▶ adjunctive study when DPL is contraindicated or cannot be performed
▶ localize very low-velocity (e.g., pellet) injury when LWE is inconclusive or contraindicated

Disposition

▶ CT evidence of contrast extravasation or free air mandates emergent surgical exploration
▶ if negative, admit for observation and serial abdominal examinations

Severe Pelvic Trauma

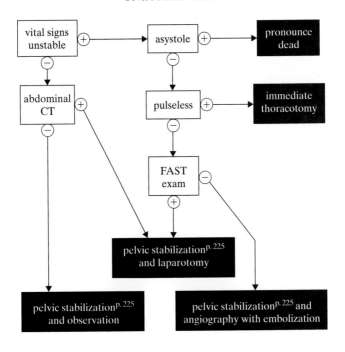

16

Pelvis

General Principles

Statistics

Etiology

- ▶ 60% motor vehicle collisions
- ▶ 30% falls

Mortality

- ▶ 15% overall
- ▶ 30% when open fracture
- ▶ 45% when hypotensive on presentation

Associated Injuries

- ▶ with severe fractures (Kane type III)
  - ▹ 50% have intraabdominal injuries
  - ▹ 15% have urethral injuries
  - ▹ 10% have bladder injuries

Anatomy

- ▶ bony pelvis comprised of
  - ▹ innominate bones
    - ▹ ilium
    - ▹ ischium
    - ▹ pubis
  - ▹ sacrum
- ▶ symphysis pubis joins the sides anteriorly
- ▶ major ligamentous unions include
  - ▹ sacroiliac
  - ▹ sacrospinatus
  - ▹ sacrotuberous

► vascular
  ► dense presacral venous plexus
  ► iliac vessel branches

Physical Examination

► check femoral pulses
► gently perform manual pelvic compressions only once, to determine if skeletally unstable by applying the following forces and checking for any "give"
  ► recommended maneuvers
    ► lateral to medial at iliac crests
    ► anterior to posterior at symphysis pubis
    ► anterior to posterior at iliac crests
  ► stop at first sign of instability
  ► these maneuvers are unreliable predictors
► do not compress the pelvis aggressively or repeatedly
  ► will increase hemorrhage if the pelvis is unstable
► rectal examination
  ► prostate position
  ► gross rectal bleeding
  ► sphincter tone
  ► lacerations or palpable fracture fragments
► urethral examination
  ► blood at the penile meatus
  ► scrotal or perineal ecchymosis/uroma
► bimanual vaginal examination
  ► lacerations
  ► tenderness
► pelvic fracture excluded if normal physical examination and confirmation of all the following
  ► normal mental status and neurologic examination
  ► no distracting pain
  ► no intoxicating substances

Fracture Classification

Important Distinctions

► determine whether likely or not to become hemodynamically unstable
  ► up to 4 liters of blood can accumulate in the retroperitoneum after a severe pelvic fracture
► determine whether skeletally stable or unstable
► determine whether closed versus open
  ► can be open to perineum, rectum, or vagina

Kane Type I

Definition

▶ fracture of one pelvic bone and no break in the pelvic ring
▶ skeletally stable

Examples (Figure 16–1)

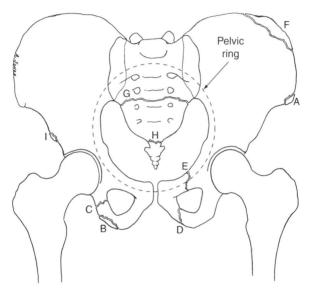

A, Anterior superior iliac spine avulsion; B, Ischial tuberosity avulsion;
C, Ischial ramus fracture; D, Inferior pubic ramus fracture; E, Superior pubic
ramus fracture; F, Iliac wing fracture; G, Sacral fracture; H, Coccyx fracture;
I, Anterior inferior iliac spine avulsion

Figure 16–1

▶ avulsions
   ▶ anterior superior iliac spine (rectus femoris attachment)
   ▶ anterior inferior iliac spine (sartorius attachment)
   ▶ ischial tuberosity (adductor magnus attachment)
▶ fracture of single ramus of pubis or ischium
▶ iliac wing (Duverney's) fracture
   ▶ due to direct trauma
▶ sacral fracture
   ▶ 80–90% associated with another pelvic fracture
   ▶ 25% with neurologic deficits
   ▶ requires CT or MRI for ideal imaging

Treatment

▶ analgesics and bed rest
▶ arrange follow-up with an orthopedic surgeon
▶ surgical fixation rarely required

Kane Type II

Definition

▶ single break in ring near pubic symphysis or sacroiliac (SI) joint
   ▶ single breaks can only occur near a mobile area
▶ skeletally stable

Examples

▶ unilateral ischiopubic rami fractures (Figure 16–2)
   ▶ comprise majority of type II fractures
   ▶ vertical fracture line
   ▶ significantly displaced fractures must be associated with second break in ring and therefore considered type III fractures

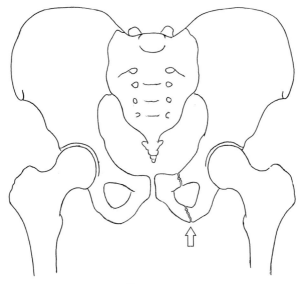

Figure 16–2

▶ fracture near or subluxation of pubic symphysis
   ▶ associated with lower genitourinary (GU) injuries
▶ fracture near or subluxation of SI joint

Treatment

▶ analgesics and bed rest
▶ need to exclude associated GU, intraabdominal, and soft tissue injuries which occur in up to 25%

Kane Type III

Definition

▶ involves two sites in the ring
▶ skeletally unstable
▶ often associated with intraabdominal, GU, and soft tissue injuries

Examples

▶ straddle fracture (Figure 16–3)
   ▶ majority of type III
   ▶ all four ischiopubic rami fractured
   ▶ one-third with lower GU injury
   ▶ treatment of fracture conservative since fracture does not involve main weight-bearing arch

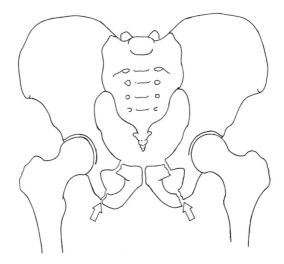

Figure 16–3

▶ Malgaigne fracture (Figure 16–4)
  ▸ called double vertical fracture/dislocation
  ▸ caused by major vertical shearing force
  ▸ 20% associated mortality
  ▸ anterior component consists of either unilateral ischiopubic rami fractures or diastasis of the pubic symphysis
  ▸ ipsilateral posterior component consists of either sacral or iliac fractures or disruption of the SI joint on the same side as the lower component
  ▸ can occur with straddle fracture

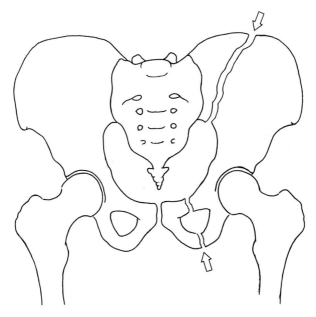

Figure 16–4

▶ "bucket handle" fracture
  ▸ same as Malgaigne except posterior component is contralateral
▶ "open book" or "sprung" pelvis (Figure 16–5)
  ▸ disruption of symphysis pubis and SI joints
  ▸ caused by AP compression
  ▸ associated with bladder rupture and retroperitoneal hematoma
▶ severe multiple fractures
  ▸ combinations of the above fracture types
  ▸ 50–70% associated mortality

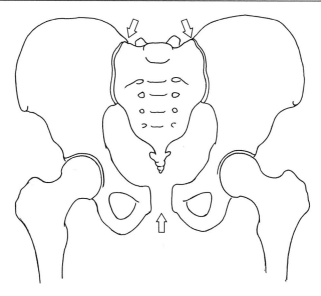

Figure 16–5

Treatment

► aggressive search for associated trauma
► stabilization of pelvis to control on-going hemorrhage
  ► external fixation
  ► surgical fixation
  ► traction
► consider urgent angiography with embolization

Kane Type IV

Definition

► acetabular fractures
► diagnosis
  ► Judet views and CT recommended

Examples

► posterior rim fracture
  ► associated with posterior hip dislocation

- ▶ transverse fracture
- ▶ ilioischial column fracture
- ▶ iliopubic column fracture

Treatment

- ▶ anatomic restoration required
- ▶ bed rest for nondisplaced fracture
- ▶ surgical fixation for displaced fractures

Young/Burgess System

- ▶ based on pattern of injury since it predicts complications and aids in applying corrective forces

Lateral Compression (LC)

- ▶ horizontal fracture of pubic rami
  - ▶ I—crush injury to sacrum
  - ▶ II—iliac wing
  - ▶ III—open book injury

A–P Compression (APC)

- ▶ diastasis of pubic symphysis or longitudinal rami fracture
  - ▶ I—diastasis but ligaments intact
  - ▶ II—widened sacroiliac joint, anterior ligaments disrupted, posterior ligaments intact
  - ▶ III—complete sacroiliac joint and ligament disruption

Vertical Shear (VS)

- ▶ vertically oriented fracture through anterior and posterior pelvis with superior displacement of injured hemipelvis

Tile System

- ▶ based on radiographic signs of stability or instability

Type A

- ▶ stable
- ▶ no pelvic ring disruption

Type B

▶ rotationally unstable, vertically stable
▶ B$_1$—open book with symphysis pubis displacement
▶ B$_2$—lateral compression causes double rami and sacral fractures

Type C

▶ rotationally and vertically unstable
▶ vertical displacement of one hemipelvis

Radiography

Plain Films

▶ screen for fracture with an AP pelvis view
   ▶ sensitivity 90%
▶ if fracture is confirmed or remains clinically suspect, obtain supplemental views, which increase sensitivity to 94%
▶ inlet view
   ▶ best visualizes posterior components
▶ outlet view
   ▶ best visualizes anterior components
▶ Judet view
   ▶ best visualizes acetabulum
   ▶ acetabular fractures are often missed

Other Studies

▶ CT or MRI are indicated when
   ▶ acetabular fracture is seen or suspected
   ▶ intraabdominal and retroperitoneal injuries are possible and the patient is hemodynamically stable
▶ retrograde urethrography is indicated when
   ▶ signs or symptoms of a urethral injury
   ▶ pelvic fracture associated with diastasis of pubic symphysis
▶ cystography indicated when
   ▶ blunt abdominal trauma with gross hematuria
   ▶ severe pelvic fracture (Kane type III)

Hemorrhage Control

General Principles

▶ hemorrhage is the most significant complication of pelvic fractures
  ▶ most pelvic bleeding is venous in origin from the bone itself and/or from disruption of the rich presacral venous plexus
  ▶ the retroperitoneal space can accommodate 4 liters of blood before tamponade occurs
  ▶ retroperitoneal hematoma is most common with posterior pelvic fractures
▶ transfuse to maintain hematocrit above 20%
  ▶ above 30% in the elderly or those with underlying cardiac or pulmonary disease
▶ avoid coagulopathy
  ▶ anticipate after massive red cell transfusion
  ▶ avoid hypothermia by using blood warmer
  ▶ transfuse sufficient fresh frozen plasma and platelets as needed to maintain adequate coagulation factors
▶ monitor vital signs and central venous pressure or pulmonary artery measurements for volume status
  ▶ maintain SBP about 100 mm Hg

Fluid Resuscitation

▶ Kane type III fracture requires blood replacement more than twice as often as other types
▶ 60% of patients that are initially hemodynamically unstable will respond to fluid resuscitation because retroperitoneal pelvic bleeding eventually tamponades

Pneumatic Anti-Shock Garments (PASG)

▶ temporizing measure to splint pelvic fractures and tamponade venous plexus bleeding
  ▶ initially inflate leg compartments then abdominal compartment
    ▶ minimum pressure is 40 mm Hg
    ▶ maximum pressure is when the Velcro slips
▶ indications
  ▶ hemodynamic instability with long transport times
▶ remove as soon as BP stabilized
  ▶ within 2 h to prevent ischemic complications
  ▶ slowly deflate one section at a time (abdomen first) watching the BP carefully
    ▶ if the SBP drops more than 5 mm Hg then stop and give fluid bolus

► contraindications
  ► concurrent severe chest or head trauma
  ► diaphragmatic rupture
  ► impalements or evisceration
  ► pulmonary edema or cardiogenic shock
  ► advanced pregnancy

Pelvis Stabilization

► external fixation techniques
  ► pins in the iliac crests fixed to a frame
  ► vacuum splinting device
  ► Ganz pelvic clamp
  ► some tie a sheet tightly around the pelvis as a temporizing measure when other stabilization means are not immediately available
► helps control ongoing hemorrhage in unstable patients
► indication
  ► Kane type III pelvic fracture, especially with hemodynamic instability
► actions
  ► limits motion
  ► decreases bleeding at fracture site and at interspinous venous plexus
  ► improves tamponade by reestablishing the dimensions of the true pelvis and controlling the size of the potential extraperitoneal space
  ► promotes early patient mobility
► does not stop arterial bleeding

Angiography with Embolization

► indications
  ► persistent hypovolemia with control of other bleeding
  ► fracture pattern not compatible with external fixation
  ► concurrent angiography for other injuries
► advantages
  ► diagnostic and temporizing for large arterial injuries
    ► common iliac, external iliac, and common femoral artery injuries that require surgical intervention may be temporized by balloon tamponade
  ► diagnostic and therapeutic for smaller arterial injuries
    ► transcatheter embolization controls bleeding and decreases blood requirements
  ► spleen is the most common extrapelvic organ injured concurrently with a severe pelvis fracture and splenic hemorrhage can be controlled with embolization

► other considerations
  ► time-consuming and highly operator-dependent
  ► GU tract evaluation should not precede angiography since extravasation of dye after a cystogram can obscure the appreciation of arterial bleeding during pelvic angiography

Direct Operative Control

► immediate operative intervention is indicated in an exsanguinating patient not responding to external fixation or angiographic embolization
  ► large arterial injuries involving proximal branches of the internal iliac must be controlled by surgical repair and/or packing

Concurrent Injuries

General Principles

► with severe pelvic fracture, do not assume hemorrhage is only retroperitoneal
► nearly one-half of patients with severe pelvic fractures have an associated intraabdominal injury

Investigation

FAST Examination

► rapid initial screening test
► in stable patients
  ► serial negative abdominal FAST and physical examinations over an 8 h observation period obviate the need for further diagnostic testing
  ► perform abdominal CT if examination is concerning
► in unstable patients
  ► positive study is indication for laparotomy
  ► negative study should point toward other sources of bleeding (retroperitoneal)

Abdomen/Pelvis CT

► study of choice for stable patients
► identifies
  ► intraabdominal injuries
  ► retroperitoneal hematoma
► defines extent of pelvic fracture

DPL

- obtain for unstable patients
- use open, supraumbilical approach
- gross aspiration of blood is an indication for immediate laparotomy
    - if indicated, perform external fixation or angiography intraoperatively
- positive result by cell count (over 100,000 RBC/mm^3)
    - 10% incidence of false positive DPLs with pelvic fractures
        - 10 times higher than blunt abdominal trauma without pelvic fracture
    - if indicated, perform external fixation or angiography preoperatively

Diagnostic Strategy

Hemodynamically Unstable Patient

- FAST examination or DPL
    - if evidence of large hemoperitoneum (i.e., intraabdominal fluid on FAST examination or positive aspiration on DPL)
        - immediate laparotomy
        - urgent intraoperative pelvic stabilization
    - if no evidence of large hemoperitoneum
        - immediate angiography
        - urgent pelvic stabilization

Hemodynamically Stable Patient

- if Kane type III fracture, notify orthopedic surgeon that stabilization is necessary
- abdominal CT
    - if patient becomes hemodynamically unstable while awaiting CT, return to the emergency department and perform FAST examination or DPL

Genitourinary Trauma

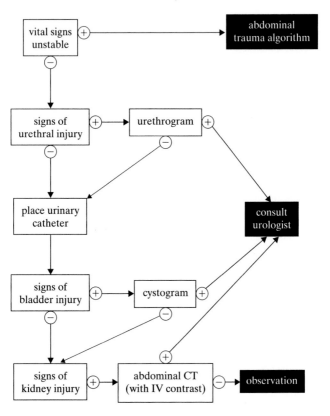

17

Genitourinary

General Principles

- ▶ prevalence
  - ▶ renal 65%
  - ▶ bladder 25%
  - ▶ urethral/ureteral 10%
- ▶ mortality directly due to renal injuries is under 3% but concurrent injuries are responsible for overall high associated mortality
  - ▶ management of head, chest, and abdominal injuries takes precedence
- ▶ work up the urinary system in a "retrograde" manner
  - ▶ injury exclusion (or confirmation) begins with the urethra, then the bladder, then the kidneys/ureters

Urethra

General Principles

Anatomy (Males) (Figure 17–1)

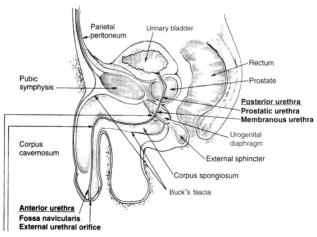

Figure 17–1

▶ the anterior urethra consists of the penile and bulbous urethra
▶ the posterior urethra consists of the membranous and prostatic urethra which contain the innervation responsible for continence and ejaculation
▶ the anterior and posterior components are divided by the urogenital diaphragm

Mechanism

▶ usually associated with blunt trauma resulting in severe pelvic fractures
▶ less often occurs with direct penetrating trauma
▶ exceedingly rare injury in women since very small structure

Clinical Findings

▶ symptoms
  ▶ perineal pain
  ▶ inability to void
▶ signs
  ▶ gross hematuria
  ▶ blood at the urethral meatus
  ▶ perineal swelling/ecchymosis
  ▶ abnormal prostate examination
    ▸ absent
    ▸ high riding
    ▸ boggy

Types

Anterior Urethral Injury

▶ mechanism
  ▶ most due to falls with straddle injuries or a blunt force to the perineum
    ▸ urethra is crushed between anterior pelvis and the impacting object
    ▸ complete disruption is unusual
  ▶ worsened by instrumentation
    ▸ passing a urinary catheter can convert a partial to a complete urethral disruption
  ▶ rarely caused by penetrating trauma
▶ relationship to Buck's fascia (see Figure 17–1)
  ▶ when intact, limits the extravasated urine to near the urethra
  ▶ when interrupted, allows extravasation into the scrotum and under the anterior abdominal wall

Posterior Urethral Injury

▶ association with severe pelvic fracture
  ▶ over 95% with posterior urethral injury due to severe pelvic fractures
  ▶ 15% with severe pelvic fractures have posterior urethral injury

▶ association with bladder rupture
 ▶ 10% with posterior urethral injury have bladder rupture

Diagnostic Testing

Retrograde Urethrography

▶ indications
 ▶ signs or symptoms of a urethral injury
 ▶ pelvic fracture associated with diastasis of pubic symphysis
▶ procedure (males) (Figure 17–2)

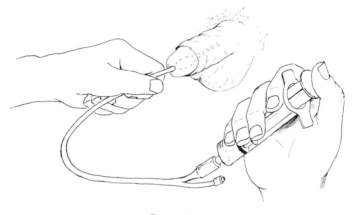

Figure 17–2

 ▶ insert an 8 Fr urinary catheter *without* lubricant 2 cm into the meatus so the balloon is at the fossa navicularis
 ▶ inflate the balloon with 1–2 ml of saline to create a seal
 ▶ administer 30 ml of contrast under gentle pressure
 ▶ obtain radiograph
 ▶ spilled contrast produces artifact if not wiped away completely

Management

▶ when the urethrogram is positive
 ▶ consult a urologist
 ▶ do not attempt urinary catheterization
 ▶ complete disruption or inability to urinate are indications for suprapubic cystostomy
  ▷ this procedure may be performed by the emergency physician or trauma surgeon when a urologist not immediately available and urgent intervention is necessary
  ▷ if the patient is able to urinate freely, urgent intervention is unnecessary

- ▶ in partial disruptions, the urologist may attempt gentle passage of a urinary catheter
  - ▷ this process is sometimes aided by filiforms and followers or urethral sounds
  - ▷ successful passage of a urinary catheter stents the injury and avoids the need for a suprapubic cystostomy

Bladder

General Principles

Mechanism

- ▶ blunt
  - ▶ accounts for 85%
  - ▶ most occur during motor vehicle collisions when a blunt force is imparted to a distended bladder
  - ▶ association with pelvic fracture
    - ▷ two-thirds with bladder disruption have a pelvic fracture
    - ▷ 15% with severe pelvic fractures (Kane type III) have a bladder disruption
  - ▶ association with urethral injury
    - ▷ 5–10% with bladder disruption also have urethral injury
- ▶ penetrating
  - ▶ accounts for 15%

Clinical Findings

- ▶ suprapubic tenderness
- ▶ inability to void
- ▶ gross hematuria almost always present

Diagnosis

Cystography

- ▶ indication
  - ▶ blunt abdominal trauma with gross hematuria
  - ▶ severe pelvic fracture (Kane type III)
  - ▶ penetrating wound near the bladder with microhematuria
- ▶ contraindication
  - ▶ urethral injury possible and not yet excluded
- ▶ technique (Figure 17–3)
  - ▶ place a urinary catheter after urethral injury is excluded clinically or radiographically
  - ▶ perform cystography via a suprapubic catheter if urethral injury is present

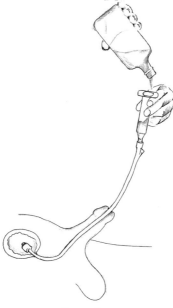

Figure 17–3

- ▶ obtain initial radiograph after 100 ml (1.5 ml/kg in children) water-soluble contrast has been administered by gravity infusion (15 cm above the patient)
  - ▷ excludes gross extravasation
  - ▷ if negative, continue
- ▶ fully distend the bladder
  - ▷ after maximum amount has been infused by gravity, use a syringe to instill an additional 50 ml in adults (0.5 ml/kg in children), then clamp the urinary catheter
  - ▷ total usually 5 ml/kg (about 350 ml contrast in adult males)
- ▶ radiographs
  - ▷ obtain AP, oblique, and lateral views of the bladder
  - ▷ always obtain a drainage or "post-void" film as 15% of bladder disruptions are seen only on this view
  - ▷ when abdominal CT is planned, one can similarly fill the bladder with contrast and clamp the catheter during the CT
- ▶ accuracy
  - ▶ approaches 100% with full distension
  - ▶ false negative studies can occur when the bladder is not fully distended or with low-velocity gunshot or stab wounds

Types

Extraperitoneal Bladder Disruption (Figure 17–4)

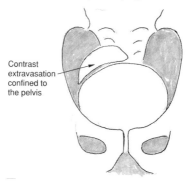

Contrast
extravasation
confined to
the pelvis

Figure 17–4

- ► 65% of bladder disruptions are limited to the pelvis
- ► mechanism in blunt abdominal trauma
  - ► one-third due to direct penetration by a bone fragment
  - ► two-thirds due to burst or shear force
- ► occurs in the anterolateral wall of the bladder near the neck
- ► extravasated bladder contrast confined to the pelvis
- ► treatment
  - ► catheter drainage and close observation
  - ► operative repair generally not required

Intraperitoneal Bladder Disruption

- ► 35% of bladder disruptions are intraperitoneal
  - ► about one-third of these also have an extraperitoneal component
- ► most are due to full bladder at time of a suprapubic blunt abdominal force
  - ► the bladder rises above the umbilicus when fully distended
- ► occurs in the fundus or posteriorly, which are the weakest walls of the bladder
- ► extravasated bladder contrast outlines intraperitoneal structures
- ► treatment
  - ► requires operative repair

Ureter

General Principles

- ► rarest of genitourinary injuries
- ► most are iatrogenic, occurring during surgical procedures

▶ when due to trauma, usually from penetrating injury
▶ blunt trauma can cause ureteropelvic junction avulsion
   ▶ most occur in children

Clinical Findings

▶ hematuria
   ▶ microscopic 60%
   ▶ absent 30%
   ▶ gross 10%
▶ symptoms/signs often obscured by associated injuries

Diagnosis

▶ confirmed by a contrast study which reveals extravasation at the site of injury

Treatment

▶ surgical repair necessary

Kidney

General Principles

Clinical Findings

▶ degree of microhematuria is not indicative of severity or nature of renal trauma
   ▶ positive dipstick correlates with over 10 red blood cells per high-power field (RBC/HPF)
   ▶ most believe there is no utility in the exact quantification of microhematuria by microscopic analysis
   ▶ others obtain contrast studies on patients with blunt trauma exceeding a certain threshold (e.g., 50 RBC/HPF)

Diagnosis

Penetrating Trauma

▶ penetrating trauma in the region of the kidney necessitates a contrast study

Blunt Trauma

▶ contrast study required when
   ▶ gross hematuria is present
   ▶ there is hemodynamic instability with microhematuria

▶ renal imaging is unnecessary when hemodynamically stable despite the presence of microhematuria
  ▶ this practice safely reduces the number of contrast studies
  ▶ it is necessary to confirm resolution of the hematuria, which occurs in the majority by repeat urinalysis a few days later
  ▶ if microhematuria is still present on reevaluation, a contrast study is indicated

Renal Contrast Studies

▶ risks
  ▶ allergic reactions occur in 2%
  ▶ when life-threatening allergy to contrast is documented, use an alternate diagnostic tool (e.g., formal ultrasound or MRI)
  ▶ otherwise, when there is known contrast or shellfish allergy
    ▶ premedicate with diphenhydramine (50 mg) and methylprednisolone (125 mg)
    ▶ use nonionic contrast media
▶ CT
  ▶ study of choice in the stable patient
  ▶ allows staging of renal injuries
  ▶ assesses other intraabdominal organs
  ▶ performed rapidly
▶ formal IVP
  ▶ can be used to screen for renal injuries in stable patients
  ▶ order if there is persistent microhematuria after blunt trauma
  ▶ confirms perfusion, defines parenchyma, and delineates the collecting system
▶ renal angiography
  ▶ the patient must be hemodynamically stable
  ▶ indications
    ▶ areas of segmental nonenhancement
    ▶ renal contrast study indeterminate
    ▶ may help plan surgical management of severe renal injuries seen on renal contrast study
▶ when renal pedicle injury is diagnosed on renal contrast study, consult urologist immediately
  ▶ if renal angiography is deemed unnecessary, time to revascularization decreases and kidney salvage rate increases
  ▶ when kidney not salvageable, embolization may be used to control bleeding

Types of Renal Injuries

Nunn Classification

▶ injuries divide into five classes
  ▶ I. contusion
  ▶ II. cortical laceration

- ▶ III. caliceal laceration
- ▶ IV. complete renal fracture ("shattered kidney")
- ▶ V. vascular pedicle injury
- ▶ distribution
  - ▶ classes I and II comprise 70%
  - ▶ class III comprises 20%
  - ▶ classes IV and V comprise 10%

Management

General Principles

- ▶ 10% of blunt injuries require surgery
- ▶ 50% of penetrating injuries require surgery

Contusion

- ▶ called Nunn Class I (Figure 17–5)

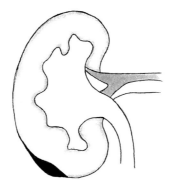

Figure 17–5

- ▶ incidence
  - ▶ most common blunt renal injury
- ▶ clinical findings
  - ▶ diagnose presumptively when blunt flank trauma is associated with hematuria
- ▶ radiographic findings
  - ▶ emergent contrast study is unnecessary when microscopic hematuria and hemodynamically stable
  - ▶ IVP is normal
  - ▶ CT may reveal a subcapsular hematoma
- ▶ management
  - ▶ discharge with plan to repeat urinalysis in a few days to ensure resolution of hematuria
  - ▶ persistent hematuria on follow-up mandates contrast study

Lacerations

▶ cortical laceration (Nunn class II) (Figure 17–6)
  ▶ contrast study reveals extrarenal extravasation

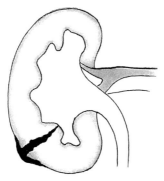

Figure 17–6

  ▶ management
    ▷ admit for observation
    ▷ no surgical intervention necessary
▶ caliceal laceration (Nunn class III) (Figure 17–7)
  ▶ contrast study reveals intrarenal extravasation
  ▶ management
    ▷ admit for observation
    ▷ need for surgical intervention debated
▶ complete renal fracture (Nunn class IV) (Figure 17–8)
  ▶ contrast study reveals intra- and extrarenal extravasation

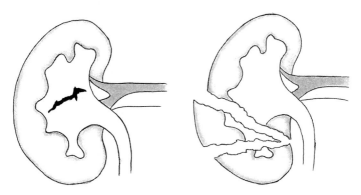

Figure 17–7   Figure 17–8

▶ management
  ▹ perform surgical intervention
  ▹ nephrectomy usually necessary

Vascular Pedicle Injury

▶ called Nunn Class V (Figure 17–9)

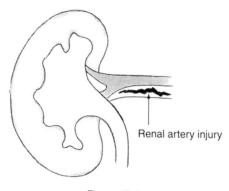

Renal artery injury

Figure 17–9

▶ incidence
  ▶ most result from penetrating trauma
  ▶ comprises only 1% of blunt renal injuries
▶ mechanism
  ▶ most occur as a result of vertical deceleration resulting in a shear force between a mobile kidney and relatively fixed vascular pedicle
▶ clinical findings
  ▶ up to 50% without hematuria
▶ radiographic findings
  ▶ renal contrast study reveals absence of renal enhancement
    ▹ time to revascularization decreases and kidney salvage rate increases when confirmatory angiography is deemed unnecessary
  ▶ inconclusive renal contrast study mandates emergent renal angiography
    ▹ when kidney is not salvageable, embolization may be used to control bleeding
▶ management
  ▶ requires surgical intervention
    ▹ surgical reperfusion within 6 h is necessary to prevent renal dysfunction
    ▹ 35% are salvageable with timely reperfusion
    ▹ overall mortality is 25% due to concurrent life threats

Reproductive Organs

Scrotum

▶ redundant tissue and dense vascularization generally make repairs technically easy and successful

Testicles

▶ obtain testicular ultrasound to rule out rupture
▶ 90% of ruptured testes are salvageable if repaired within 72 h

Penis

▶ complete amputations must be microsurgically reattached within 6 h to attain any chance of success
▶ impotence is common with extensive penile injuries
▶ exclude urethral injuries before repairing penile lacerations

Vagina

▶ vaginal wall injuries
  ▶ occur directly from straddle mechanism
  ▶ occur secondarily from pelvic fractures
    ▷ laceration caused by sharp fracture edges
    ▷ perform careful digital examination to determine if there is vulvo-vaginal communication
▶ obtain gynecologic consultation when significant injuries are found
▶ prophylactic antibiotics are recommended with penetrating injuries and open pelvic fractures

Part III

EXTREMITY TRAUMA

18

Soft Tissue

Penetrating

Arterial Injury

Clinical Findings

▶ strong clinical evidence of vascular injury ("hard signs")
  ▶ pulsatile bleeding
  ▶ expanding hematoma
  ▶ palpable thrill or audible bruit
  ▶ evidence of distal ischemia—commonly known as the "six P's"
    ▹ pain
    ▹ pallor
    ▹ pulselessness
    ▹ paralysis
    ▹ paresthesia
    ▹ poikilothermia (cool to touch)
▶ moderate clinical evidence of vascular injury ("soft signs")
  ▶ diminished ankle–brachial indices (ABI)
    ▹ utilized in evaluating lower-extremity injuries
    ▹ defined as ratio of ankle SBP (by doppler of dorsalis pedis or posterior tibial artery) to brachial artery SBP
    ▹ ABI under 0.9 is abnormal and when asymmetric mandates angiography

Table 18–1 Peripheral Nerves

Upper Extremity Nerves	Sensory	Motor
Ulnar	Little finger pad	Spread fingers (interossei)
Median	Index finger pad	Pinch thumb to little finger
Radial	First dorsal webspace	Wrist extension
Axillary	Lateral shoulder (over deltoid)	Deltoid (abduct arm)
Lower Extremity Nerves		
Femoral	Anterior knee	Knee extension
Obturator	Medial thigh	Hip adduction
Posterior tibial	Sole of foot	Plantarflexion of toes
Superficial peroneal	Dorsal–lateral foot	Evert ankle
Deep peroneal	First dorsal webspace	Dorsiflexion of toes
Sciatic	Foot	Dorsi-/plantarflexion at ankle

- ► asymmetrically absent or weak distal pulse
- ► history of moderate hemorrhage and wound proximate to a major artery
- ► peripheral nerve (Table 18–1) deficit

Management

▶ emergent surgery is necessary (with or without intraoperative angiography) when there is evidence of distal ischemia
▶ perform immediate angiography when there is strong clinical evidence of vascular injury ("hard signs")
▶ perform urgent color duplex scan or angiography when there is moderate clinical evidence of vascular injury ("soft signs")
▶ when there is asymptomatic penetrating injury in proximity to a major artery without clinical evidence of injury
- ► significant arterial injury present in up to 1%
- ► requires observation, serial physical exams, and close follow-up
- ► urgent color duplex scan or angiography appropriate with high-velocity missile injury or an unreliable patient

Blunt

Reduction Principles

▶ reduce immediately if there is neurovascular compromise
▶ surgical reduction is indicated when dislocations cannot be reduced by closed means
▶ obtain adequate analgesia and muscle relaxation
- ► use a nerve block whenever possible
- ► titrate a combination of opiates and benzodiazepines until the patient can tolerate the procedure
▶ arrange follow-up with an orthopedic surgeon
▶ see p. 469 for post-reduction splinting techniques

Open Fractures

▶ control active hemorrhage with direct pressure
▶ assume any proximate skin interruption is an open fracture and manage in the following manner
- ► paint skin about wound with povidone-iodine (Betadine)
- ► administer parenteral antibiotic
  - ► first-generation cephalosporin or equivalent
  - ► many recommend adding an aminoglycoside as a second agent
- ► update tetanus immunization if necessary
- ► immediately notify an orthopedic surgeon
  - ► operative wound debridement and irrigation should take place urgently unless other life-threatening problems take precedence
▶ obtain urgent orthopedic consultation

▶ immobilize, elevate, and apply ice pack as soon as possible to minimize swelling

Neurovascular Complications (Table 18–2)

Table 18–2 Neurovascular Complications

Skeletal injury	Neurovascular injury
Anterior shoulder dislocation	Axillary nerve
Humeral shaft fracture	Radial nerve
Supracondylar humeral fracture	Brachial artery
Distal radius fracture	Median artery
Posterior hip dislocation	Sciatic nerve
Supracondylar femur fracture	Popliteal artery
Knee dislocation	Popliteal artery
Proximal fibular fracture	Peroneal nerve

▶ angiography is indicated when objective evidence of vascular injury is present and for knee dislocations

Compartment Syndrome

Clinical Findings

▶ common in crush injuries or fractures with marked swelling
  ▶ much more often in lower (rather than upper) extremities (Figure 18–1)

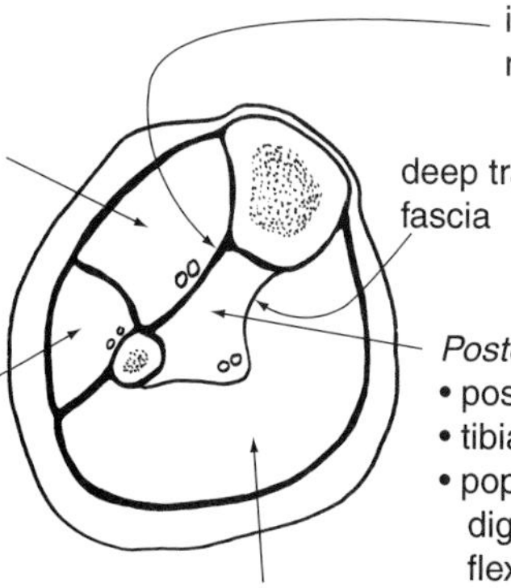

Anterior (most common site of compartment syndrome)
• anterior tibial artery
• deep peroneal nerve
• tibialis anterior, extensor digitorum longus, peroneus tertius, and extensor hallucis longus muscles

interosseous membrane

deep transverse fascia

Posterior (deep)
• posterior tibial artery
• tibial nerve
• popliteus, flexor digitorum longus, flexor hallucis longus, and tibialis posterior muscles

Lateral
• peroneal artery branches
• peroneal nerve
• peoneus longus and peroneus brevis muscles

Posterior (superficial)
• gastrocnemius, plantaris, and soleus muscles

Figure 18–1

Table 18–3 Pain by Compartment

Compartment	Involved muscles
Hand interosseus	Interosseus
Dorsal forearm	Digit extensors
Volar forearm	Digit flexors
Upper arm flexor	Biceps
Upper arm extensor	Triceps
Anterior leg	Toe extensor/tibialis anterior
Superficial posterior leg	Soleus-gastrocnemius
Deep posterior leg	Toe flexor/tibialis posterior
Foot	Foot intrinsics—flexors/extensors

▶ determine the presence or absence of each of the six "P's" (p. 243)
  ▶ the most common sign is pain with passive stretch of muscles within the affected compartment (Table 18–3)
  ▶ distal pulses often intact

Management

▶ remove compressive dressings or casts
▶ apply ice to the affected extremity and do not elevate
  ▶ keeping the area dependent will increase the perfusion pressure
▶ suspicion mandates immediate measurement of compartmental pressures
  ▶ methods
    ▶ hand-held transducer (Stryker Surgical)
    ▶ needle-manometer technique (p. 468)
  ▶ normal pressure under 20 mm Hg
▶ notify an orthopedic surgeon immediately
  ▶ treatment is emergent fasciotomy

Amputations

Initial Management

Stump Care

▶ irrigate with saline to decontaminate
▶ cover with saline-moistened sterile gauze
▶ splint and elevate
▶ do not apply tourniquet or clamp arterial bleeders
  ▶ use pressure to control bleeding

Amputated Part Preparation

▶ irrigate with saline to decontaminate
▶ wrap in saline-moistened gauze
▶ place in water-tight plastic bag
▶ immerse bag in container of ice water

Replantation

General Principles

▶ immediate surgical consultation
  ▷ delay of reimplantation worsens outcome
▶ sharp distal wounds with little associated damage have highest success rates
▶ children have better outcomes than adults because of their superior regeneration and rehabilitation capabilities

Hand Injuries

▶ thumb
  ▷ deserves aggressive attempt at replantation since loss results in severe hand disability
▶ multiple fingers
  ▷ deserve aggressive attempts at replantation
▶ single finger
  ▷ replantation believed unnecessary
  ▷ best outcome with amputations proximal to distal interphalangeal (DIP) joint and distal to insertion of flexor digitorum superficialis

Facial Injuries

▶ ear and nose reimplantations heal well

Relative Contraindications

▶ prolonged warm ischemia
  ▷ over 6 h
  ▷ over 12 h for a digit
▶ contamination
▶ lower extremity

Absolute Contraindications

▶ severe crush injury
▶ inability to withstand long surgical procedure due to concurrent medical conditions

19

Hand

Phalanx Fracture

Comminuted Tuft

▶ frequent nailbed involvement
  ▶ the presence of a large (over 50%) subungual hematoma indicates a nailbed injury
    ▹ evacuate using heated cautery or by boring a hole with a large hollow needle
  ▶ if the nail is avulsed, either trim and replace its base or place an artificial stent between the eponychial fold and germinal nail matrix
    ▹ prevents adhesions and subsequent nail deformities

Distal Shaft

Nondisplaced (Figure 19–1)

▶ protective (hairpin) splint for 2–4 weeks
  ▶ until fracture site is painless and stable

Displaced (Figure 19–2)

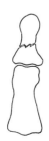

Figure 19–1

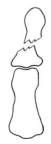

Figure 19–2

- ▶ reduce with longitudinal traction
- ▶ volar splint for 4–6 weeks
- ▶ nonreducible fractures may require pinning
    - ▶ often due to interposed adipose tissue

Intraarticular/Distal Interphalangeal Joint (DIP)

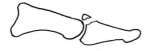

Figure 19–3

- ▶ dorsal surface of base (Figure 19–3)
    - ▶ "bony" Mallet finger
        - ▶ intraarticular avulsion fracture of the dorsal surface of the distal phalanx causing loss of full extension at DIP joint
    - ▶ "nonbony" Mallet finger
        - ▶ avulsion of the extensor tendon from the base of the distal phalanx without a fracture
    - ▶ treatment
        - ▶ when under 33% joint surface, splint with DIP joint in slight hyperextension for 6 weeks
        - ▶ do not "test" the joint before 6 weeks
        - ▶ when over 33% joint surface (Figure 19–4), surgical fixation is recommended by some while others splint (as above)

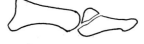

Figure 19–4

- ▶ volar surface of base (Figure 19–5)
    - ▶ treatment
        - ▶ when under 33% joint surface, splint with DIP joint in 5–10° of flexion for 6 weeks

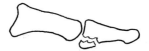

Figure 19–5

- do not "test" the joint before the 6-week point
- when over 33% joint surface, surgical fixation is recommended by some while others splint (as above)

Middle and Proximal Phalanx Shaft

▶ rotational deformity
  - ▶ leads to functional compromise especially in the second and third digits
  - ▶ rotational deformity can be appreciated on clinical examination
    - flex metacarpophalangeal (MCP) and proximal interphalangeal (PIP) joints while extending DIPs and the fingers should point to the same spot on the wrist and certainly not overlap one another (Figure 19–6)
    - slightly flex fingers and view finger nails to make sure planes are level and similar to the opposite hand
▶ angulation deformity
  - ▶ can occur in any direction but is most common in the volar direction

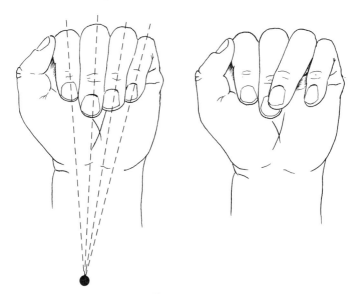

Figure 19–6

- ▶ always obtain a true lateral radiograph for metacarpal and phalangeal fractures to determine the degree of angulation
▶ initial treatment
  - ▶ volar aluminum splint with
    - MCP joint in 70° flexion
    - PIP joint in 15° flexion
    - DIP joint in 10° flexion

▶ definitive treatment
  ▶ volar aluminum splint for 2 weeks followed by dynamic splinting (i.e., "buddy taping") for 1 week if
    ▷ greenstick fracture
    ▷ nondisplaced fracture
  ▶ reduction followed by splinting if
    ▷ displaced fracture (Figure 19–7)
    ▷ angulated fracture
    ▷ rotational deformity
  ▶ surgical fixation necessary if
    ▷ failure to maintain reduction
    ▷ spiral fracture (Figure 19–8)
    ▷ over 15° angulation in plane of motion
    ▷ multiple fractures
    ▷ open fracture
    ▷ comminuted fracture

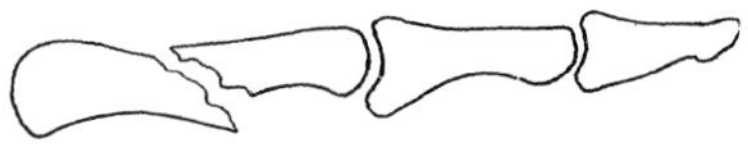

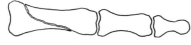

Figure 19–7

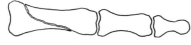

Figure 19–8

Intraarticular/Middle and Proximal Phalanx

▶ initial treatment
  ▶ volar aluminum splint
▶ definitive treatment
  ▶ dynamic splint if
    ▷ nondisplaced fractures

▶ surgical fixation if
  ▷ displaced condylar fractures (Figure 19–9)
  ▷ displaced volar lip fracture with over 25% joint surface involved (Figure 19–10)
  ▷ displaced dorsal lip fracture of DIP joint with over 25% joint surface involved (Figure 19–11)
  ▷ comminuted fracture

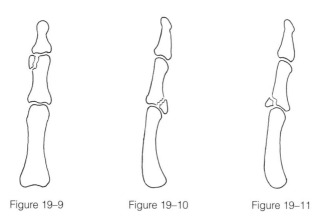

Figure 19–9   Figure 19–10   Figure 19–11

Dislocation

DIP

▶ perform digital nerve block for pain control
▶ longitudinal traction with manipulation back into joint
▶ test collateral ligament stability post reduction
  ▷ when stable, splint for 2 weeks
  ▷ when unstable, splint in 30° flexion for 3 weeks

PIP

Posterior

▶ digital nerve block for pain control
▶ longitudinal traction with manipulation back into joint
▶ splint in 15° flexion for 3 weeks followed by dynamic splinting for 3 weeks

Anterior

▶ digital nerve block for pain control
▶ longitudinal traction with manipulation back into joint
▶ splint with the PIP and DIP joints in extension and the MP joint in 50° flexion
▶ associated with injury of central slip
   ▶ may lead to Boutonniere deformity
▶ refer to hand surgeon for follow-up

MCP

▶ dorsal dislocation of the MCP joint is most common
▶ reduction technique
   ▶ metacarpal nerve block anesthesia
   ▶ longitudinal traction with manipulation back into place
▶ post reduction, immobilize MCP joint in 50–70° flexion for 7 days followed by dynamic splint
▶ closed reduction may fail due to interposition of the volar plate between the base of the proximal phalanx and head of the metacarpal

Metacarpal Fracture

Shaft of 1st Metacarpal

▶ can be transverse (more common) (Figure 19–12) or oblique
▶ nonsurgical treatment
   ▶ under 30° of rotational deformity or angulation requires thumb spica splint or cast for 4 weeks
   ▶ over 30° of rotational deformity or angulation requires reduction followed by thumb spica splint or cast
▶ surgical fixation if
   ▶ oblique fracture
   ▶ rotational deformity
   ▶ fracture over 30° angulation that is unstable after reduction

Base of 1st Metacarpal

▶ Bennett's fracture/dislocation (Figure 19–13)
   ▶ oblique intraarticular fracture at the base of the 1st metacarpal
   ▶ 1st metacarpal subluxed by pull of the abductor pollicis brevis and longus
   ▶ initial treatment
      ▶ immobilization in thumb spica splint
   ▶ definitive treatment
      ▶ surgical fixation with percutaneous pinning

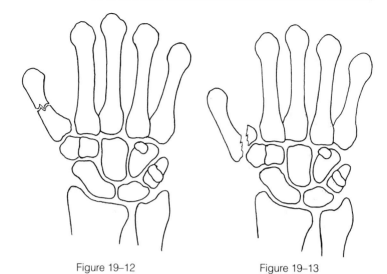

Figure 19–12   Figure 19–13

▶ Rolando's fracture (Figure 19–14)
  ▶ comminuted intraarticular fracture of the base of 1st metacarpal
  ▶ initial treatment
    ▷ immobilization in thumb spica splint
  ▶ definitive treatment
    ▷ surgical fixation

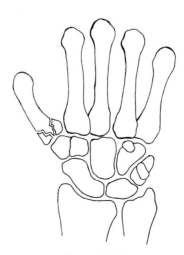

Figure 19–14

▶ "gamekeeper's thumb"
  ▶ mechanism
    ▹ radially directed stress at 1st MCP joint (a common ski pole injury) causes disruption of its ulnar collateral ligament
  ▶ apply valgus stress to 1st MCP joint with joint at 40° flexion to check for laxity (Figure 19–15)

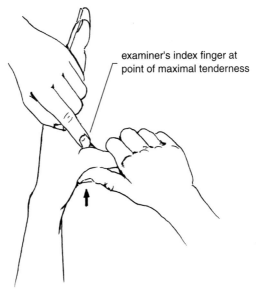

examiner's index finger at point of maximal tenderness

Figure 19–15

▶ initial treatment
  ▹ immobilization in thumb spica splint
▶ definitive treatment
  ▹ for partial tears use thumb spica cast for 4–6 weeks
  ▹ for complete tears perform surgical repair of ulnar collateral ligament

2nd–5th Metacarpals

General Treatment

▶ initial
  ▶ reduce displaced fractures
  ▶ immobilize in gutter or volar splint extending from DIP joint to elbow with
    ▹ MCP flexed at 70°
    ▹ PIP and DIP flexed at 15–20°
    ▹ wrist dorsiflexed at 15°
▶ definitive
  ▶ nondisplaced fractures (Figure 19–16)
    ▹ splint or cast for 3–6 weeks
  ▶ unstable or poor anatomic reduction
    ▹ surgical reduction (see specific indications below)

Head

▶ indications for internal fixation
  ▶ large displaced intraarticular fragments
  ▶ comminuted fractures that cannot be adequately reduced (Figure 19–17)

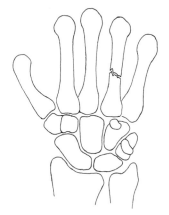

Figure 19–16

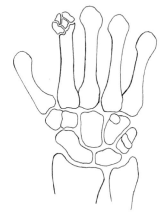

Figure 19–17

Neck

▶ commonly results from striking surface with closed fist
  ▶ 5th metacarpal commonly referred to as a "boxer's fracture" (Figure 19–18)

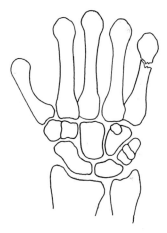

Figure 19–18

▶ indications for internal fixation
  ▶ rotational deformity
  ▶ angulation of 4th or 5th metacarpal over 40°
  ▶ angulation of 2nd or 3rd metacarpal over 10–15°

Shaft

▶ transverse fracture prone to angulate dorsally due to pull of the interosseus muscles (Figure 19–19)

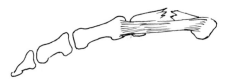

Figure 19–19

▶ oblique fracture prone to rotational deformity (Figure 19–20)
▶ indications for internal fixation
  ▶ shortening over 5 mm
  ▶ rotational deformity (see p. 251)
  ▶ angulation
    ▷ over 30°, for 4th or 5th metacarpal
    ▷ over 10°, for 2nd or 3rd metacarpal

Base (Figure 19–21)

▶ splint or apply bulky hand dressing in neutral position
  ▶ wrist in 30° extension
  ▶ MCP joint free

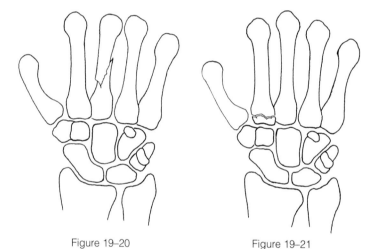

Figure 19–20   Figure 19–21

▶ indications for close follow-up and possible surgical fixation
  ▶ isolated, nondisplaced fracture of 4th metacarpal associated with displacement
    ▷ expect movement of fracture fragments
  ▶ intraarticular fracture of 5th metacarpal due to subluxation of metacarpal hamate joint (Figure 19–22)
    ▷ acts similar to a Bennett's fracture since 5th metacarpal subluxed by pull of the extensor carpi ulnaris (called "reverse" Bennett's fracture)
  ▶ rotational deformity (see p. 251)
    ▷ leads to functional compromise, especially in the second and third digits

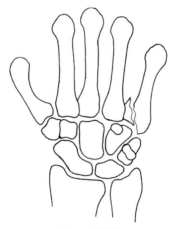

Figure 19–22

20

Wrist

Scaphoid Fracture

General Principles

▶ also called the navicular bone
▶ most common carpal fracture
  ▶ the distal radius is actually the most common wrist fracture
▶ most commonly occurs after a fall onto an outstretched hand and presents with pain over radial aspect of wrist
▶ radiography
  ▶ 60% through middle third
  ▶ 20% through proximal third
    ▹ this fracture site has greatest risk of avascular necrosis since blood supply enters distally
  ▶ 10% through distal third
  ▶ 10% not radiographically apparent
▶ clinically suspect when anatomic "snuff box" tenderness is present, regardless of radiographic confirmation
  ▶ "snuff box" landmarks
    ▹ ulnar border is the extensor pollicis longus
    ▹ radial border is the extensor pollicis brevis/abductor pollicis longus
    ▹ proximal border is the distal radius
    ▹ distal border is the base of the 1st metacarpal

Treatment

▶ when clinically suspected
  ▶ short arm thumb spica splint
  ▶ follow-up examination and radiograph in 7–10 days
▶ nondisplaced (Figure 20–1)
  ▶ long arm thumb spica cast for 2–4 weeks
  ▶ followed by short arm thumb spica for 4–6 weeks

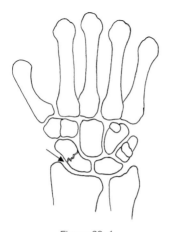

Figure 20–1

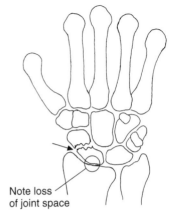

Note loss of joint space

Figure 20–2

▶ displaced (Figure 20–2)
  ▶ over 1 mm separation
  ▶ initial therapy
    ▸ thumb spica splint
    ▸ orthopedic referral
  ▶ definitive therapy
    ▸ closed reduction followed by a thumb spica cast
    ▸ surgical fixation if closed reduction unsuccessful

Triquetrum Fracture

General Principles

▶ tenderness present over dorsal wrist just distal to the ulnar styloid

Dorsal Chip

▶ seen on the lateral wrist view just dorsal to the lunate (Figure 20–3)
▶ short arm volar splint for 4–6 weeks with wrist at 15° extension

Nondisplaced Transverse

▶ short arm cast for 4–6 weeks

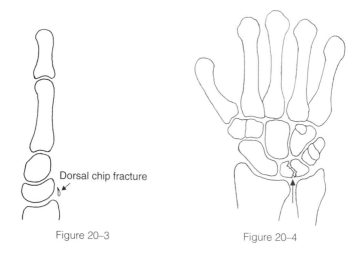

Dorsal chip fracture

Figure 20–3

Figure 20–4

Displaced Body

▶ surgical fixation

Lunate Fracture

General Principles

▶ highest incidence of avascular necrosis (Keinbock's disease) of any carpal
fracture
▶ suspect when there is tenderness in the lunate fossa regardless of whether
or not confirmed by radiograph (Figure 20–4)
  ▶ palpate just distal to the center of the distal radius
  ▶ wrist flexion causes the lunate to move against the examiner's finger
  and increases tenderness
▶ when clinically suspected
  ▶ short arm thumb spica splint
  ▶ follow-up examination and radiograph in 7–10 days

Nondisplaced

▶ short arm cast for 4–6 weeks

Displaced

▶ surgical fixation

Lunate Dislocation

General Principles

▶ most commonly dislocated carpal bone
▶ volar displacement most common
▶ dorsal displacement can occur
  ▸ associated with median nerve injury

Radiographic Appearance

▶ posterior-anterior (PA) view
  ▸ lunate takes on a triangular "piece of pie" appearance
▶ lateral view (see Figure 40–27, p. 491)
  ▸ lunate volarly or dorsally displaced in relation to lunate fossa of radius and not associated with proximal surface of capitate
  ▸ takes on a "spilled teacup" appearance

Treatment

▶ immobilize in neutral position
▶ request urgent orthopedic referral as most require surgical reduction and fixation
▶ closed reduction technique (volar dislocation) (Figure 20–5)
  ▸ dorsiflexion of wrist while applying volar to dorsal force on lunate to reduce into lunate fossa of distal radius
  ▸ followed by palmar flexion of wrist to reduce capitate into concavity of distal lunate

Perilunate Dislocation

General Principles

▶ dorsal dislocation is most common
▶ radiographic appearance
  ▸ PA view
    ▸ distal carpal row overrides proximal carpal row and creates the "crowded carpal sign"
  ▸ lateral view (see Figure 40–28, p. 491)
    ▸ lunate in lunate fossa of distal radius
    ▸ capitate proximal surface dorsally or volarly displaced out of concavity of distal lunate

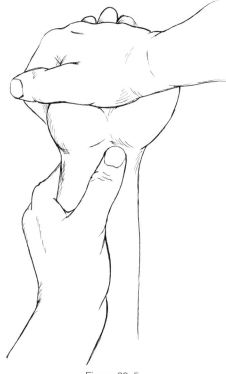

Figure 20–5

Treatment

▶ immobilize in neutral position
▶ urgent orthopedic referral for closed reduction followed by cast immobilization
▶ technique for reducing a dorsal dislocation
    ▶ finger trap distraction for 5–10 min with muscle relaxation/pain control
    ▶ dorsiflexion of wrist
    ▶ longitudinal traction
    ▶ volar flexion so capitate can reduce over dorsal rim of lunate
▶ surgical fixation is usually necessary since closed reduction is usually unstable

Scapholunate Dislocation

General Principles

▶ most commonly from a fall onto an outstretched hand in slight ulnar deviation
▶ represents instability of the scapholunate ligament
▶ radiographic appearance
　▶ PA view
　　▸ suspected when scapholunate joint space is over 2 mm
　　▸ confirmed when scapholunate joint space is over 4 mm

Treatment

▶ immobilize initially in thumb spica splint
▶ orthopedic referral for closed reduction followed by either
　▶ three-point pressure cast on volar scaphoid, dorsal capitate, and dorsal distal radius to maintain reduction
　▶ percutaneous pinning
▶ alternatively
　▶ arthroscopically controlled reduction and percutaneous pinning
　▶ surgical fixation and ligament repair
　▶ intercarpal fusion

Radiocarpal Dislocation

General Principles

▶ radiographic appearance
　▶ lateral view
　　▸ carpus and hand displaced volar or dorsal to radius
　　▸ frequently associated with carpal fractures

Treatment

▶ immobilized initially in neutral position
▶ urgent orthopedic referral
▶ closed reduction attempted when there is no associated carpal injury
　▶ finger trap traction
　▶ manipulation of carpal row back into place
▶ open reduction for
　▶ failed closed reduction
　▶ if associated carpal fracture or instability

Capitate Fracture

General Principles

▶ usually occurs in combination with a scaphoid fracture

Nondisplaced (Figure 20–6)

▶ short arm thumb spica cast

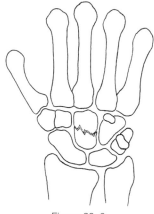

Figure 20–6

Displaced

▶ closed reduction followed by short arm thumb spica cast
▶ if reduction is unsuccessful, surgical fixation is necessary

Hamate Fracture

General Principles

▶ usually fracture is of the "hook" of the hamate, a palmar bony prominence
▶ point tenderness is appreciated over the base of the hypothenar eminence, 1–2 cm medial to the pisiform

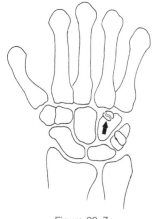

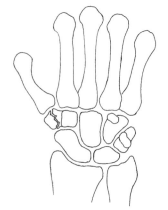

Figure 20–7   Figure 20–8

Nondisplaced (Figure 20–7)

▶ short arm cast for 6 weeks

Displaced

▶ surgical fixation or excision of the "hook"

Trapezium Fracture

General Principles

▶ point tenderness appreciated over the base of the thenar eminence

Nondisplaced (Figure 20–8)

▶ short arm thumb spica cast for 6 weeks

Displaced

▶ surgical fixation

Pisiform Fracture

General Principles (Figure 20–9)

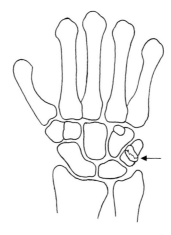

Figure 20–9

▶ point tenderness over its bony prominence at the base of the hypothenar eminence
▶ immobilization in short arm cast for 6 weeks
▶ if symptomatic after a period of immobilization, may require excision

21

Forearm

Distal Fractures

Nondisplaced Radius or Ulna Fractures

▶ immobilize with short arm cast for 4–6 weeks
▶ percutaneous pinning may be indicated for intraarticular fractures

Colles' Fracture (Figure 21–1)

▶ most common wrist fracture due to forceful wrist extension usually by fall on outstretched hand
▶ dorsal displacement of fragments

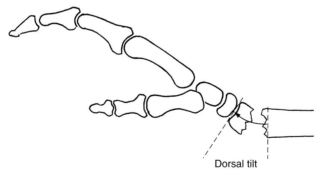

Dorsal tilt

Figure 21–1

▶ indications for closed reduction
  ▶ over 5 mm loss in radial length (shortening)
  ▶ over 10° dorsal tilt (angulation)
    ▹ normally there averages 14° of volar tilt and 22° of radial inclination

▶ method for closed reduction (Figure 21–2)
  ▶ hematoma block
  ▶ attach fingertraps and apply counterweight (10–20 lb) hanging from arm
  ▶ manipulate by applying pressure dorsally to restore the normal length and volar tilt
  ▶ afterward apply a cylindrical short arm cast and immobilize with wrist in slight flexion and ulnar deviation

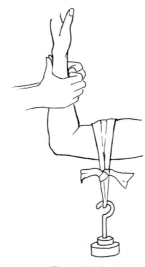

Figure 21–2

▶ indications for surgical fixation
  ▶ after closed reduction there remains
    ▹ over 5 mm loss in radial length
    ▹ over 15° dorsal tilt
  ▶ open fracture
  ▶ comminuted fracture
  ▶ intraarticular fracture

Smith's Fracture (Figure 21–3)

▶ flexion fracture with volar displacement of distal radius
▶ treatment
  ▶ closed reduction
    ▹ often unsuccessful due to flexor muscle pull
  ▶ surgical fixation usually necessary

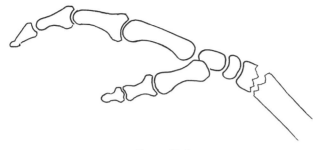

Figure 21–3

Barton's Fracture

▶ intraarticular rim fracture of distal radius
▶ dorsal Barton's fracture (Figure 21–4A)

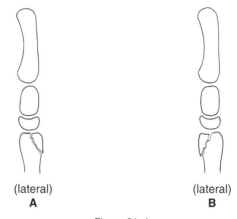

| (lateral) | (lateral) |
| A | B |

Figure 21–4

   ▶ dorsal rim fracture of distal radius
   ▶ treatment
      ▷ for small nondisplaced fracture, apply a short arm cast with wrist in neutral position
      ▷ for displaced fracture, attempt closed reduction and casting
      ▷ surgical fixation is necessary when over 50% articular surface is involved or fragment is inadequately reduced
▶ volar Barton's fracture (Figure 21–4B)
   ▶ volar rim fracture of distal radius
   ▶ treatment
      ▷ closed reduction is difficult to maintain because of flexor muscle pull
      ▷ surgical fixation is usually necessary

Radial Styloid (Chauffeur's Fracture)

▶ originally named for an injury sustained when an automobile backfires while it is being hand-cranked
▶ when nondisplaced (Figure 21–5), managed with cast immobilization
▶ when displaced, requires surgical fixation

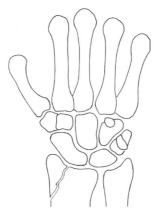

Figure 21–5

Radius Shaft Fracture

General Principles

▶ because of protection by the surrounding musculature, most radial shaft fractures require significant force and most are associated with ulna fractures
▶ nondisplaced fractures are rare

Proximal Radial Shaft

▶ nondisplaced (Figure 21–6)
  ▶ long arm cast with elbow in 90° flexion and forearm supinated
▶ displaced proximal one-third (Figure 21–7)
  ▶ fractures tend to displace due to supinating force exerted on proximal fragment and pronating force exerted on distal fragment

- ► initial treatment
  - ► long arm anterior–posterior (AP) splint with elbow in 90° flexion and forearm supinated
- ► definitive treatment
  - ► surgical fixation
- ► displaced proximal one-fifth (Figure 21–8)
  - ► initial treatment
    - ► long arm AP splint with elbow in 90° flexion and forearm supinated
  - ► definitive treatment
    - ► reduction and immobilization with elbow in 90° flexion and forearm supinated
    - ► surgical fixation is difficult

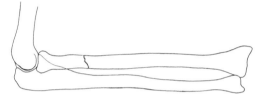

Figure 21–6

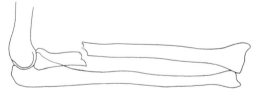

Figure 21–7

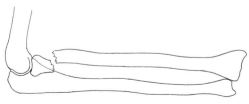

Figure 21–8

Midshaft Radius

▶ nondisplaced
  ▶ initial treatment
    ▹ posterior splint
  ▶ definitive treatment
    ▹ long arm cast with elbow in 90° flexion and forearm supinated
▶ displaced (Figure 21–9)
  ▶ initial treatment
    ▹ long arm AP splint in position of comfort
  ▶ definitive treatment
    ▹ surgical fixation

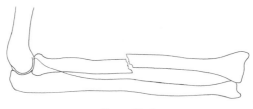

Figure 21–9

Distal Radial Shaft

▶ nondisplaced
  ▶ initial treatment
    ▹ posterior splint
  ▶ definitive treatment
    ▹ long arm cast with elbow in 90° flexion and forearm pronated
    ▹ may be associated with radioulnar joint subluxation
▶ displaced
  ▶ initial treatment
    ▹ posterior long arm splint with elbow in 90° flexion and forearm neutral
  ▶ definitive treatment
    ▹ surgical fixation
▶ Galeazzi fracture/dislocation (Figure 21–10)
  ▶ displaced distal radius fracture with associated distal radioulnar joint (DRUJ) dislocation
  ▶ fracture at junction of middle and distal 1/3 of radius is more commonly associated with DRUJ dislocation than not
  ▶ requires surgical fixation
  ▶ always obtain wrist radiographs in displaced shaft fractures to avoid missing a Galeazzi fracture/dislocation

- ▶ to determine DRUJ dislocation, look for
    - ▷ over 5 mm shortening of radius
    - ▷ fracture of ulnar styloid
    - ▷ DRUJ space widened over 2 mm

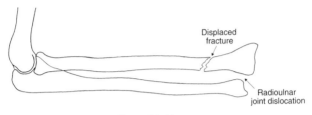

Displaced
fracture

Radioulnar
joint dislocation

Figure 21–10

Ulna Shaft Fracture

General Principles

- ▶ solitary fracture of the ulna often called "nightstick fracture" since it can be caused when struck with a blunt object while protecting one's head

Types

- ▶ nondisplaced
    - ▶ proximal one-third (Figure 21–11)
        - ▷ posterior splint initially
        - ▷ requires open reduction and internal fixation

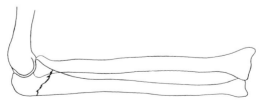

Figure 21–11

- ▶ distal two-thirds (Figure 21–12)
  - ▷ long arm volar splint

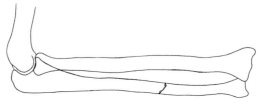

Figure 21–12

▶ displaced (Figure 21–13)
  - ▶ initially apply posterior long arm splint with elbow in 90° flexion and forearm neutral
  - ▶ requires open reduction and internal fixation

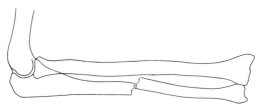

Figure 21–13

▶ Monteggia's fracture/dislocation (Figure 21–14)
  - ▶ proximal one-third of ulnar shaft with radial head dislocation
  - ▶ always obtain elbow radiographs in displaced shaft fractures to avoid missing a Monteggia fracture/dislocation (see p. 000 for radiograph interpretation method)
  - ▶ treatment
    - ▷ surgical fixation in adults
    - ▷ closed reduction in children

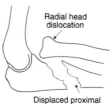

Radial head
dislocation

Displaced proximal
one-third ulnar fracture

Figure 21–14

Combined Radius/Ulna Fractures

Nondisplaced Radius/Ulna (Figure 21–15)

▶ rare since generally unstable
▶ long arm cast with elbow in 90° flexion and forearm neutral

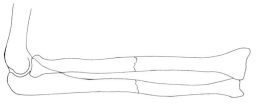

Figure 21–15

Displaced Radius/Ulna (Figure 21–16)

▶ options
  ▶ surgical fixation
  ▶ closed reduction and immobilization
    ▸ appropriate in pediatric greenstick and torus fractures
    ▸ goal is to achieve under 15° angulation

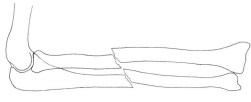

Figure 21–16

22

Elbow

Olecranon Fracture

General Principles

► usually intraarticular

Nondisplaced (Figure 22–1)

► treatment
   ► posterior long arm splint with elbow in 90° flexion and forearm neutral
   ► immobilize for 6–8 weeks
   ► begin elbow range of motion at 2–3 weeks in older adults

Displaced (Figure 22–2)

► pull of triceps displaces proximal fragment proximally
► treatment
   ► initially immobilize with elbow in 50–90° flexion and forearm neutral
   ► followed by surgical fixation

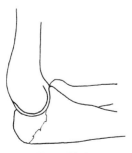

Figure 22–1

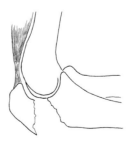

Figure 22–2

Radial Head Fracture

Nondisplaced (Figure 22–3)

▶ under one-third of articular surface
▶ under 1 mm separation
▶ treatment
  ▶ sling
  ▶ some aspirate hemarthrosis and then inject the joint with bupivicaine
  ▶ start early motion

Displaced (Figure 22–4)

▶ initial treatment
  ▶ posterior long arm splint
▶ definitive treatment
  ▶ no mechanical block of joint motion and less than one-third of articular surface involved
    ▶ long arm posterior splint followed by early motion
  ▶ mechanical block of joint motion, over 3 mm depression of one-third of articular surface or over 1 mm displacement
    ▶ elderly patients require excision of radial head followed by early range of motion
    ▶ younger patients require surgical fixation

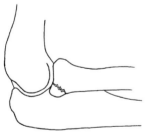

Figure 22–3

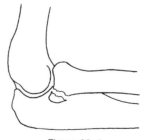

Figure 22–4

Severely Comminuted (Figure 22–5)

▶ treatment
  ▶ initially apply posterior long arm splint
  ▶ consider surgical excision of radial head

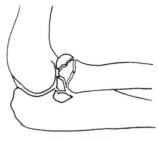

Figure 22–5

Essex Lopresti Fracture

▶ radial head fracture with distal radioulnar joint (DRUJ) dislocation
▶ treatment
  ▶ surgical fixation

Supracondylar Fracture

General Principles

▶ most occur in children after fall on outstretched hand
  ▶ 25% are of greenstick variety
▶ disposition and complications
  ▶ displaced fractures require hospitalization and close observation for neurovascular checks
    ▶ delayed swelling may cause subsequent neurovascular compromise
    ▶ brachial artery and median nerve may be interrupted by sharp fracture edge
    ▶ always consider the possibility of compartment syndrome in children with displaced supracondylar fractures
    ▶ untreated compartment syndrome can result in Volkmann's ischemic contracture and a nonfunctional arm

Treatment

▶ nondisplaced, which implies under 20° angulation (Figure 22–6)
  ▶ posterior long arm splint for 1–2 weeks
  ▶ early range of motion

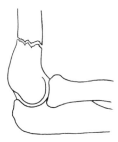

Figure 22–6

▶ displaced types are extension (Figure 22–7) or flexion (Figure 22–8)
  ▶ closed reduction followed by posterior long arm splint for 4–6 weeks
  ▶ overhead olecranon traction
  ▶ surgical fixation for failed closed reduction, associated injuries, or to allow early motion

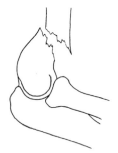

Figure 22–7

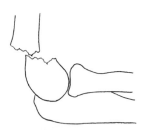

Figure 22–8

Condylar Fracture

Transcondylar (Figure 22–9)

General Principles

▶ fracture through both condyles and into the joint capsule

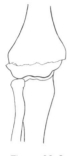 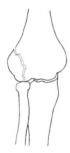

Figure 22–9 Figure 22–10

Treatment

▶ apply long arm posterior splint initially without repositioning the arm
  ▶ flexion or extension of joint may result in vascular compromise
▶ nondisplaced fracture
  ▶ long arm cast for 3–4 weeks
  ▶ then apply removable splint and begin active range-of-motion exercises for another 3–4 weeks
▶ displaced fracture
  ▶ surgical fixation

Lateral Condylar Fractures (Figure 22–10)

Treatment

▶ apply long arm posterior splint initially with elbow flexed at 90°, forearm in supination, and wrist in extension
  ▶ this position minimizes distraction by the pull of extensor muscles on lateral epicondyle
▶ nondisplaced
  ▶ long arm cast for 3 weeks followed by active range-of-motion exercises
▶ displaced
  ▶ surgical fixation

Medial Condylar Fracture (Figure 22–11)

General Principles

▶ less common than lateral condylar fracture

Treatment

▶ apply long arm posterior splint with elbow in 90° flexion, forearm
  pronated, and wrist flexed
  ▶ this position minimizes distraction by pull of flexor muscles on the me-
    dial epicondyle
▶ nondisplaced fracture
  ▶ long arm cast for 3 weeks followed by active range-of-motion exercises
▶ displaced fracture
  ▶ surgical fixation

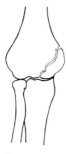

Figure 22–11

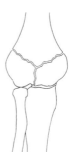

Figure 22–12

Intercondylar Fractures (Figure 22–12)

General Principles

▶ occur in elderly with brittle bones
▶ associated with neurovascular compromise

Treatment

▶ apply long arm posterior splint initially
▶ nondisplaced fracture
  ▶ long arm cast for 3 weeks followed by active range-of-motion exercises

▶ displaced fracture
  ▶ surgical fixation or olecranon traction

Elbow Dislocation

Posterior

General Principles

▶ olecranon displaced posteriorly
  ▶ most common (85%)
  ▶ presents with elbow flexed at 45° and prominent olecranon with palpable notch
  ▶ 20% with ulnar and/or median neuropraxia
  ▶ brachial artery injury is possible

Reduction Techniques

▶ palm–palm technique (recommended)
  ▶ grasp patient's hand with palm to palm and fingers interlocked (Figure 22–13)
  ▶ place examiner's elbow in patient's antecubital fossa
  ▶ distract dislocation by pushing downward on patient's distal humerus with examiner's elbow
  ▶ pull posteriorly dislocated elbow back into anatomic position

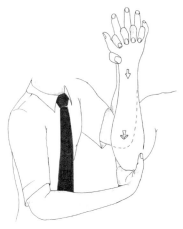

Figure 22–13

- hanging technique
  - place prone on stretcher with the elbow hanging over side
  - suspend weights off of the wrist
  - begin with 2 kg and increase as needed till reduction is successful
- traction–countertraction technique
  - with an assistant providing countertraction to the arm, apply traction along the long axis of the forearm followed by progressive flexion to 90°

Postreduction Treatment

- immobilize in long arm splint with elbow in 90° flexion for 1 week
- arrange orthopedic follow-up
- begin active range of motion exercises in 1 week

Anterior

General Principles

- olecranon displaced anteriorly
  - least common (15%)
  - presents with elbow fully extended
  - neurovascular injuries are common
  - associated with triceps avulsion

Reduction Technique

- partial extension and distal traction of the wrist with backward pressure on forearm

23

Humerus

Shaft Fracture

General Principles (Figure 23–1)

▶ displace differently depending on level of fracture and pull of attached
  muscles

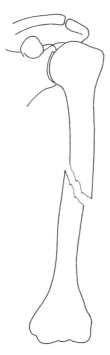

Figure 23–1

Treatment

▶ most successfully managed nonoperatively and options include
  ▶ coaptation splint with a sling and swathe (see p. 471)
    ▸ initial and definitive treatment for nondisplaced fractures
  ▶ hanging cast
  ▶ Velpeau dressing
  ▶ functional brace
  ▶ consider surgical fixation when
    ▸ segmental, spiral, bilateral, pathologic, comminuted, or open fractures
    ▸ failed closed reduction
    ▸ ipsilateral elbow dislocation
    ▸ ipsilateral forearm fracture ("floating elbow")
    ▸ multisystem trauma
    ▸ vascular compromise

Head/Neck Fracture

Neer System

▶ used for fracture classification and treatment
▶ four segments of the proximal humerus are assessed for relationship to each other (Figure 23–2)
  ▶ anatomic neck
  ▶ surgical neck

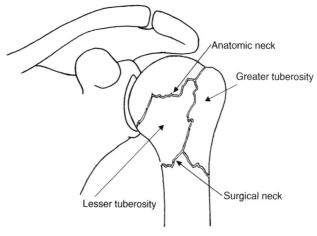

Figure 23–2

- ▶ greater tuberosity
- ▶ lesser tuberosity
▶ displacement implies that one of the four parts is either over 45° angulated from its normal alignment or over 1 cm separated from its normal anatomic position
  - ▶ one-part means no fragments displaced
  - ▶ two-part means one fragment displaced
  - ▶ three-part means two fragments displaced
  - ▶ four-part means three fragments displaced

Treatment

▶ a major complication of proximal humeral fractures is stiffness from immobilization
  - ▶ advise patient to discontinue sling and start pendulum exercises within 1–3 days
▶ one-part fracture (nondisplaced)
  - ▶ sling and early motion
▶ two-part fracture
  - ▶ all must be reduced
  - ▶ anatomic neck (Figure 23–3)
    - ▹ surgical fixation in young patient
    - ▹ hemiarthroplasty in elderly patient

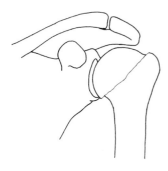

Figure 23–3

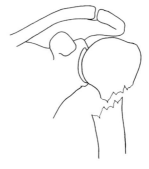

Figure 23–4

  - ▶ surgical neck (Figure 23–4)
    - ▹ closed reduction followed by sling and swath
    - ▹ surgical fixation for inadequate reduction
  - ▶ greater tuberosity
    - ▹ surgical fixation
  - ▶ lesser tuberosity
    - ▹ sling
    - ▹ often occurs with posterior shoulder dislocation
    - ▹ surgical fixation if fracture fragment blocks medial rotation

▶ three-part fracture
  ▶ surgical fixation
▶ four-part fracture (Figure 23–5)
  ▶ surgical fixation in young patient
    ▻ high incidence of avascular necrosis
  ▶ hemiarthroplasty for active elderly patient
    ▻ results in a strong, painless shoulder with limited motion
  ▶ sling for inactive elderly patient
    ▻ mobility and strength of shoulder will be limited

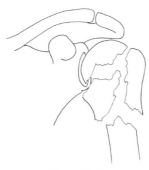

Figure 23–5

▶ fracture with dislocation
  ▶ can attempt closed reduction in case of dislocation and two-part fracture of the greater tuberosity
  ▶ open reduction and surgical fixation are necessary for all other fracture types and when closed reduction is unsuccessful
    ▻ hemiarthroplasy considered for active, elderly patients

24

Shoulder and Clavicle

Scapular Fracture

General Principles

- ▶ scapular pain or tenderness
- ▶ bony crepitus
- ▶ decreased shoulder motion

Treatment

- ▶ shoulder immobilizer and sling are adequate for most
- ▶ consult orthopedic surgeon
  - ▶ operative repair is necessary for severely displaced fractures
- ▶ exclude associated injuries aggresively since significant force is required to fracture the scapula

Shoulder Dislocation

General Principles

- ▶ most frequently dislocated joint
- ▶ analgesia and muscle relaxation essential

Anterior

General Principles

- ▶ 95% of shoulder dislocations
- ▶ 90% recurrence rate
- ▶ presents with
  - ▶ fullness anteriorly, with the humeral head palpable below the midclavicle
  - ▶ "squared off" shoulder due to loss of the deltoid contour laterally
- ▶ minimal range of motion with inability to touch hand on affected side to the opposite shoulder

▶ 10% have axillary neuropraxia
  ▶ decreased sensation over the deltoid
▶ associated with a Hill–Sachs deformity in about half
  ▶ posterolateral compression fracture of the humeral head

Reduction Techniques

▶ scapular manipulation (Figure 24–1)
  ▶ positioning options
    ▹ while patient sitting, assistant applies mild anterior traction to the arm
    ▹ while patient is lying supine with affected arm hanging off table
  ▶ inferior tip of scapula is rotated medially
  ▶ superior lateral aspect of scapula rotated laterally and inferiorly
▶ Hennepin or Milch method
  ▶ flex elbow to 90° and support the arm (Figure 24–2A)
  ▶ grasp the wrist and slowly externally rotate the humerus (Figure 24–2B)
  ▶ after full external rotation is achieved, abduct the arm (Figure 24–2C)

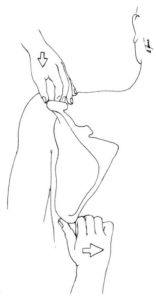

Figure 24–1

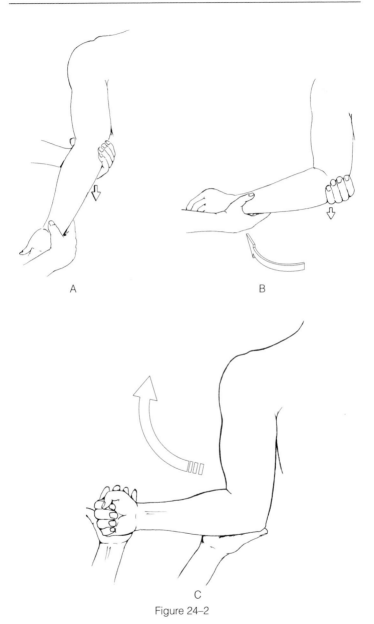

A

B

C

Figure 24–2

▶ traction–countertraction or modified Hippocratic method
  ▶ apply sheet wrapped around upper chest for countertraction
    ▷ tie patient to bed rail for one-person reduction
  ▶ with patient's elbow flexed, grasp affected arm and apply traction (Figure 24–3)
    ▷ can utilize sheet around arm and physician's waist to make traction easier (Figure 24–4)
  ▶ gentle internal and external rotation assists in reduction

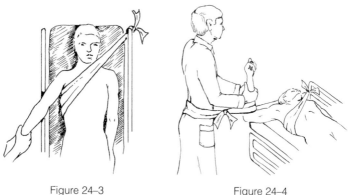

Figure 24–3   Figure 24–4

▶ Stimson (Figure 24–5)
  ▶ patient prone with affected arm hanging off the side
  ▶ suspend 10-lb weight from the wrist
  ▶ modification of this technique is to perform scapular manipulation (as above) while the weight is suspended

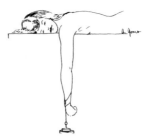

Figure 24–5

Posterior

General Principles

▶ 5% of shoulder dislocations
▶ up to 75% misdiagnosed as "frozen shoulder"
▶ associated with generalized tonic–clonic seizure or electrical injury as causative event
▶ arm adducted and internally rotated
▶ spasm of strong anterior musculature causes impact of humeral head on posterior scapular neck
▶ most frequently missed dislocation
▶ inability to reduce is more common than with anterior dislocations

Reduction Techniques

▶ traction–countertraction
  ▹ use same technique as for anterior dislocation (see Figures 24–3 and 24–4)
  ▹ in addition, apply anterior directed pressure on humeral head
▶ Stimson
  ▹ same technique as for anterior dislocation (see Figure 24–5)

Inferior (Luxatio Erecta)

General Principles

▶ rare
▶ patient presents with arm in full abduction at 180° of elevation
  ▹ looks like an eager student raising hand to get the teacher's attention
▶ humeral head forced through inferior capsule
  ▹ rotator cuff torn
  ▹ neurovascular injuries prevalent

Reduction Technique (Figure 24–6)

► traction applied to arm
► countertraction applied to shoulder
► while maintaining traction, rotate the arm inferiorly in an arc toward position of complete adduction

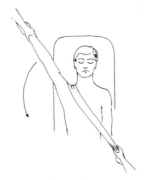

Figure 24–6

Postreduction Treatment

► applies to all dislocation types not associated with fractures
► under 30 years old
  ► shoulder immobilization for 3 weeks
  ► followed by gentle range-of-motion exercises for 3 weeks
    ► avoid abduction and external rotation
► over 30 years old
  ► shoulder immobilization for 1 week
  ► followed by gentle range-of-motion exercises
    ► avoid abduction and external rotation
    ► early range of motion prevents stiffness

Clavicle Fracture

Middle Third (Figure 24–7)

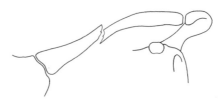

Figure 24–7

General Principles

▶ comprise 80% since the middle third of the clavicle is the weakest portion

Treatment Options

▶ sling and early motion
▶ many use "figure of 8" clavicular strap for improved pain control (see p. 472)
▶ can be followed by a primary care provider if the injury is isolated, closed, and without neurovascular compromise

Lateral Third

General Principles

▶ comprise 15%

Treatment

▶ nondisplaced (Figure 24–8)
   ▶ sling and early motion

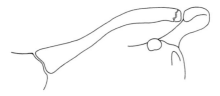

Figure 24–8

▶ displaced, which implies coracoclavicular ligament disrupted (Figure 24–9)
   ▶ nonunion occurs in 25% and usually results in a stable, nonpainful shoulder
   ▶ orthopedic referral for possible surgical fixation

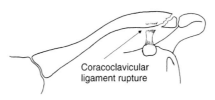

Coracoclavicular
ligament rupture

Figure 24–9

▶ articular surface (Figure 24–10)
   ▶ sling and early motion

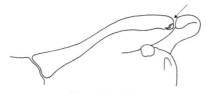

Figure 24–10

Medial Third

General Principles

▶ comprise 5%

Treatment

▶ nondisplaced (Figure 24–11)
   ▶ sling

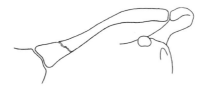

Figure 24–11

▶ displaced (Figure 24–12)
   ▶ orthopedic referral for possible surgical reduction

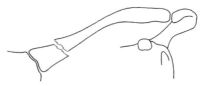

Figure 24–12

Indications for Surgical Fixation

▶ neurovascular injury that persists after closed reduction
▶ fracture fragments that threaten skin penetration (e.g., cause tenting)
▶ displaced lateral third fracture
▶ concurrent fracture of shoulder girdle
▶ nonreducible displacement
▶ open fracture

Acromioclavicular Injury

General Principles

▶ mechanisms
  ▶ fall directly onto the apex of the shoulder (with arm adducted)
  ▶ classic football block
▶ uncommon injury in children

Type I

Injury Pattern (Figure 24–13)

▶ acromioclavicular (AC) ligament sprained
▶ coracoclavicular (CC) ligament intact
▶ clavicle undisplaced
▶ tender over AC joint
▶ normal radiograph

Treatment

▶ sling and daily range-of-motion exercise

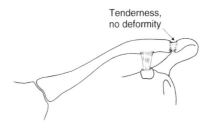

Figure 24–13

Type II

Injury Pattern (Figure 24–14)

▶ AC ligament disrupted
▶ CC ligament sprained
▶ tenderness over AC joint with slight separation

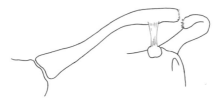

Figure 24–14

Treatment

▶ sling immobilization for 2 weeks then begin daily range-of-motion exercises
▶ may resume lifting heavy objects after 6 weeks

Type III

Injury Pattern (Figure 24–15)

▶ AC ligament disrupted
▶ CC ligament disrupted
▶ detachment of deltoid and trapezius insertion on the clavicle
▶ tender over AC joint with widening and step-off
▶ complete disruption of joint seen radiographically

Treatment

▶ younger, active patients
   ▶ surgical fixation

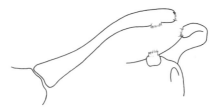

Figure 24–15

▶ older, inactive patients
  ▶ sling immobilization
    ▷ consider Kenny Howard shoulder harness since reduces separation though uncomfortable
  ▶ may resume lifting heavy objects after 8 weeks

Type IV

Injury Pattern (Figure 24–16)

▶ AC ligament disrupted
▶ CC ligament disrupted
▶ detachment of deltoid and trapezius insertion on the clavicle
▶ clavicle displaced posteriorly into trapezius muscle

Treatment

▶ surgical fixation

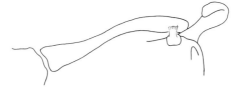

Figure 24–16

Type V

Injury Pattern (Figure 24–17)

▶ AC ligament disrupted
▶ CC ligament disrupted
▶ detachment of deltoid and trapezius insertion on the clavicle
▶ clavicle displaced superiorly (elevated)

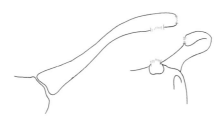

Figure 24–17

Treatment

► surgical fixation

Type VI

Injury Pattern (Figure 24–18)

► AC ligament disrupted
► CC ligament disrupted
► detachment of deltoid and trapezius insertion on the clavicle
► clavicle displaced inferiorly (behind the biceps and coracobrachialis tendons) and locked below the coracoid
  ► rare

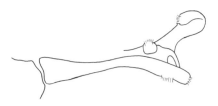

Figure 24–18

Treatment

► surgical fixation

Sternoclavicular Dislocation

General Principles

► rare condition
► requires significant lateral force to the shoulder or directly to the medial clavicle
  ► generally occurs from vehicular trauma
► present with hematoma over the sternoclavicular joint and severe pain with shoulder movement

Anterior

General Principles

▶ more common than posterior

Reduction Technique

▶ with the patient supine, place a rolled towel between the scapulae
▶ apply lateral traction to the abducted arm (Figure 24–19A)
▶ push the clavicle back into place (Figure 24–19B)

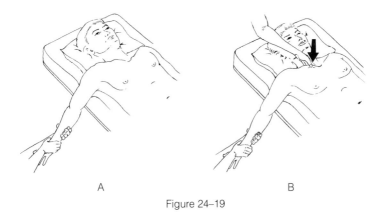

A   B

Figure 24–19

Postreduction Treatment

▶ joint is often unstable after reduction and many recur
▶ "figure of 8" splint and sling for 4 weeks (see p. 472)
▶ surgical fixation is not recommended

Posterior

General Principles

▶ about 25% associated with severe intrathoracic injuries
  ▶ tracheal compression
  ▶ pneumothorax
  ▶ angiography or helical CT is indicated to exclude injury to underlying vascular structures

Reduction Technique

▶ with the patient supine, place a rolled towel between the scapulae
▶ apply lateral traction to the abducted arm
▶ after infiltrating local anesthesia, grasp the clavicle with towel clip and pull back into position

Postreduction Treatment

▶ joint is usually unstable after reduction
▶ "figure of 8" splint and sling for 4 weeks (see p. 472)

25

Hip and Femur

Hip Dislocation

General Principles

▶ mechanism
  ▶ forceful blow to knee with hip and knee in flexion
  ▶ commonly occurs when knee strikes dash in motor vehicle collision
▶ associated with other, more serious injuries
▶ likelihood of avascular necrosis of the femoral head is directly related to the length of time before reduction

Posterior Dislocation

General Principles

▶ 90% of hip dislocations
▶ presentation
  ▶ leg internally rotated and thigh adducted
  ▶ femoral head palpable in the buttock
  ▶ marked knee flexion

Reduction Techniques

▶ prone or Stimson maneuver
  ▶ initiate conscious sedation
  ▶ affected hip flexed over end of table
  ▶ assistant stabilizes the pelvis by applying pressure on sacrum
  ▶ flex involved hip and knee to 90°
  ▶ apply downward pressure behind flexed knee
  ▶ hip rotated internally and externally while assistant pushes greater trochanter forward toward acetabulum

▶ supine or Allis maneuver (Figure 25–1)
  ▶ initiate conscious sedation
  ▶ assistant immobilizes the pelvis
  ▶ apply traction in the same linear direction as the deformity
  ▶ flex hip to 90°
  ▶ pull hip anteriorly and place force on the trochanter
  ▶ hip rotated internally and externally during traction until reduced

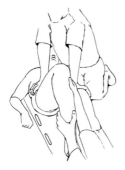
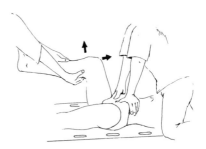

Figure 25–1

Anterior Dislocation

General Principles

▶ 10% of hip dislocations
▶ presentation
  ▶ leg externally rotated and thigh abducted
  ▶ femoral head palpable over the anterior iliac crest or inguinal region
  ▶ slight knee flexion
▶ often requires general/spinal anesthesia for reduction
▶ orthopedic referral for reduction

Reduction Technique

▶ supine maneuver
  ▶ initiate conscious sedation
  ▶ assistant stabilizes pelvis
  ▶ apply strong longitudinal traction in conjunction with a lateral force to proximal thigh
  ▶ pull femoral head distal to acetabulum
  ▶ rotate hip internally to reduce dislocation

Postreduction Treatment

▶ admission for traction and neurovascular checks
▶ obtain hip CT to determine whether there is associated acetabular fracture, which occurs in up to half

Hip Fracture

Femoral Head (Figure 25–2)

General Principles

▶ mechanism is high-energy sheer
▶ associated with hip dislocation

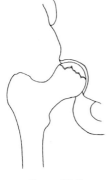

Figure 25–2

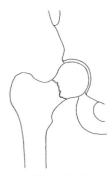

Figure 25–3

Treatment Options

▶ surgical fixation
▶ hemiarthroplasty

Femoral Neck

Nondisplaced (Figure 25–3)

▶ uncommon
▶ occurs as a stress fracture in athletes
  ▶ patients ambulatory with antalgic gait

▶ treatment for elderly
  ▶ require surgical fixation
▶ treatment for younger patients
  ▶ crutches, non–weight-bearing for 6–12 weeks
  ▶ surgical fixation occasionally necessary

Displaced (Figure 25–4)

▶ common and especially prevalent in elderly, white women
▶ severe pain elicited with any hip motion
▶ presents with an externally rotated hip and an abducted, shortened leg
▶ treatment options
  ▶ emergency surgical fixation (within 12 h) to prevent avascular necrosis
  ▶ prosthetic hip replacement preferred in the elderly

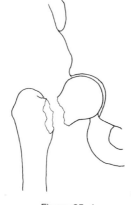

Figure 25–4

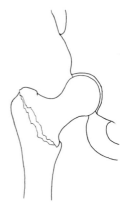

Figure 25–5

Intertrochanteric (Figure 25–5)

General Principles

▶ most common type of hip fracture
▶ presentation same as displaced femoral neck fracture (above)

Treatment

▶ surgical fixation

Trochanteric

Greater Trochanter (Figure 25–6)

▶ nondisplaced
  ▶ treatment
    ▸ bed rest followed by crutch walking
▶ displaced
  ▶ treatment options
    ▸ surgical fixation for over 1 cm displacement of the fragment in young patients
    ▸ bed rest followed by crutch walking in others

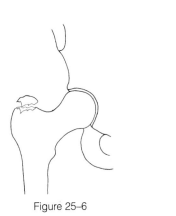

Figure 25–6

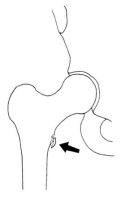

Figure 25–7

Lesser Trochanter (Figure 25–7)

▶ nondisplaced
  ▶ treatment
    ▸ bed rest followed by crutch walking
▶ displaced
  ▶ treatment options
    ▸ surgical fixation for over 2 cm displacement of the fragment in young patients
    ▸ bed rest followed by crutch walking in others

Subtrochanteric

General Principles

- ▶ requires great force
- ▶ common and especially prevalent in elderly, white women
- ▶ severe pain elicited with any hip motion
- ▶ presents with an externally rotated hip and an abducted, shortened leg

Treatment

- ▶ surgical fixation

Femur Fracture

General Principles

- ▶ clinically apparent with focal pain, swelling, and deformity
- ▶ can result in over 1 liter of blood loss into the thigh

Shaft

Transverse or Spiral (Figure 25–8)

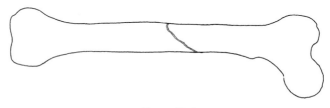

Figure 25–8

▶ initial treatment
  ▶ immobilize with Hare or Buck traction device (Figure 25–9)
  ▶ use long leg posterior splint if traction device is unavailable
▶ definitive treatment
  ▶ surgical fixation using intramedullary nailing
  ▶ young children treated with 4 weeks of traction followed by body spica casting

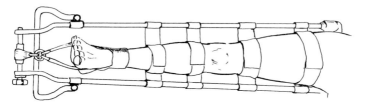

Figure 25–9

Open

▶ treatment
  ▶ emergency operative debridement with delayed intramedullary nailing
  ▶ prophylaxis for infection
    ▶ first-generation cephalosporin and aminoglycoside

26

Knee

Distal Femur Fracture

▶ initial treatment for all types
  ▶ immobilization
  ▶ assess vascular status
  ▶ traction before delayed surgical fixation

Supracondylar

▶ nondisplaced (Figure 26–1)
  ▶ definitive treatment options
    ▶ surgical fixation
    ▶ traction casting
▶ displaced (Figure 26–2)
  ▶ definitive treatment
    ▶ surgical fixation

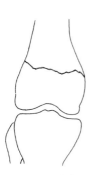

Figure 26–1

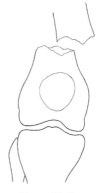

Figure 26–2

► comminuted (Figure 26–3)
  ► definitive treatment options
    ► surgical fixation
    ► skeletal traction

Intercondylar (Figure 26–4)

► definitive treatment
  ► surgical fixation

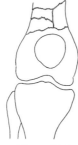

Figure 26–3

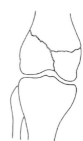

Figure 26–4

Condylar (Medial or Lateral)

► nondisplaced (Figure 26–5)
  ► definitive treatment depends on fragment size and options include
    ► cast
    ► cast–brace
    ► skeletal traction
    ► surgical fixation
► displaced (Figure 26–6)
  ► definitive treatment
    ► surgical fixation

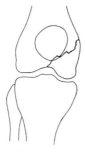

Figure 26–5

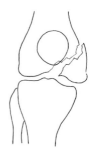

Figure 26–6

Patellar Fracture

Nondisplaced (Figure 26–7)

Initial Treatment

▶ some aspirate hemarthrosis if it is large to relieve pain and intraarticular tension

Definitive Treatment Options

▶ knee immobilizer in full extension
▶ long leg cylinder cast well molded around the patella with knee in full extension

Displaced Transverse (Figure 26–8)

General Principles

▶ categorize as displaced when over 2 mm
▶ most common type

Definitive Treatment

▶ surgical fixation

Comminuted or Stellate (Figure 26–9)

Definitive Treatment Options

▶ surgical fixation
▶ patellectomy

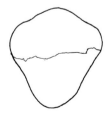

Figure 26–7

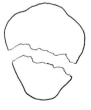

Figure 26–8

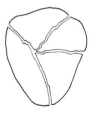

Figure 26–9

Knee Dislocation

General Principles

▶ presents with leg extended and loss of landmarks
▶ associated with severe ligament disruption
　▶ assume a spontaneously reduced dislocation when knee is unstable with laxity in two directions
　　▷ implies both cruciate ligaments acutely disrupted
▶ neurovascular injuries common

Anterior Dislocation

▶ tibia anterior to femur
▶ reduction technique
　▶ initiate conscious sedation
　▶ place longitudinal traction on tibia
　▶ femur is lifted anteriorly to reduce dislocation
　▶ avoid hyperextension of knee joint

Posterior Dislocation

▶ tibia posterior to femur
▶ reduction technique
　▶ initiate conscious sedation
　▶ longitudinal traction on tibia
　▶ proximal tibia is lifted anteriorly to reduce dislocation
　▶ avoid hyperextension of knee joint

Postreduction Treatment

▶ immobilize knee in 15° flexion
▶ consult orthopedic surgeon
▶ angiography is recommended in suspected and confirmed knee dislocations to exclude popliteal artery injury
▶ admit for neurovascular checks

Patellar Dislocation

General Principles

▶ lateral dislocation is the norm
▶ presents with knee flexed and dislocation clinically obvious
▶ when patella reduces before arrival, one can appreciate recent dislocation with "apprehension test"
　▶ when patella is moved laterally, patient responds with resistance and fear

Reduction Technique

▶ initiate conscious sedation
▶ flex hip
▶ slowly extend knee
▶ gently apply direct pressure to distract the patella medially

Postreduction Treatment

▶ knee immobilizer

Knee Strain

General Principles

▶ grading system
  ▶ I. stretch
  ▶ II. partial tear
  ▶ III. disruption
▶ hemarthrosis
  ▶ marked swelling with loss of normal joint indentations
  ▶ ballottement of patella present
  ▶ decreased range of motion
    ▶ normal 0–140°
  ▶ immediacy associated with severity (e.g., grade III injury)

Injury Patterns

Medial Collateral Ligament (MCL)

▶ most common ligamentous knee injury
▶ stress and palpation
  ▶ application of valgus stress and palpation of the medial joint line causes focal pain

Lateral Collateral Ligament (LCL)

▶ stress and palpation
  ▶ application of varus stress and palpation of the lateral joint line causes focal pain

Anterior Cruciate Ligament (ACL)

▶ common cause of severe knee injury
  ▶ usual mechanism is running and sudden stop, often during pivoting

▶ often associated with MCL injury
▶ immediate hemarthrosis
▶ Lachman test
  ▶ flex knee 20° and hold distal femur firmly with nondominant hand
  ▶ dominant hand grasps proximal leg
  ▶ laxity consistent with ACL disruption
▶ anterior drawer test
  ▶ flex hip 45° and knee 90° while grasping proximal leg with thumbs over anterior joint line of proximal tibia
  ▶ laxity with gentle *pull* indicates ACL disruption

Posterior Cruciate Ligament (PCL)

▶ usually occurs with ACL injury and in conjunction with knee dislocation
▶ suspect spontaneous reduction if dislocation is not apparent
▶ posterior drawer test
  ▶ flex hip 45° and knee 90° while grasping proximal leg with thumbs over anterior joint line of proximal tibia
  ▶ laxity with gentle *push* indicates PCL disruption

Medial Meniscus

▶ most common type is "bucket handle" tear, which creates an intraarticular flap of cartilage
▶ often the mechanism seems relatively minor compared to the pain provoked
▶ McMurray test
  ▶ flexed knee is slowly extended while applying *external* rotatory stress, resulting in a "popping" sensation
▶ medial joint line tenderness may be present
▶ delayed hemarthrosis common

Lateral Meniscus

▶ less frequently involved
▶ McMurray test
  ▶ flexed knee is slowly extended while applying *internal* rotatory stress, resulting in a "popping" sensation
▶ lateral joint line tenderness may be present
▶ delayed hemarthrosis common

Radiography

▶ plain radiography is unhelpful unless fracture needs to be excluded
▶ MRI reliably diagnoses most injuries, though it is not necessary to perform it urgently

Treatment

▶ Jones dressing
▶ knee immobilization device
▶ ice and elevation
▶ crutches
  ▶ allow partial weight bearing when tolerable
▶ analgesics
▶ consider aspiration of hemarthrosis to relieve pain, although this increases infection risk
▶ orthopedic referral
  ▶ operative repair is necessary if the knee is unstable and the patient is active

Proximal Tibia Fracture

Tibial Plateau

Nondisplaced Condylar (Figure 26–10)

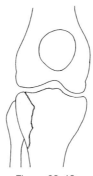

Figure 26–10

▶ treatment when ligaments stable
  ▶ long leg cast for 4–8 weeks
    ▶ knee stiffness is common

Local Compression (Figure 26–11)

▶ localized depression in articular surface
▶ tenderness to palpation adjacent to tibial tuberosity
  ▶ consider this diagnosis until proven otherwise
▶ treatment options
  ▶ immobilization in a posterior splint, non–weight-bearing and close follow-up
  ▶ surgical intervention for
    ▹ depression over 8 mm
    ▹ depression located on anterior or middle tibial plateau
    ▹ associated ligamentous injuries

Split Condylar Compression (Figure 26–12)

▶ lateral plateau most frequently involved
▶ associated fracture of fibular head or neck common
▶ treatment options
  ▶ cast immobilization
    ▹ under 4 mm articular depression
    ▹ split fragment able to be restored to anatomic position by closed reduction
  ▶ surgical fixation
    ▹ over 4 mm articular depression
    ▹ unsuccessful closed reduction

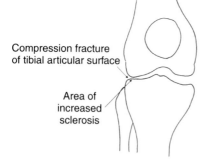

Compression fracture of tibial articular surface

Area of increased sclerosis

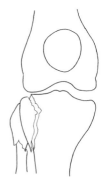

Figure 26–11   Figure 26–12

Total Depression (Figure 26–13)

▶ oblique fracture beginning near intercondylar eminence and extending to cortex of medial or lateral tibial flare
▶ treatment
    ▶ under 4 mm depression
        ▻ closed reduction and cast immobilization
    ▶ over 4 mm depression
        ▻ options include skeletal traction to restore displaced condyle followed by long leg cast and surgical fixation

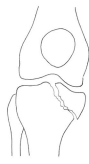

Figure 26–13

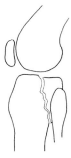

Figure 26–14

Split Fracture (Figure 26–14)

▶ large articular fragment separates from posterior position of medial tibial plateau
▶ treatment options
    ▶ closed reduction and cast immobilization when
        ▻ fragment reduction successful
        ▻ knee stable in extension
    ▶ surgical fixation when
        ▻ nonreducible fragments
        ▻ unstable knee ligaments

Bicondylar (Figure 26–15)

▶ treatment options
  ▶ nonoperative treatment preferred
    ▶ cast–brace
    ▶ skeletal traction
  ▶ some advocate surgical fixation

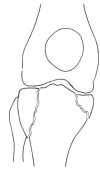

Figure 26–15

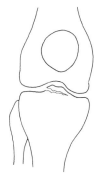

Figure 26–16

Tibial Spine

Incomplete Avulsion (Figure 26–16)

▶ can occur with or without displacement
▶ treatment options
  ▶ closed reduction followed by long leg cast immobilization in full extension for 4–6 weeks
  ▶ surgical fixation when these are associated ligamentous injuries or incomplete reduction

Complete Avulsion (Figure 26–17)

▶ treatment
  ▶ surgical fixation when displaced

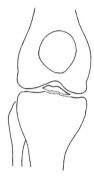

Figure 26–17

27

Leg and Ankle

Tibial Shaft Fracture

Treatment

- ▶ closed reduction and long leg cast for 12 weeks if
  - ▶ nondisplaced (Figure 27–1)
  - ▶ low-energy longitudinal spiral fractures
- ▶ surgical fixation if
  - ▶ displaced or unstable (Figure 27–2)
    - ▶ compartment syndrome can develop
  - ▶ intraarticular extension
  - ▶ open fracture
  - ▶ bilateral fractures

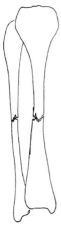

Figure 27–1

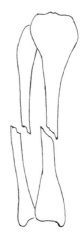

Figure 27–2

Fibular Shaft Fracture

Treatment

▶ applies to isolated fibular shaft fracture (Figure 27–3)
▶ ace wrap
▶ posterior splint or walking cast for comfort

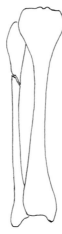

Figure 27–3

Ankle Anatomy

▶ considered a closed ring surrounding the talus (Figure 27–4) consisting of
  ▶ interosseous membrane (a)
  ▶ lateral malleolus (b)
  ▶ lateral ligaments (c)—allow significant movement (inversion)
    ▹ anterior talofibular ligament (ATFL)
    ▹ calcaneofibular ligament (CFL)
    ▹ posterior talofibular ligament (PTFL)
  ▶ calcaneus (d)
  ▶ deltoid ligament (e)—allows limited movement (eversion)
  ▶ medial malleolus (f)
  ▶ tibial articular surface (g)

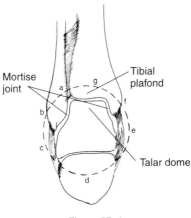

Mortise joint

Tibial plafond

Talar dome

Figure 27–4

▶ breaks in the ring consist of either fractures or ligament disruption (grade III injuries)

Ankle Sprain

General Principles

▶ grading system
  ▶ I. stretch
  ▶ II. partial tear
  ▶ III. disruption
▶ lateral sprains are most common
  ▶ lateral ligaments are typically injured from anterior to posterior
    ▹ ATFL alone (usually a grade I)
    ▹ ATFL and CFL
    ▹ ATFL, CFL, and PTFL (usually a grade II or III)

Presentation

▶ usual mechanism is forced inversion for lateral sprain and eversion for deltoid sprain
▶ patient often remembers a "popping" sensation followed by progressive pain and swelling
▶ tenderness is appreciated over the affected ligaments
▶ gentle stress testing provokes less pain and more laxity in grade III injuries

► hemarthrosis
  ► marked swelling with loss of normal joint indentations
  ► decreased range of motion
  ► immediacy associated with severe problems (e.g., grade III injury)

Radiographs

► obtain whenever fracture is suspected
► Ottawa resource utilization rules for ankle radiography
  ► can safely avoid in patients between 18 and 55 years old when the following coexist
    ► no tenderness of the posterior edge of the distal 6 cm or the tip of either malleolus
    ► ability to bear weight (for four steps) both immediately after injury and in the emergency department

Treatment

► ice and elevation
► analgesics
► grade I
  ► apply an air splint/stirrup
  ► allow partial weight bearing when tolerable
  ► refer to primary care physician
► grades II and III
  ► apply a posterior splint
  ► crutches with no weight bearing for at least one week
  ► refer to orthopedic surgeon, who determines when to begin weight bearing

Malleolar Fracture

Single Ring Break

► stable injury
► examples
  ► isolated, nondisplaced fibular fractures (Figure 27–5)
  ► isolated deltoid ligament rupture
► initial treatment
  ► short leg splint
► definitive treatment
  ► short leg walking cast

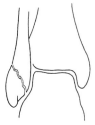

Figure 27–5

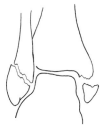

Figure 27–6

Double Ring Break

- ▶ unstable injury
- ▶ ankle "stress" radiographs may aid in diagnosing a ligamentous injury when tenderness is present opposite the fracture
- ▶ examples
    - ▶ two fractures in ring
        - ▹ bi- or trimalleolar fracture (Figure 27–6)
    - ▶ one fracture and one ligamentous injury in ring
        - ▹ fracture of lateral malleolus with medial joint widening due to del- toid ligament rupture
    - ▶ displaced fracture in ring which implies a ligamentous injury
        - ▹ single malleolus fracture with asymmetric ankle mortise
    - ▶ two ligaments ruptured in ring
        - ▹ medial and lateral
- ▶ initial treatment
    - ▶ long leg posterior splint
- ▶ definitive treatment
    - ▶ long leg cast for 6 weeks
        - ▹ when successful, closed anatomic reduction is maintained
    - ▶ surgical therapy is indicated when
        - ▹ closed reduction fails
        - ▹ closed reduction requiring abnormal or forced foot positioning
        - ▹ bi- and trimalleolar fractures
        - ▹ other unstable fractures that result in displacement of talus or widening of mortise by more than 2 mm

Maisoneuve Fracture

Definition

- medial malleolar fracture or deltoid ligament tear
- oblique fracture of proximal fibula
    - palpate the proximal fibula in all ankle injuries and radiograph when tender
- disruption of tibiofibular ligament complex

Treatment

- long leg posterior splint followed by long leg cast for 6–12 weeks
- surgical fixation necessary when
    - medial malleolar fracture
    - medial joint space abnormal

Pilon Fracture

- comminution of distal tibia
- often confused with trimalleolar fractures
- mechanism is high-energy axial compression
- requires surgical repair

Plafond Fracture

- mechanism is external rotation and abduction
- represents avulsion of anterolateral piece of the distal tibia attached to the ATFL
    - Salter III injury in children
- requires surgical repair

Tillaux Fracture

- mechanism is high-energy impact of talus on medial aspect of the tibia during dorsiflexion
- requires surgical repair

Ankle Dislocation

Lateral

▶ most common
▶ associated with fracture of malleoli or distal fibula
▶ reduction technique
  ▸ longitudinal traction of foot
  ▸ countertraction on the leg
  ▸ foot manipulated into place
▶ postreduction therapy
  ▸ long leg splint
  ▸ surgical repair when there are associated fractures or instability

Posterior

▶ reduction technique
  ▸ plantar flexion of foot
  ▸ foot pulled anteriorly
▶ postreduction therapy
  ▸ posterior splint
  ▸ surgical repair of capsular injuries

Anterior

▶ reduction technique
  ▸ dorsiflexion of foot to disengage talus
  ▸ downward traction of foot
  ▸ push foot posteriorly to reduce dislocation
▶ postreduction therapy
  ▸ exclude talar dome fracture
  ▸ initial immobilization in splint
  ▸ many require ligamentous repair

28

Foot

Talus Fracture

Types and Treatment

Body and Neck

- ▶ most common type
- ▶ associated dislocation requires emergency reduction
- ▶ nondisplaced fracture (Figure 28–1)
  - ▶ non–weight-bearing in a short leg cast for 6–10 weeks
- ▶ displaced fracture (Figure 28–2)
  - ▶ surgical fixation

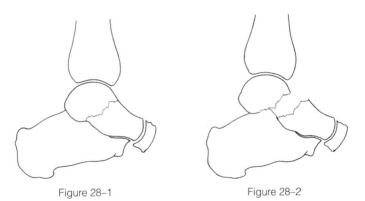

Figure 28–1   Figure 28–2

Posterior Process (Shepherd's Fracture)

- ▶ often confused with os trigonum tarsi, an accessory bone

Dome

▶ rare fracture that presents as a nonhealing ankle sprain

Calcaneus Fracture

General Principles

▶ usual mechanism is a high fall
▶ the "lovers triad" is named for what can occur after jumping from an upper floor window and consists of the following
  ▶ calcaneal fracture
  ▶ vertebral compression fracture(s)
    ▹ occur concomitantly in 80% of calcaneal fractures
  ▶ forearm fracture(s)
    ▹ occur concomitantly in 15% of calcaneal fractures

Types and Treatment

Extraarticular

▶ nondisplaced body/neck (Figure 28–3)
  ▶ compressive dressing, bed rest, elevation
  ▶ progressive weight bearing
  ▶ active exercise for 8–12 weeks
▶ displaced body/neck (Figure 28–4)
  ▶ nonsurgical approach
    ▹ compressive dressing
    ▹ bed rest and elevation initially
    ▹ progressive weight bearing and active exercise for 8–12 weeks
  ▶ surgical fixation indicated for young, active patients with severe displacement

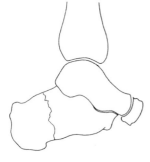

Figure 28–3

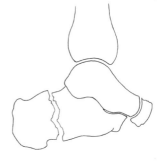

Figure 28–4

▶ posterior tuberosity
  ▶ avulsed by Achilles tendon
  ▶ nondisplaced (Figure 28–5)
    ▷ non–weight-bearing cast with foot in equinus for 6–8 weeks
  ▶ displaced (Figure 28–6)
    ▷ surgical fixation

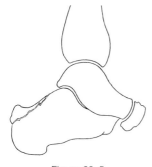

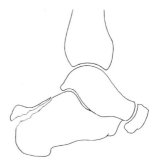

Figure 28–5   Figure 28–6

Intraarticular

▶ nondisplaced body/neck (Figure 28–7)
  ▶ non–weight-bearing for 4–8 weeks
  ▶ casting leads to stiffness
▶ displaced body/neck (Figure 28–8)

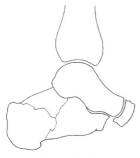

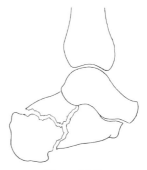

Figure 28–7   Figure 28–8

- ▶ surgical fixation when
  - ▹ Bohler's angle under 10° (Figure 28–9)
  - ▹ loss of articular congruity of posterior facet
  - ▹ over 4 mm shortening of tuberosity seen on axial projection
  - ▹ loss of parallelism between the posterior facets of the calcaneus and talus

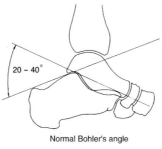

Normal Bohler's angle

Figure 28–9

Navicular Fracture

Types and Treatment

Dorsal Avulsion (Figure 28–10)

- ▶ caused by ligamentous pull
- ▶ short leg walking cast for 4 weeks
- ▶ large chips may require surgical fixation

Tuberosity (Figure 28–11)

- ▶ inactive patients require compressive dressing
- ▶ active patients require short leg walking cast for 4 weeks

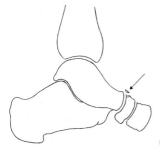

Figure 28–10

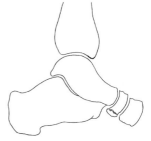

Figure 28–11

Body

▶ high incidence of avascular necrosis
▶ nondisplaced (Figure 28–12)
   ▶ short leg non–weight-bearing cast for 4 weeks followed by walking cast
▶ displaced (Figure 28–13)
   ▶ surgical fixation

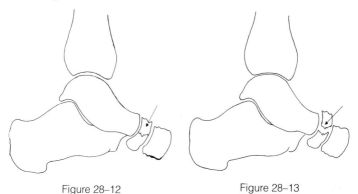

Figure 28–12   Figure 28–13

Cuboid Fracture

Types and Treatment

Nondisplaced (Figure 28–14)

▶ short leg walking cast for 6 weeks

Displaced (Figure 28–15) or Dislocated

▶ surgical fixation

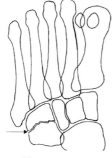 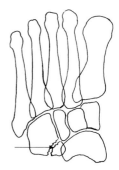

Figure 28–14   Figure 28–15

Cuneiform Fracture

Types and Treatment

Nondisplaced (Figure 28–16)

▶ short leg walking cast for 6 weeks

Displaced (Figure 28–17) or Dislocated

▶ surgical fixation

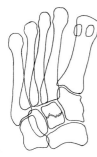

Figure 28–16

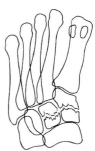

Figure 28–17

Lisfranc's Injury

General Principles

▶ the Lisfranc joint consists of a six-bone arch
  ▶ 3 cuneiforms distally and 1st through 3rd metatarsals proximally
  ▶ 2nd metatarsal serves as the cornerstone of the arch
▶ Lisfranc's injury refers to a tarsometatarsal dislocation with or without fracture

► displaced fracture of the base of the 2nd metatarsal and diffuse soft-tissue swelling is a spontaneously reduced Lisfranc's fracture/dislocation until proven otherwise
► Lisfranc's dislocation is not always readily evident on radiographs
  ► remains the most common misdiagnosed foot fracture
  ► look for the following radiographic findings (Figure 28–18)
    ► fracture base of the 2nd metatarsal
    ► diastasis of the 1st and 2nd metatarsals
    ► diastasis of the middle and medial cuneiforms
  ► consider stress views if there is significant foot pain/swelling with "normal" initial radiographs

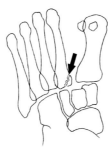

Figure 28–18

Treatment

► surgical fixation
► warn of complications, which include arthritis and reflex sympathetic dystrophy

Metatarsal Fracture

Types and Treatment

Nondisplaced (Figure 28–19)

▶ short leg cast for 2–4 weeks

Displaced (Figure 28–20)

▶ closed reduction with axial traction
▶ short leg cast
▶ open reduction needed if closed reduction is unsuccessful

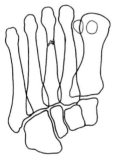

Figure 28–19

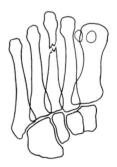

Figure 28–20

Jones Fracture (Figure 28–21)

▶ transverse fracture of base of 5th metatarsal within 1–3 cm distal to the proximal tuberosity
▶ short leg cast for 6 weeks
▶ one-third develop nonunion and may require surgical fixation and bone grafting

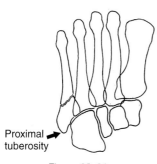

Proximal
tuberosity

Figure 28–21

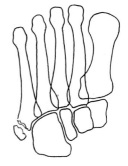

Figure 28–22

Avulsion Base of 5th Metatarsal or Tennis Fracture (Figure 28–22)

► caused by same mechanism as inversion ankle injuries
► avulsion occurs at attachment of peroneus brevis tendon
► treatment
  ► compressive dressing
  ► hard sole shoe
  ► crutches for 2–3 weeks
  ► rapid progression to full ambulation

Stress or March Fracture

► usually of 2nd and/or 3rd metatarsals
► seen in athletes
► treat by cessation of aggravating activity for 2–4 weeks

Phalange Fracture

Types and Treatment

Nondisplaced

► dynamic splint (buddy taping)
► hard sole shoe

Displaced Great Toe (Figure 28–23)

▶ attempt closed reduction followed by short leg cast extended to include great toe
▶ surgical fixation

Displaced Other Toes

▶ reduce after digital nerve block
▶ dynamic splint (buddy taping)
▶ non–weight-bearing until tolerated

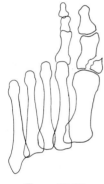

Figure 28–23

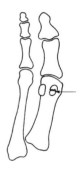

Figure 28–24

Sesamoid Fracture

General Principles

▶ located within the flexor hallucis brevis tendon (Figure 28–24)
▶ caused by direct strike or repetitive stress

Treatment

▶ short leg walking cast for 3–4 weeks
▶ followed by hard sole shoe with metatarsal pad

Part IV

SPECIAL GROUPS

29

Children

General Principles

Statistics

Mortality

▶ trauma is the leading cause of death in children
  ▶ 85% blunt
  ▶ 15% penetrating
▶ males are victims twice as often

Pediatric Trauma Centers

▶ recommended in urban areas
▶ improved survival rates documented
▶ differences include
  ▶ medical and nursing staff more experienced in pediatric trauma
  ▶ pediatric surgeon and other sub-specialists available
  ▶ pediatric intensive care unit available

Key Differences

General Principles

▶ this section covers important differences between the management of pediatric trauma and that of adults
  ▶ use a systematic approach to determining tube sizes and drug doses based on weight and age
▶ Broselow tape and/or color-coded equipment and drug carts are recommended

Anatomic

▶ children have greater relative body surface area, causing greater heat loss
▶ head-to-body ratio is greater, brain is less myelinated, and cranial bones are thinner—thus a higher incidence of head injury
▶ spleen and liver are more anteriorly placed with less protective musculature—thus they are more susceptible to injury
▶ kidney is less well protected and more mobile
  ▶ more susceptible to deceleration injury
▶ growth plates are not yet closed
  ▶ Salter-type fractures occur, with possible limb-length abnormalities in healing

Prehospital Immobilization

▶ often difficult since traumatized children are generally uncooperative and combative
▶ infants still in car seat after motor vehicle collision can be left in place with head stabilized as long as more exposure in the field is unnecessary

Airway/Breathing

General Principles

▶ infants are obligate nose breathers
  ▶ the tongue is relatively large and easily obstructs the oropharynx
  ▶ carefully clear nasal mucus and/or obstruction
    ▶ place oropharyngeal airway when the patient is unconscious
▶ administer supplemental oxygen
  ▶ restlessness and/or change in mentation is often due to hypoxia

Manual Ventilation

▶ use an appropriate-size bag with a pressure valve to prevent barotrauma
▶ avoid submandibular pressure when applying the mask
  ▶ causes an iatrogenic airway obstruction

Endotracheal Intubation

▶ estimation of ideal tube size
  ▶ 4 + (age/4)
  ▶ same caliber as child's little-finger nail width (Figure 29–1)
  ▶ always have available one size above and below the size predicted to be best prepared

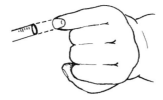

Figure 29–1

▶ epiglottis is floppy, shorter, and more "U"-shaped in children
  ▶ use straight blade in young children to lift the epiglottis
▶ larynx is more cephalad and anterior in children
  ▶ look upward to visualize the cords
▶ cricoid ring is the narrowest portion of airway in children
  ▶ may be able to pass the tube past the cords but not further due to cricoid ring resistance
    ▹ forceful insertion can cause a laryngotracheal injury
  ▶ use uncuffed tubes in children under 10 years old
    ▹ the cricoid ring creates a natural seal with the appropriate size tube
    ▹ cuffed tubes can cause tracheal stenosis in children
  ▶ perfect fit implies no resistance during placement and no air leak afterward
▶ because children have a proportionately larger head than adults, they are normally in the "sniffing" position when supine
  ▶ there is no need to elevate the occiput during orotracheal intubation
▶ shorter tracheal length in children
  ▶ 4–5 cm in newborn
  ▶ 7–8 cm in 18-month-old
  ▶ can lead to
    ▹ intubation of right mainstem bronchus if too deep
    ▹ easy dislodgement if too shallow

Cricothyrotomy/Tracheostomy

▶ surgical cricothyrotomy is contraindicated in children under 5–10 years (depending on the size of the child)
▶ needle cricothyrotomy is recommended as a temporizing measure before further attempts at endotracheal intubation
  ▶ jet insufflation of oxygen through a 14-gauge needle allows for adequate oxygenation
  ▶ expect hypercarbia as ventilation is usually inadequate
▶ tracheostomy is difficult
  ▶ narrow tracheal diameter and short distance between the rings

Impediments to Ventilation

▶ restraining straps
▶ gastric distension
  ▶ common due to aerophagia
  ▶ mimics intraabdominal injury
  ▶ increases the likelihood of aspiration
  ▶ relieved with the passage of an orogastric tube
▶ chest injuries
  ▶ can severely impair ventilation
  ▶ mediastinum shifts easily in children to the contralateral hemithorax
    ▹ causes compression of the ipsilateral and contralateral lung
    ▹ may result in respiratory failure

Cervical Spine

General Principles

▶ infant head is relatively larger than the body, so the neck becomes flexed when supine
  ▶ place a towel under the upper back for neutral position of the neck
▶ injuries
  ▶ ligamentous injuries are more common than fractures
  ▶ upper cervical spine is more vulnerable
  ▶ spinal cord injury without radiographic abnormalities (SCIWORA) is common
    ▹ cord (rather than ligament) injury occurs since it is securely tethered in children
    ▹ associated with paresthesias and generalized weakness
    ▹ symptoms delayed in 25%
    ▹ MRI helps confirm diagnosis

Radiographic Differences

▶ incomplete ossification makes interpretation of bony alignment difficult
  ▶ basilar odontoid synchondrosis fuses at 3–7 years old
  ▶ apical odontoid epiphysis fuses at 5–7 years old
  ▶ posterior arch of C1 fuses at 4 years old
  ▶ anterior arch of C1 fuses at 7–10 years old
  ▶ epiphyses of spinous process tips may mimic fractures
▶ increased predental space
  ▶ 5 mm in children (3 mm in adults)
▶ pseudo-subluxation of C2 on C3 is seen in 40% of children
▶ prevertebral space size may change depending on respiration

Circulation

General Principles

▶ difficult to diagnose early hemorrhagic shock since children compensate better than adults
  ▶ high catecholamine levels cause intense vasoconstriction
  ▶ children can lose up to 50% blood volume before blood pressure falls
▶ clinical shock in children is best diagnosed by
  ▶ cool, clammy, mottled, slow capillary refill (over 2 s)
  ▶ tachycardia
  ▶ tachypnea
  ▶ decreased responsiveness
  ▶ decreased urine output
▶ amount of blood loss is frequently underestimated
▶ bradycardia in an injured child is an ominous sign
  ▶ cardiac output is dependent on heart rate since the stroke volume is fixed in young children and infants

Measuring Vital Signs

▶ always use an appropriately sized blood pressure cuff
▶ usual measurements by age (Table 29–1)

Table 29–1 Vital Sign Measurements by Age

Age (years)	Average weight (kg)	RR (/min)	HR (/min)	SBP (mm Hg)	Fluid bolus (ml)	Urine Output (ml/h)
Newborn	3.5	40	125	80	70	2.0
1	10	35	120	85	200	1.5
5	20	20	100	90	400	1.0
10	30	16	80	100	600	0.5

▶ age-specific formulas for estimating blood pressure
  ▶ SBP = 80 mm Hg + (2 times age)
  ▶ DBP = 2/3 of SBP

Hypothermia

▶ increased body surface area-to-weight ratio promotes heat loss
▶ prevention measures
  ▶ overhead heaters or lights
  ▶ blankets
  ▶ warmed fluids
  ▶ warm packs
▶ monitor core temperature closely

Disability

▶ use pediatric Glasgow Coma Scale (GCS) (Table 29–2)

Table 29–2 Glasgow Coma Scale

Eye-Opening Response

Score	Over 1 year	Under 1 year
4	Spontaneous	Spontaneous
3	To verbal commands	To shout
2	To pain	To pain
1	None	None

Motor Response

Score	Over 1 year	Under 1 year
6	Obeys commands	Spontaneous
5	Localizes pain	Localizes pain
4	Withdraws to pain	Withdraws to pain
3	Abnormal flexion (decorticate)	Abnormal flexion (decorticate)
2	Abnormal extension (decerebrate)	Abnormal extension (decerebrate)
1	None	None

Verbal Response

Score	Over 5 years	2–5 years	Under 2 years
5	Oriented and converses	Appropriate words	Babbles, coos
4	Confused conversation	Inappropriate words	Cries, but consolable
3	Inappropriate words	Persistent cry/scream	Persistent cry/scream
2	Incomprehensible sounds	Grunts or moans to pain	Grunts or moans to pain
1	None	None	None

Tube Sizes

Endotracheal Tube

▶ use the formula 4 + (age/4) to estimate
▶ same caliber as patient's little-finger nail width

Nasogastric Tube or Urinary Catheter

▶ double the estimated endotracheal tube size

Chest Tube

▶ quadruple the estimated endotracheal tube size
▶ smaller sizes can be used for isolated pneumothoraces

Vascular Access

Sites

▶ antecubital vein
  ▶ good first site
  ▶ limit repeat attempts if urgent access is necessary
▶ intraosseous (see p. 446)
  ▶ placed in an uninjured extremity (usually proximal anterior tibia)
  ▶ fast and safe in patients under 6 years old
  ▶ high success rate
  ▶ more rapidly performed than cut-downs or central lines during circulatory collapse
▶ venous cut-down (see p. 445)
  ▶ permissible at any age
▶ central veins
  ▶ not recommended for children under 2 years old

Fluids

Resuscitation

Isotonic Crystalloid

▶ bolus in 20 ml/kg increments when crystalloid resuscitation is indicated
  ▶ warmed solution is ideal

▶ use the "3:1 rule," whereby the volume of crystalloid replacement is triple the estimated blood loss
▶ begin blood transfusion after the second bolus if hemodynamic instability persists

Blood Transfusion

▶ give PRBCs in 10 ml/kg increments
  ▶ each raises the hematocrit by about 9%

Maintenance

Type

▶ when under 2 years old, use D5/0.2NS
▶ when over 2 years old, use D5/0.45NS

Amount

▶ for the total amount of maintenance fluid necessary over 24 h use the following formula
  ▶ 100 ml/kg for the first 10 kg
  ▶ 50 ml/kg for the second 10 kg
  ▶ 20 ml/kg for every kg over 20 kg
  ▶ for example, a 25-kg child requires 1600 ml/24 h or 67 ml/h of D5/0.45NS

Injury Mechanisms

Motor Vehicle Collisions

▶ account for half of all pediatric trauma
▶ child safety seats
  ▶ could have prevented up to three-quarters of deaths of those under 4 years old who were unrestrained

Pedestrians Struck by Vehicles

▶ leading cause of death for children 5–9 years old

Bicycle Falls

▶ helmets prevent 85% of the morbidity and mortality of head injuries

Drownings

▶ common in children under 5 years old
▶ surround pool with a 5-foot fence and utilize a self-closing and self-latching gate

Burns

▶ 80% from house fires
▶ children under 4 years old commonly sustain scalds and electrical burns

Firearms

▶ rising sharply because of the availability of handguns

Child Abuse

General Principles

▶ consider child abuse in all cases of pediatric trauma
▶ more common in young children and infants
  ▶ two-thirds are under 3 years old
  ▶ one-third are under 6 months
▶ when abuse is missed
  ▶ 1 in 3 will experience further abuse
  ▶ 1 in 10 will die as a result of further abuse
▶ classification
  ▶ intentional injury
    ▷ physical or emotional assault
  ▶ unintentional injury
    ▷ unrestrained passenger in MVC
    ▷ lack of supervision at time of injury

Common Injury Patterns

Head Injury

▶ leading cause of fatal child abuse
▶ 85% under 2 years old
▶ skull fracture
  ▶ second most common skeletal injury associated with abuse
  ▶ be suspicious when there is a complex fracture (i.e., comminuted, diastatic, depressed) and a history inconsistent with a plausible mechanism
▶ shaken infant syndrome
  ▶ external signs of injury often absent
  ▶ retinal hemorrhages in 50–80%
  ▶ intracranial hemorrhage

Blunt Abdominal Trauma

▶ second leading cause of fatal child abuse
▶ often no external evidence
▶ nonoperative management of solid visceral injuries is the rule in hemodynamically stable pediatric patients

Bruises

▶ nonsuspicious
   ▶ expected over bony prominences (e.g., shins, forehead) once cruising/walking
   ▶ unilateral and focal
▶ suspicious
   ▶ found on face, neck, abdomen, back, buttocks, thighs
   ▶ present on infant not yet cruising/walking
   ▶ distinctive marks
      ▸ hand or teeth
      ▸ belt or cord

Burns

▶ nonsuspicious
   ▶ child-initiated splash or spill
▶ suspicious
   ▶ immersion
      ▸ extremity or buttocks/genitalia dipped in scalding water
   ▶ cigarette burn pattern

Fractures

▶ suspicious types
   ▶ direct strike
      ▸ e.g., ulnar nightstick fracture, a common defense injury
   ▶ torsion
      ▸ e.g., spiral femur fracture
▶ prevalence of child abuse in children presenting with fractures decreases with age
   ▶ 50% under 1 year old
   ▶ 30% under 3 years old

Clinical Evaluation

Determining Level of Suspicion

▶ observe for unnatural interaction between the child and parent
▶ talk with the child without the parent present to get details of the injury

- ▶ focus on aspects of the story that are unusual or changing
- ▶ unnecessary or unexplained delays in obtaining treatment should heighten concern
- ▶ higher-risk children
  - ▶ premature infant
  - ▶ learning-disabled or physically handicapped
  - ▶ step-child

Management

Reporting

- ▶ immediately report to the local Child Protective Services (CPS) whenever there is reasonable suspicion of abuse
- ▶ document carefully on the medical record all pertinent historical and physical findings

Evaluation

- ▶ carry out a detailed physical examination for evidence of old injuries
- ▶ perform skeletal survey to uncover occult healing fractures

Disposition

- ▶ lower threshold to admit children when there is suspicion of abuse
- ▶ in a nonaccusatory fashion, explain to the parents that reporting is required procedure given certain clinical scenarios
  - ▶ CPS workers must complete an evaluation of anyone felt to be at risk of further abuse before the child may be released to parents
- ▶ protective custody
  - ▶ invoke when parents wish to take their child from the hospital despite your reasonable suspicion of potential for further harm
  - ▶ immediately involve CPS
  - ▶ have security/local police stand by to prevent escape
  - ▶ maintain a professional demeanor and try to remain unemotional
  - ▶ explain that this is a legal matter beyond your control

30

Pregnancy

General Principles

▶ blunt trauma
   ▶ occurs in 6% of all pregnancies and most due to MVCs
   ▶ most common in the third trimester
   ▶ lap belts, when not worn below the uterus, increase risk to the fetus after a MVC
▶ obtain a pregnancy test on all female trauma patients who are capable of child bearing
▶ resuscitate term pregnant women aggressively
   ▶ do not turn attention to the fetus until the mother either stablizes or arrests
▶ essential trauma management does not change in pregnant patients
▶ consider the fetus potentially viable after 22 weeks of gestation
   ▶ correlates to the uterine fundus just above the umbilicus
▶ perform at least 4 h of fetal cardiotocographic monitoring in all pregnant trauma patients with a potentially viable fetus

Key Differences

Estimated Gestational Age (Figure 30–1)

Fundal Height

▶ at 12 weeks the uterine fundus is palpable just at the pubic symphysis
▶ at 20 weeks the uterine fundus is palpable at the umbilicus
▶ at 36 weeks the uterine fundus is palpable at the xiphoid process
▶ between 20 and 40 weeks the height (in cm) of the fundus above the pubic symphysis correlates with the number of weeks gestation

Dates

▶ gestational age in weeks is measured starting from the first day of the last menstrual period (LMP)

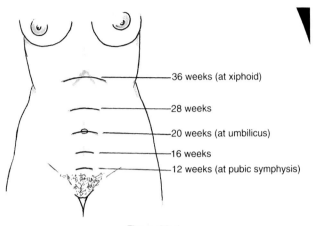

Figure 30–1

▶ the delivery date can be estimated by subtracting 3 months and adding 7 days to the LMP
  ▶ for instance, if the LMP is 12/30, term delivery is expected on 10/6

Fetal Heart Tones (FHTs)

▶ FHTs can be reliably detected by transabdominal doppler after 12 weeks of gestation
  ▶ documentation of presence or absence is mandatory after trauma
  ▶ apply a fetal monitor or measure every 10 min in major trauma victims
▶ the normal range is 140 ± 20 bpm
  ▶ sustained bradycardia occurs with placental abruption or fetal head trauma and is associated with poor fetal outcome

Maternal Ventilation

▶ in the third trimester, tidal volume and minute ventilation each rise by 50% and result in a P_{CO_2} of 30 mm Hg
  ▶ pH should be normal due to metabolic compensation for the chronic respiratory alkalosis
  ▶ "normocarbia" (e.g., P_{CO_2} of 40 mm Hg) in term pregnancy may actually represent ventilatory failure
▶ there is a 15% increase in oxygen consumption which diminishes the oxygen reserve
▶ the diaphragm rises by up to 4 cm, which decreases functional reserve and makes hemothoraces or pneumothoraces even more life-threatening
  ▶ insert tube thoracostomy no lower than the 4th intercostal space to ensure placement above the diaphragm

Maternal Hemodynamics

Averages	Nonpregnant	Term pregnancy
HR (/min)	80	95
BP (/min)	110/70	100/60
Blood volume (ml)	4200	6000
Hematocrit (%)	37	32
Tidal volume (ml)	500	700
ABG:		
pH	7.40	7.43
P_{CO_2}	40	30
P_{O_2}	100	105

▶ blood volume gradually increases 50% by term
  ▶ because red cell mass increases 25%, physiologic anemia occurs
    ▶ hematocrit averages 32%
  ▶ results in lowered plasma oncotic pressure, causing an increased risk of maternal pulmonary edema from any etiology
▶ cardiac output increases by 40% at term, with 10% shunted to the uterus
  ▶ primarily due to increased stroke volume
▶ blood pressure decreases by 10 mm Hg and HR increases by 15 bpm above baseline during pregnancy
  ▶ hypotension or tachycardia in the setting of trauma should never be attributed solely to these physiologic changes until occult hemorrhage is excluded
▶ since uterine blood flow decreases to compensate for maternal shock, evidence of fetal distress may be the first sign of occult maternal hemorrhage
  ▶ up to 30% blood volume (1500 ml) can be lost before maternal shock is clinically evident
  ▶ maternal shock is associated with an 80% fetal mortality rate
▶ inferior vena caval compression occurs when the mother is supine
  ▶ causes supine hypotension syndrome (see below)
  ▶ pelvic and lower-extremity veins become engorged
  ▶ venous return is improved by positioning in a manner that takes the weight of the uterus off the vena cava

Supine Hypotension Syndrome

▶ after 20 weeks of gestation, maternal hemodynamic instability and decreased fetal oxygenation may occur when supine

▶ results from decreased venous return when the uterus compresses the inferior vena cava

    ▶ reduces maternal SBP by 25 mm Hg and cardiac output by 25% as a result of decreased preload

▶ temporization techniques

    ▶ turn the patient on her left side by placing a wedge under the right hip or under the right side of the backboard (if the patient is immobilized)

    ▶ manually displace the uterus to the left

Placental Abruption

Pathophysiology (Figure 30–2)

▶ direct blow to the uterus or rapid deceleration can cause a shearing force between the placenta and uterus, causing the placenta to fracture or detach

    ▶ occurs because the uterus is elastic whereas the placenta is relatively inelastic and friable

    ▶ results in a variable amount of bleeding between the uterus and placenta

▶ occurs in 3% with minor and 30% with major blunt trauma

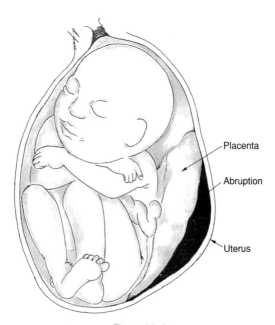

Placenta

Abruption

Uterus

Figure 30–2

Clinical Findings

▶ vaginal bleeding occurs in 80%
▶ abdominal pain occurs in 65%
▶ uterine irritability occurs in 35%
▶ all of the above, the classic triad, occurs in 25%
▶ other findings
  ▶ uterine tenderness or firmness on palpation
  ▶ low back pain
  ▶ premature contractions may occur
  ▶ an amniotic fluid leak may be evident
    ▷ nitrazine paper turns blue in the presence of amniotic fluid, which has a pH over 7 but can be falsely positive when blood or urine is present
    ▷ ferning is seen when amniotic fluid dries on a slide and is examined under a microscope
▶ maternal hypovolemia may occur as up to 2 liters of blood can accumulate in the uterus
▶ fetal distress occurs due to decreased uterine blood flow and may not be evident until over 50% abruption has occurred
▶ DIC can develop when the uterus releases thromboplastin stores
  ▶ measure coagulation factors, platelets, fibrinogen, and fibrin degradation products
  ▶ the fibrinogen level at term is expected to double, so a value reported as "normal" may be consistent with DIC

Diagnosis

Formal Ultrasound

▶ only 50% sensitive
▶ cannot adequately rule out placental abruption

Fetal Cardiotocographic Monitoring (Figure 30–3)

▶ also called a "nonstress test"
▶ most sensitive modality for detecting abruption and occult maternal shock
▶ for any trauma in a pregnant woman with a potentially viable fetus (over 20 weeks of gestation), initiate fetal cardiotocographic monitoring
  ▶ in minor trauma, even with no clinical evidence of injury, monitor for at least 4 h
  ▶ in major trauma or when there are uterine contractions or vaginal bleeding, monitor for at least 24 h
▶ fetal distress and consideration of emergency abdominal delivery when
  ▶ fetal bradycardia (under 120 bps) or tachycardia (over 160 bps)
  ▶ flat variation of fetal heart beat
  ▶ late decelerations

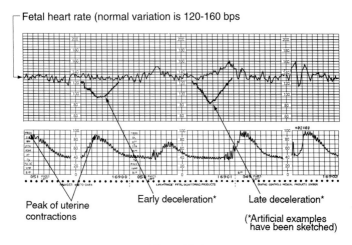

Fetal heart rate (normal variation is 120-160 bps

Peak of uterine contractions

Early deceleration*

Late deceleration*

(*Artificial examples have been sketched)

Figure 30–3

Prognosis

▶ maternal mortality is under 1%
▶ fetal mortality
  ▸ averages 30%
  ▸ if over 50% placenta abrupted, the fetus will usually die unless an emergency abdominal delivery is performed

Other Obstetrical Complications

Preterm Labor

▶ uterine contusions cause release of arachidonic acid, resulting in uterine irritability
▶ occurs in about one-quarter of blunt uterine trauma cases
▶ stops spontaneously in 90%

Uterine Rupture

▶ uncommon
▶ associated with prior abdominal deliveries
▶ due to blunt force directed to the uterus
▶ diagnosed clinically with uterine asymmetry, peritoneal signs, maternal shock, and palpation of fetal parts during abdominal examination
▶ maternal mortality is 10% and fetal mortality approaches 100%

Rh Sensitization

▶ an Rh-positive fetus causes sensitization of an Rh-negative mother after just a few drops of fetal blood enter the maternal circulation
▶ following abdominal trauma, especially when associated with vaginal bleeding, all Rh-negative pregnant women should receive RhoGAM because of the possibility of occult fetal–maternal hemorrhage
  ▶ usual dose is 300 mcg IM
  ▶ higher dose necessary with massive fetal–maternal hemorrhage, which can be determined by the Kleihauer–Betke assay

Physical Abuse

▶ occurs in up to one in six pregnancies, especially with teenagers
▶ ask about this possibility whenever a pregnant woman presents with trauma

Considerations by Mechanism

Chest Trauma

▶ tube thoracostomy during term pregnancy should never be placed below the 4th intercostal space

Abdominal Trauma

Clinical Findings

▶ peritoneal signs from hemoperitoneum are often blunted in late pregnancy

FAST Examination

▶ rapid, safe, and over 90% accurate in detecting hemoperitoneum
▶ can also use ultrasound for determining the presence of fetal movement or fetal heart activity

DPL

▶ rapid, safe, and 95% accurate
▶ use a supraumbilical open technique when the uterus is palpated above the pubic symphysis (over 12 weeks)
▶ in advanced pregnancy, upper abdominal stab wounds more frequently cause hollow viscus perforations, so use a lower DPL cell count to define a positive study

CT

▶ consider shielding the pelvis and limiting to the upper abdomen in early pregnancy
  ▶ will detect hemoperitoneum and liver/spleen injuries

Pelvic Fractures

▶ in late pregnancy, as a result of compression of the inferior vena cava by the uterus, there is marked pelvic venous congestion, which can result in severe hemorrhage after pelvic fracture
▶ the normal symphyseal distance of under 5 mm may increase to 20 mm by term pregnancy and cause an erroneous diagnosis of traumatic "open book" pelvic disruption
  ▶ make clinical determination based on presence of both mechanism and tenderness

Radiographic Considerations

▶ necessary radiographs must never be withheld out of concern for fetal radiation
▶ use a lead shield to avoid exposure to scatter radiation
▶ cervical spine and chest radiographs can be safely ordered using the same criteria as for nonpregnant patients
▶ trauma radiographs associated with high fetal radiation doses include
  ▶ plain radiographs of the pelvis, hips, proximal femurs, lumbar spine, or abdomen (e.g., IVP)
    ▶ about 0.5 rad each
  ▶ abdominal/pelvic CT
    ▶ about 2.5 rads
▶ limit uterine exposure to under 10 rads, especially before 15 weeks of gestation
▶ MRI and contrast agents have not been shown to be deleterious to the fetus

Postmortem Cesarean Section

▶ resuscitation of the mother takes priority over the fetus, and an abdominal delivery should not be contemplated until the mother has arrested
▶ a pregnant woman in traumatic arrest, with the fundus above the umbilicus, may simultaneously undergo immediate thoracotomy and abdominal delivery
  ▶ evacuation of the uterus improves maternal hemodynamics during CPR
  ▶ neonatal survival is likely when less than 5 min have elapsed between maternal death and abdominal delivery

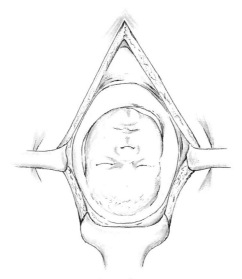

Figure 30–4

▶ there is no chance of fetal survival when the mother has been pulseless over 25 min before abdominal delivery
▶ procedure (Figure 30–4)
  ▶ place urinary catheter to decomress the bladder
  ▶ make a vertical xiphoid to pubis incision along the linea alba
  ▶ transect all layers of the abdominal wall and peritoneum
  ▶ carefully open the uterus by making a midline vertical incision across the upper segment using one's hand to shield the baby
    ▶ if there is an anterior placenta, cut through it and address bleeding after the baby is delivered
  ▶ remove the infant and suction the mouth and nose
  ▶ cut and clamp the cord
  ▶ begin the neonatal resuscitation

31

Elderly

General Principles

▶ there will be 65 million people in the U.S.A. over 65 years old by the year 2030
  ▶ this group currently represents 15% of trauma patients
▶ trauma is the fifth leading cause of death in those over 65 years old
  ▶ mortality is 5 times greater when age is over 70 years for a given severity score
  ▶ mortality is 25 times greater when age is over 80 years for a given severity score

Key Differences

Head Injury

▶ increased incidence of subdural hematoma
  ▶ because of increased dural vein fragility and less elasticity with age
  ▶ atrophy of the brain allows for greater movement of the brain within the cranium
▶ maintain a lowered threshold for CT scanning in the elderly
▶ those with intracranial injury have a poorer prognosis
  ▶ two-thirds over 65 years old presenting unconscious will die

Chest Injury

▶ thorax is less compliant and more susceptible to injury
  ▶ flail chest can occur from a simple fall, due to osteopenia, and has high associated morbidity
▶ reducing pulmonary reserve occurs with the aging process
▶ anticipate progressive pulmonary compromise and admit elderly patients with
  ▶ multiple rib fractures since splinting often causes ventilatory failure and pneumonia
  ▶ single rib fracture if there is advanced chronic obstructive pulmonary disease (COPD) or congestive heart failure

Cardiovascular Injury

▶ less able to increase cardiac output on demand in the elderly since
  ▶ decreased compliance and limited degree of compensatory tachycardia for a decrease in stroke volume
  ▶ less able to increase myocardial oxygen delivery during stress
  ▶ more likely to be taking beta-blockers or diuretics
▶ a relatively inelastic aorta is more vulnerable to transection
▶ in the traumatized geriatric patient, keep the hematocrit at least 30% and the SpO_2 over 90% to maximize the oxygen-carrying capacity

Abdominal Injury

▶ signs of peritoneal irritation are more subtle
▶ elderly are far more susceptible to postoperative complications
▶ impaired renal function complicates recovery

Orthopedic Injury

▶ osteoporotic bones are more vulnerable to fracture
▶ there is decreased pain perception and subtle fractures may be missed
▶ pelvic fractures carry an extremely high mortality rate
▶ perform a bone scan if there is high clinical suspicion of a significant fracture that is not seen radiographically

Resuscitation

▶ lower threshold for early invasive hemodynamic monitoring
▶ perform careful input–output monitoring
  ▶ although creatinine clearance drops with aging, so does muscle mass; thus serum creatine level may remain stable despite worse renal function
  ▶ older kidneys no longer concentrate urine as well
▶ maintain good oxygenation, but be wary of the possibility of hypercarbia-associated narcosis in patients with COPD
▶ consider transfusion to keep hematocrit above 30% to maximize oxygen-carrying capacity (especially if there is underlying cardiac or pulmonary disease)
▶ lower the threshold for intubation and do so with less delay whenever necessary
▶ artificial pacemakers, beta-blockers, and calcium channel-blockers blunt the usual chronotropic response to hemorrhage

Injury Mechanisms

Falls

Statistics

▶ 25% over 70 years fall at least once each year
▶ 50% who fall do so repeatedly
▶ nursing homes experience up to two falls per patient annually

Morbidity/Mortality

▶ fractures and other serious injuries occur in 25%
  ▶ 50% will die within 1 year of a serious fall
▶ a fall is often due to an underlying medical problem and this mandates a complete medical evaluation

Burns

Pathophysiology

▶ dermis much thinner
  ▶ decreased epidermal replacement
  ▶ takes longer to heal
▶ more difficult to judge fluid requirements
  ▶ use central catheter hemodynamic monitoring liberally

Morbidity/Mortality

▶ burns over 20% of total body surface area
  ▶ 50% will die if over 60 years
  ▶ 10% will die if under 60 years
▶ burn survivors generally do not experience a shortened life expectancy or significant loss in level of function

Elder Abuse

▶ underreported by the victims due to
  ▶ denial or acceptance as "normal"
  ▶ fear of abandonment
  ▶ failure of healthcare workers to inquire

▶ look for the following clinical evidence
  ▶ injuries of varying age (as in child abuse)
  ▶ unexplained medication overdoses
  ▶ physical neglect

Part V:

ENVIRONMENTAL ISSUES

32

Burns

Thermal

Pathophysiology

▶ burns cause
  ▶ cellular necrosis
  ▶ denaturation of collagen in dermis
  ▶ vascular occlusion
  ▶ edema formation
  ▶ 20-fold increase in evaporative water loss
  ▶ excellent growth medium for opportunistic bacteria
▶ release of mediators initiates an inflammatory response
  ▶ mediators include
    ▶ histamine
    ▶ serotonin
    ▶ prostaglandin
    ▶ complement
  ▶ when burn is under 10% of total body surface area (TBSA), mediators act locally
  ▶ when burn is over 20% TBSA, mediators act systemically

Burn Classification

Partial Thickness

▶ first degree
  ▶ only epidermis involved
  ▶ no blister
  ▶ skin appears red and painful, like a "mild sunburn"
  ▶ injured epithelium desquamates (peels) after 3–4 days
▶ second degree (superficial)
  ▶ involves epidermis and upper dermis
  ▶ blisters with fluid collection at epidermal–dermal interface may occur within hours post injury
  ▶ base of blister is pink, wet, and painful and blanches to touch
  ▶ with proper care wound heals spontaneously in 3 weeks

Full Thickness

- second degree (deep)
  - extends toward base of dermis
  - base of blisters mottled pink and white with slow capillary refill after pressure applied
  - minimally painful
  - wound is less sensitive to touch than surrounding normal skin
  - with proper care, wound heals spontaneously in 3–9 weeks with scar formation
  - grafting often required
- third degree
  - involves all layers of dermis including hair follicles and sweat glands
  - mottled or waxy appearance
  - rarely blanches with pressure
  - painless due to nerve destruction
  - heals by wound contracture, epithelialization from wound margin, or skin grafting
- fourth degree
  - extends to subcutaneous tissues, muscle, or bone
  - usually results in some loss of function
  - always requires grafting

Burn Size

"Rule of Nines" (Figure 32–1)

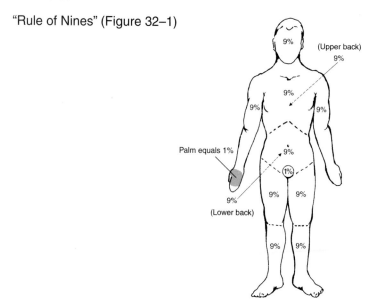

Figure 32–1

- applies to adults
  - entire head 9%
  - *each* arm/forearm 9%
  - anterior chest 9%
  - abdomen 9%
  - upper back 9%
  - buttock and lower back 9%
  - *each* thigh 9%
  - *each* leg 9%
  - perineum 1%
- infants
  - head larger in proportion to body
    - 18% TBSA
  - lower extremities smaller in proportion to body
    - *each* lower extremity 13.5% TBSA
  - other areas similar to adult proportions
- "Rule of Palms"
  - patient's palm area (not including fingers) equals 1% body surface area

Clinical Findings

- airway may reveal thermal injury with edema formation
- carbon monoxide or cyanide toxidrome may be clinically evident
- hypotension
- paralytic ileus
- constricting eschar

General Management

Airway

- prophylactic intubation is necessary with significant pharyngeal thermal injury

Escharotomy

- perform when necessary
  - circumferential thoracic burns impede ventilation
  - circumferential extremity burns impede perfusion

Fluid Resuscitation

- Parkland formula
  - estimates the amount of crystalloid necessary in the first 24 h to replace fluid lost into the extracellular space
  - total requirement (ml) = 4 times patient weight (in kg) times total body surface burn (in %)
    - half given in the first 8 h
    - rest given over the next 16 h
  - initiate when full thickness burn is over 10% TBSA

▶ objective measures of normovolemia supersede the Parkland formula estimate and include
  ▶ urine output over 0.5 ml/kg/h
  ▶ central venous pressure over 10 mm Hg

Wound Care

▶ apply cool fluids to reduce pain in low-TBSA burns
  ▶ with hot tar burns, cool immediately to halt the burning process
  ▶ omit cooling with large-TBSA burns (over 20%) due to risk of hypothermia
▶ gently cleanse with surgical detergent
▶ for second-degree blisters
  ▶ debride nonviable tissue and ruptured blisters
  ▶ leave small blisters intact
▶ to remove adherent tar, use a petroleum solvent (e.g., neosporin ointment or Vasoline)
▶ antibiotic ointment
  ▶ silver sulfadiazine 1% cream (Silvadene)
  ▶ bacitracin ointment
▶ cover with sterile dressing or sheets

Medications

▶ do not administer prophylactic parenteral antibiotics
  ▶ their use promotes organism resistance
▶ tetanus prophylaxis
▶ adequate analgesia

Other Interventions

▶ nasogastric tube
▶ urinary catheter

Disposition

Admission/Transfer Criteria

▶ partial thickness
  ▶ over 15% TBSA in adults
  ▶ over 10% TBSA in children
▶ full thickness
  ▶ over 5% TBSA
  ▶ involving face, eyes, ears, hands, feet, or perineum
▶ high-voltage electrical
▶ transfer to regional burn center whenever feasible and the patient is hemodynamically stable

Electrical

Physics

▶ voltage
  ▶ equivalent to the force driving the electrons that constitute the current
  ▶ directly proportional to both amperage (I) and resistance (R)
    ▶ Ohm's law states $V = I \times R$
▶ amperage is analogous to the number of electrons flowing
▶ resistance varies with type of tissue
  ▶ from least to most resistance (i.e., best to worst conductor): nerve, blood, muscle, skin, tendon, fat, bone
▶ alternating current causes sustained muscle contraction, which can prevent the victim from releasing a live wire
▶ direct current requires greater voltage to impart injury
▶ lightning imparts direct current
  ▶ typically up to two billion volts for under 100 milliseconds
  ▶ majority of current passes outside of body, so deep-tissue injury uncommon due to this "flash-over phenomenon"
  ▶ entrance/exit wounds rare

Clinical Findings

▶ cardiac arrest
  ▶ direct current often causes asystole
  ▶ alternating current often causes ventricular fibrillation
▶ respiratory arrest
  ▶ common in lightning injury
  ▶ due to paralysis of medullary respiratory center
  ▶ may lead to hypoxic cardiac arrest
▶ ECG abnormalities commonly include
  ▶ sinus tachycardia
  ▶ atrial fibrillation
  ▶ transient ST elevation
  ▶ bundle branch blocks
▶ burns
  ▶ at entry or exit sites of current
  ▶ may appear to be "kissing" due to flexor surface arcing
  ▶ usually much more extensive than they appear on the surface
  ▶ lightning injury burns
    ▶ usually superficial because of flash-over phenomenon
    ▶ deep muscle damage is rare
▶ myonecrosis ("crush-like" physiology)
  ▶ hyperkalemia
  ▶ acidosis
  ▶ rhabdomyolysis causing myoglobinuria

- neurologic sequellae
  - loss of consciousness
  - seizures
  - paralysis or spinal cord syndromes
  - confusion and coma
- orthopedic injuries
  - vertebral column fractures
  - posterior shoulder dislocation(s) secondary to seizures
- other
  - tympanic membrane rupture in 50%
  - cataracts often develop

Therapy

- ACLS maneuvers as necessary
- fluid resuscitation
  - adequate amount of crystalloid to maintain urine output over 0.5 ml/kg/h
  - may have larger fluid requirements than standard burn formulas indicate due to extensive third spacing in injured muscle
- for rhabdomyolysis or myoglobinuria
  - hydration
  - alkalization
  - consider mannitol or furosemide
- cardiac monitoring during a 6–24 h observation period after high-voltage injury or when initial ECG is abnormal
  - household electricity sources are generally not high-voltage
- tetanus prophylaxis

Admission Criteria

- high-voltage current or lightning injury
- sustained loss of consciousness
- dysrhythmias or abnormal ECG
- elevated CK-MB index (over 2.5%)
- indication of rhabdomyolysis/myoglobinuria from myonecrosis
  - elevated total CK
  - urinary heme proteins
    - positive urine dip stick for blood without RBCs on microscopic specimen
- acidemia
- significant skin burns (see p. 378)

Chemical

Pathophysiology

▶ caused by strong acids or alkalis
▶ damage progresses until chemicals are inactivated by reaction with tissues or are diluted
▶ alkalis are generally more dangerous than acids

Clinical Findings

▶ may initially appear benign
▶ continue to penetrate for 24–48 h
▶ full thickness burns appear deceptively superficial

Treatment

▶ immediately irrigate with copious fluids
  ▶ at least 15 min
  ▶ longer for alkaline agents
  ▶ for eye exposure, see p. 99.
▶ fluid resuscitation may be required for large burns
▶ antidotes for
  ▶ hydrofluoric acid
    ▶ 10% calcium gluconate (topical, subcutaneous, or intraarterial)
  ▶ phenols
    ▶ swab with polyethylene glycol and industrial methylated spirits in 2:1 mixture
  ▶ phosphorus
    ▶ 1% copper sulfate solution identifies residual phosphorus (by causing an insoluble black precipitate),which can then be removed

33

Near Drowning

Pathophysiology

Suffocation

▶ "wet drowning" (85%)
  ▶ aspiration occurs
▶ "dry drowning" (15%)
  ▶ aspiration is absent
  ▶ asphyxia is due to laryngospasm
▶ profound hypoxemia is the final common pathway

Fresh Versus Salt Water

General Principles

▶ most victims do not aspirate enough water to cause life-threatening changes in blood volume or serum electrolytes
  ▶ over 10 ml/kg aspiration is required before significant changes in intravascular volume occur
  ▶ over 20 ml/kg aspiration is required before changes in electrolytes occur
▶ water impurities are the most important factor in determining patient outcome

Fresh Water

▶ hypotonic to plasma and readily passes through the lungs into the pulmonary vasculature
▶ blood volume increases 3–4 min after aspiration, decreasing the concentration of serum electrolytes
▶ serum potassium levels may rise due to lysis of red blood cells
▶ causes "wash-out" of surfactant, which leads to atelectasis, ventilation perfusion imbalance, and hypoxia
▶ direct destruction of alveolar cells may lead to accumulation of fluid in the lung and decreased compliance

Salt Water

▶ osmolarity over 3 times that of plasma
  ▶ fills the alveoli and pulls protein-rich fluid from the pulmonary capillaries into the alveoli and interstitium
▶ blood volume decreases and serum electrolyte concentrations increase

Clinical Findings

Pulmonary

▶ atelectasis and pulmonary edema lead to hypoxia
▶ ventilatory insufficiency secondary to aspiration pneumonia may also develop hours to days after the initial resuscitation
▶ presence of coughing, dyspnea, or tachypnea indicates some pulmonary involvement

Neurologic

▶ hypoxia results in severe neurologic damage in up to a quarter of near-drowning victims
  ▶ hypothermia provides limited protection from hypoxia

Management

Survival Factors

Environmental

▶ water temperature
  ▶ affects the degree of hypothermia
  ▶ improved chance of survival if water is under 60°F (16°C)
▶ duration submerged
▶ water contamination

Age

▶ younger victims have better outcomes
  ▶ usually survive if submersion is
    ▶ less than 3 min
    ▶ less than 10 min if water is under 60°F (16°C)

Resuscitation Considerations

▶ prompt and effective prehospital resuscitation
▶ supplemental oxygen
▶ intubate when
  ▸ airway protective reflexes are absent
  ▸ wide A-a gradient exists despite high supplemental oxygen
    ▹ use positive end-expiratory pressure (PEEP)
▶ obtain chest radiograph (CXR)
  ▸ absence of abnormalities on initial radiograph does not ensure normal pulmonary status
▶ measure arterial blood gas
▶ nasogastric tube and suction to evacuate stomach contents
  ▸ massive amounts of water may be swallowed and then vomited and aspirated during resuscitation
▶ prophylactic antibiotics and steroids are not indicated
▶ hypothermia is managed in the standard fashion (see p. 390)
▶ evaluate cervical spine since there is high association with diving injuries
  ▸ near drowning may result when the person cannot swim because of a spinal cord syndrome

Prognosis

▶ depends on the degree of brain anoxia sustained
▶ 95% young victims survive with, at most, mild neurologic impairment when less than 10 min of CPR required before spontaneous return of circulation

Disposition

Admission Criteria

▶ pulmonary symptoms
▶ abnormal vital signs
▶ widened A–a gradient
▶ abnormal CXR or ECG

Discharge Criteria

▶ asymptomatic or symptoms resolve
▶ normal radiographic and laboratory studies
▶ may be discharged after a 4 h observation period if adequate follow-up assured

34

Temperature Extremes

Pathophysiology

Mechanisms

Heat Loss

▶ radiation
  ▶ heat transfer via electromagnetic waves
  ▶ 65% of heat loss in cool environments
  ▶ major source of heat gain in warm environments
▶ evaporation
  ▶ conversion of a liquid to a gas consumes heat energy
  ▶ accounts for 30% of cooling at rest
  ▶ greatest in dry/cool/windy climates
  ▶ at ambient temperatures over 95° (35°C), evaporation of sweat accounts for all heat loss
  ▶ evaporative heat loss is limited by humidity
    ▶ if humidity is over 90%, no evaporation occurs
    ▶ sweat simply drips off the skin
▶ conduction
  ▶ transfer of heat energy from warmer to cooler objects by direct physical contact
  ▶ water conducts heat 32 times more efficiently than air
    ▶ immersion in cold water and wet clothes increase loss
▶ convection
  ▶ heat loss to air circulating around the body
  ▶ varies significantly with wind velocity
▶ factors accelerating heat loss
  ▶ burns
  ▶ alcohol
    ▶ modifies the protective behavior
    ▶ impairs thermoregulation at both high and low temperatures
    ▶ impairs shivering thermogenesis

- ▶ impaired thermoregulation
  - ▷ central nervous system conditions may affect the hypothalamus
  - ▷ spinal cord transection
  - ▷ sedatives like barbiturates, phenothiazines, and benzodiazepines

Heat Gain

- ▶ normal body heat production at rest would result in a rise of 1°C/h if no cooling mechanisms interceded
- ▶ hard work increases heat production 12 times
- ▶ as ambient temperature rises above 90°F (33°C), the incidence of heat stroke rises dramatically
- ▶ conditions of high humidity and high ambient temperature block body defenses against heat production and lead to severe forms of heat illness

Physiologic Compensation

Skin Blood Flow

- ▶ important step in regulation of body temperature
- ▶ blood flow virtually ceases during cold exposure because of extreme vasoconstriction

Cardiovascular System

- ▶ most important in dissipating heat
- ▶ since 97% of cooling takes place at the skin, cutaneous vessel dilatation maximizes the cooling surface
  - ▶ cardiac output must double or quadruple to maintain the blood pressure

Sweating

- ▶ increases during heat load
- ▶ maximum rate
  - ▶ 1.5 L/h in unacclimatized individuals
  - ▶ double in acclimatized individuals

Hyperthermia

Heat Exhaustion

General Principles

- ▶ nonspecific syndrome resulting from volume depletion occurring under conditions of heat stress

Clinical Findings

▶ headache
▶ anorexia
▶ nausea/vomiting
▶ malaise
▶ orthostatic hypotension
▶ tachycardia
▶ muscle cramps
▶ temperature usually elevated but generally under 104°F (40°C)
▶ mental status remains intact

Treatment

▶ rest
▶ cool environment
▶ IV or oral rehydration
▶ symptoms resolve in 12 h with no permanent sequelae

Heat Stroke

General Principles

▶ heat control is lost and body temperature rises precipitously to levels that damage cells and organs throughout the body
▶ damage results both from the elevated temperature and from the length of time of exposure to the temperature
▶ complete recovery has been reported despite core temperatures as high as 115°F (46°C)

Clinical Findings

▶ essentials for diagnosis
  ▶ exposure to heat load
  ▶ temperature elevated over 104°F (40°C)
  ▶ major form of CNS dysfunction
▶ CNS signs
  ▶ delirium, coma, bizarre behavior
  ▶ seizures
  ▶ cerebellum is the most sensitive to heat and to permanent damage
▶ cardiovascular
  ▶ hyperdynamic
  ▶ low peripheral vascular resistance
  ▶ tachycardia
  ▶ increased cardiac index
▶ sweating may be present or absent
  ▶ depends on the degree of dehydration

▶ acute renal failure due to dehydration and rhabdomyolysis
▶ disseminated intravenous coagulation
▶ hepatic damage with cellular necrosis

Treatment

▶ secure the ABCs
▶ remove clothes and begin cooling immediately to prevent continued cellular damage

Immediate Cooling

▶ evaporative cooling
  ▶ spray skin with a fine mist of water
  ▶ use fans to accelerate evaporation
  ▶ cooling rates about 0.2°F (0.1°C)/min
  ▶ shivering can be prevented by
    ▸ spraying with warm water
    ▸ chlorpromazine
▶ ice packs applied to areas of maximal heat transfer
  ▶ scalp
  ▶ axilla
  ▶ groin
  ▶ neck
▶ iced peritoneal lavage
  ▶ high rate of cooling
  ▶ invasive, so reserve for extreme cases
▶ iced gastric lavage
  ▶ minimal effect because of the small surface area involved
▶ stop cooling when the body temperature drops to 102°F (39°C)

Hypothermia

Stages of Hypothermia (Table 34–1)

Physiologic Response

▶ 90–95°F (32–35°C)—thermogenesis preserved via
  ▶ shivering
  ▶ endocrine mechanisms
  ▶ vasoconstriction
▶ 75–95°F (24–32°C)
  ▶ vasoconstriction preserved
  ▶ shivering and endocrine mechanisms fail
▶ under 75°F (24°C)
  ▶ all heat conservation mechanisms fail

Table 34–1 Stage of Hypothermia

Stage	Temp. (°F/°C)	Characteristics
Mild	99/37	Normal temperature
	95/35	Maximum shivering thermogenesis
	93/34	Amnesia and dysarthria
	91/33	Ataxia and apathy develop
Moderate	90/32	Stupor 25% decrease in oxygen consumption
	88/31	Extinguished shivering thermogenesis
	86/30	Atrial fibrillation
	82/28	Ventricular fibrillation susceptibility; 50% decrease in oxygen consumption
Severe	80/27	Loss of reflexes and voluntary motion
	75/24	Significant hypotension
	72/22	Maximum risk of ventricular fibrillation 75% decrease in oxygen consumption
	66/19	Flat EEG
	64/18	Asystole
	59/15	Lowest accidental hypothermia survival

Clinical Findings

CNS

▶ linear decrease in cerebral metabolism
  ▶ 7% per degree from 95°F (35°C) to 75°F (24°C)
  ▶ EEG becomes silent at 66°F (19°C)

Cardiovascular

▶ early tachycardia followed by progressive bradycardia
  ▶ 50% decrease in the HR at 82°F (28°C)
  ▶ bradycardia
    ▹ caused by decreased spontaneous depolarization of pacemaker cells
    ▹ refractory to atropine
▶ conduction system is more sensitive to the cold than myocardium
  ▶ increased PR, QRS, and QT intervals
▶ Osborn or "J" Wave
  ▶ also called the "hypothermic hump"
  ▶ repolarization abnormality seen at the junction of the QRS and ST segments at under 90°F (32°C)
▶ dysrhythmias
  ▶ atrial and ventricular dysrhythmias encountered at under 90°F (32°C)
  ▶ spontaneous ventricular fibrillation and asystole may develop at under 77°F (25°C)

Pulmonary

▶ progressive ventilatory failure
  ▶ carbon dioxide retention and respiratory acidosis develop in severe hypothermia

Laboratory/Radiology

▶ blood glucose
▶ complete blood count
  ▶ hematocrit rises due to decreased plasma volume
  ▶ thrombocytopenia common
▶ electrolytes
  ▶ change during rewarming
  ▶ must be continuously rechecked
▶ BUN/creatinine
▶ blood cultures
▶ urinalysis
▶ coagulation profile
  ▶ prolonged clotting time with thrombocytopenia is common
▶ chest radiograph

Treatment

General Information

▶ faster rewarming rates (over 2°F [1°C]/h) generally have better prognosis than slower rewarming rates
▶ inaccurate core temperature measurement results in missed diagnosis of hypothermia
  ▶ rectal temperature is accurate unless the probe placed in cold feces
  ▶ tympanic membrane temperature most closely approximates hypothalamic temperature
  ▶ esophageal or bladder temperatures are accurate and probes are incorporated into special catheters to accommodate this measurement

Initial Therapy

▶ remove clothing
▶ insulate with blankets
▶ monitor and oxygen
▶ fluid resuscitation (warmed)
  ▶ D5/0.9NS is recommended
  ▶ avoid lactated Ringer's, since a cold liver cannot metabolize lactate

Airway Management

- ▶ indications for endotracheal intubation in hypothermia are identical to those for normothermia
    - ▶ careful oral intubation does not increase rate of cardiac arrest
    - ▶ nasotracheal intubation is safe when indicated

Cardiovascular Management

Resuscitation

- ▶ factors that result in induction of ventricular fibrillation include
    - ▶ rough handling of the patient
    - ▶ hypoxia
    - ▶ acid/base changes
    - ▶ cardiovascular instability
- ▶ CPR is less effective because of decreased chest wall elasticity

Defibrillation

- ▶ rarely successful at under 86°F (30°C)
- ▶ direct current from defibrillation results in myocardial damage
    - ▶ perform up to three times then repeat after rewarming

Arrhythmia

- ▶ atrial fibrillation
    - ▶ common below 86°F (30°C)
    - ▶ usually converts spontaneously with rewarming
    - ▶ use of digoxin or diltiazem is not indicated
        - ▹ ventricular rate is usually slow
- ▶ ventricular arrhythmia
    - ▶ do not treat transient ventricular arrhythmias
    - ▶ low temperatures result in abnormal responses to many cardiac medications
        - ▹ may increase ventricular fibrillation

Passive Rewarming

- ▶ ideal technique for the majority of healthy patients with mild hypothermia (over 90°F [32°C])
    - ▶ cover the patient with dry insulating material and ensure a warm environment

▶ endogenous thermogenesis must generate an acceptable rate of rewarming for this technique to be successful
▶ rewarming rate about 0.8°F (0.4°C)/h

Active Rewarming

General Information

▶ required when moderate-severe hypothermia (under 90°F [32°C])
  ▶ shivering thermogenesis ceases below 90°F (32°C)
  ▶ humans are poikilothermic below 86°F (30°C)
  ▶ body's metabolic heat generation under 50% below 82°F (28°C)

External

▶ deliver heat directly to the skin using a warming device
▶ apply preferentially to trunk
  ▶ when extremities are actively rewarmed
    ▶ vasodilation of the extremities provokes hypotension
    ▶ sudden circulation of cold pooled blood causes the core temperature to precipitously drop ("afterdrop" phenomenon)
▶ safe in previously healthy, young, acutely hypothermic victims
▶ rewarming rate about 2°F (1°C)/h

Airway

▶ administer oxygen with complete humidification warmed up to 106°F (41°C)
▶ indicated for all patients with temperature of under 90°F (32°C)
▶ rewarming rate about 2°F (1°C)/h

Intravenous

▶ administer fluids warmed up to 106°F (41°C)
▶ high flow rates must be maintained to deliver warmed fluid
  ▶ for pediatric patients or those with slow infusion rates
    ▶ fluid warmer must be close to the patient
    ▶ IV tubing must be insulated
▶ microwave warming of IV solution
  ▶ warm 1 liter with microwave set at high for 1 min
  ▶ shake the bag after heating to mix the cool and warm saline within the bag

Gastric Irrigation

▶ limited effects because of the small surface area

► risk of aspiration when the airway is not secured
► not recommended

Pleural Irrigation

► technique
  ► place a left-sided chest tube
    ▹ 3rd intercostal space at the midclavicular line (inflow)
    ▹ 5th intercostal space at the posterior axillary line (outflow)
  ► use saline warmed up to 106°F (41°C)
► do not initiate in patients who have an organized cardiac rhythm
  ► chest tube may induce ventricular fibrillation
► rewarming rate about 20°F (10°C)/h

Heated Peritoneal Lavage/Dialysis

► indications
  ► unstable hypothermic patients
  ► stable patients with severe hypothermia whose rewarming rates are under 2°F (1°C)/h
► technique
  ► place catheters in the abdominal cavity in the same manner as for a DPL
  ► fluid warmed to 106°F (41°C) should be instilled and then removed via the same catheter or via a second catheter
► rewarming rate about 6°F (3°C)/h
► advantages over other techniques
  ► overdose—may remove toxic substances
  ► rhabdomyolysis—"peritoneal dialysis" effect may be helpful
  ► rewarms liver

Cardiopulmonary Bypass

► major advantage
  ► preservation of flow if mechanical cardiac activity is lost
► treatment of choice in severe hypothermia especially with cardiac arrest
► initiated through median sternotomy or femoral artery/vein bypass
  ► femoral bypass is preferred in the severely, unstable hypothermic patient
► core temperature may be elevated by 1°F (0.5°C)/min
► for patients with suspected coagulopathies/contraindications to heparinization
  ► can be performed without heparin by using nonthrombogenic atraumatic centrifugal pumps and in exceptional cases with standard pumps

Prognosis

▶ consider terminating resuscitative efforts when
  - ▶ temperature under 59°F (15°C)
  - ▶ asystole without CPR over 2 h
  - ▶ submerged over 1 h
  - ▶ initial serum potassium over 7 mmol/L

35

Terrorism Preparation

Agent Types

Nuclear

► degree of illness related to the strength of the radiation source and time exposed
► scenarios
  ► conventional bomb used to disperse radioactive material
    ► long half-life of radioactive materials creates a significant environmental clean-up problem
    ► relatively few will experience acute radiation syndrome
  ► nuclear reactor tampering
  ► nuclear device detonation
    ► mass casualties and widespread damage
    ► technologically difficult and unlikely
► production
  ► radioactive materials available on the black market
  ► difficult to transport

Biologic

► small volumes are highly lethal, stored as a powder, and easy to carry and hide
► scenarios
  ► spores can be dispersed as a powder or aerosol in a contained space in a population-dense area (e.g., subway)
  ► can also be put into a food or water source
► the emergency department will become the site where most patients first present since exposure occurs days before illness develops
► unless the terrorist announces the agent beforehand, identification is delayed
► if biologic agents are even remotely suspected, inform the authorities immediately
► production
  ► bacterial agents can be easily cultured in large quantities and dispersed in a liquid broth using a spraying device

► viral agents are more deadly, though less likely since they are technically difficult to produce

Chemical

► small volumes are highly lethal, stored as a liquid, and easy to carry or hide
► scenarios
  ► can be disseminated as an aerosol or gas in a contained space in a population-dense area (e.g., subway)
  ► can also be put into a food/water source
► degree of illness is related to the concentration and time exposed
► some decontamination will likely be done at the scene by EMS staff, though many victims will flood local emergency departments
► production
  ► most are technically difficult to produce
  ► many are currently available on the black market

Equipment

► incorporate nuclear–biologic–chemical (NBC) treatment plans into hospital disaster drills
  ► practice setting up a large outdoor decontamination area
    ► disrobing alone decontaminates the overwhelming majority
    ► showering should be set up in a manner that can accommodate non-ambulatory patients
  ► do not depend on the local EMS service to help at the hospital as they may be simultaneously overwhelmed
► consider stockpiling the following resources, supplies of which are most likely to become exhausted in a real event
  ► barrier devices
    ► water-impermeable gowns, face shields, shoe covers, long gloves
  ► certain medications
    ► for instance, atropine, doxycycline, and ciprofloxacin

Identification

► early awareness that a terrorist event has occurred and rapid identification of the agent will minimize risk to human life
► understand the various clinical presentations of the main NBC agents and how each should be managed
  ► maintain hospital resources that include pathophysiology, management protocols, and contact numbers

▶ emergency department staff will be impacted most and its staff should be best prepared
▶ promptly identify the agent to initiate treatment and prevent further dissemination
  ▶ clues
    ▷ sharp rise in the number of people seeking care for fever, respiratory or GI complaints
    ▷ patients coming from a single location or with a "common denominator"
    ▷ many unexpected deaths
    ▷ a disease highly associated with terrorism (e.g., anthrax)

Management

Internal Notification

▶ invoke the hospital disaster plan if more staff are needed
▶ consult a radiation oncologist for nuclear agents
▶ consult an infectious disease specialist for biologic agents
▶ consult a toxicology specialist for chemical agents
▶ notify hospital administration and public affairs

External Notification

▶ local and state health department
▶ local FBI field office
▶ CDC Emergency Response office
  ▶ (770) 488-7100
▶ CDC Hospital Infections Program
  ▶ (404) 639-6413
▶ US Public Health Service
  ▶ (800) 872-6367
▶ Domestic Preparedness Information line
  ▶ (800) 368-6498
▶ National Response Center
  ▶ (800) 424-8802
▶ US Army Medical Research Institute of Infectious Diseases
  ▶ (301) 619-2833
▶ Radiation Emergency Assistance Center/Training Site (REAC/TS)
  ▶ (865) 576-3131 (weekdays)
  ▶ (865) 481-1000 (nights and weekends)

Treatment

▶ decontaminate patients
  ▶ large open outdoor space is ideal
  ▶ the ideal system would
    ▶ be rapidly activated
    ▶ accommodate a large number of ambulatory patients who must disrobe, shower, don gowns or paper clothing, and proceed to a remote holding area
  ▶ removal of clothing alone reduces contamination by 80%
  ▶ whenever possible, contain clothing and wash water, label as contaminated, and leave outside for environmental clean up crews to manage
  ▶ hospital staff wearing full barrier gear should be available to shower patients on backboards or otherwise unable to help themselves
  ▶ enact hazardous materials decontamination plan and set up the equipment
▶ protect staff from transmissible diseases
  ▶ implement full barrier precautions
    ▶ water-impermeable gown
    ▶ gloves
    ▶ eye shield
    ▶ shoe covers
  ▶ implement respiratory precautions
    ▶ HEPA mask
  ▶ wash hands and carefully clean the environment between cases
    ▶ use 0.5% hypochlorite solution (add 1 part household bleach to 9 parts water) to clean equipment
  ▶ self-contained breathing apparatus
    ▶ felt by many to be unnecessary and may delay important treatment
    ▶ does allow an extra layer of safety to properly trained staff and may alleviate their anxiety
▶ if there are space constraints within the emergency department
  ▶ cohort patients with similar symptoms in the same rooms
  ▶ do not let the exposed and asymptomatic patients overrun the clinical area
    ▶ expect many "emotionally" symptomatic patients (exhibiting panic, anger, or fear) for each significantly exposed patient
▶ notify the appropriate authorities

36

Nuclear

Radiation Physics

Electromagnetic Rays

Nonionizing

- ▶ long-wavelength and low-frequency
  - ▶ includes ultraviolet rays, visible light, infrared, radiowaves, and microwaves
- ▶ mechanism of injury
  - ▶ heat production
    - ▹ microwaves, lasers, visible light
  - ▶ delayed skin cancer
    - ▹ ultraviolet rays
  - ▶ eye injuries
    - ▹ ultraviolet rays, lasers, visible light

Ionizing

- ▶ short-wavelength and high frequency as well as particulate radiation
  - ▶ alpha particles, beta particles, and gamma rays emitted during the decay of unstable isotopes
  - ▶ machine-generated X-rays and particle beams
- ▶ mechanism of injury
  - ▶ acute radiation syndrome (short term)
  - ▶ gene mutations and chromosomal changes (long term)

Radioactive Substances

General Principles

- ▶ radioisotopes are substances that emit radiation
- ▶ irradiation implies that radiation has been absorbed by an object
- ▶ radioactive contamination of a person refers to the presence of radioactive material on the skin or clothing
- ▶ measuring radiation exposure

- ▶ one radiation-absorbed dose (rad) refers to a fixed amount of energy imparted to matter
  - ▹ 1 rad = 100 ergs/g
- ▶ the gray (Gy) is the SI (International System of Units) measure
  - ▹ 1 Gy = 100 rads (1 J/kg)

Types of Ionizing Radiation

- ▶ alpha particles
  - ▶ equivalent to a helium nucleus
  - ▶ derived from the decay of certain nuclides of heavy elements, including plutonium (Pu), radium (Ra), polonium (Po), radon (Rn), uranium (U), and strontium (Sr)
  - ▶ most are blocked by the skin's stratum corneum and therefore only partially penetrate the epidermis
  - ▶ alpha-emitting materials can contaminate skin wounds and are removed by skin cleansing
- ▶ beta particles
  - ▶ are electrons derived from the decay of numerous nuclei
  - ▶ are able to penetrate the skin and over time cause skin injury resembling thermal burns
  - ▶ beta-emitting materials can be removed by skin cleansing
    - ▹ check the adequacy of removal with survey meter readings
    - ▹ radiation survey meter can be found in the nuclear medicine department
- ▶ gamma rays
  - ▶ essentially the same as X-rays
    - ▹ gamma rays are produced in the nuclei of atoms
    - ▹ X-rays are produced by orbital interaction (e.g., a heavy metal target is bombarded by accelerated electrons)
  - ▶ possible sources of hazard include
    - ▹ explosion dispersing nuclear material (terrorist attack)
    - ▹ malfunction of an industrial radiography device
    - ▹ mishap with radioisotopes for medical and research use
    - ▹ nuclear reactor disasters
  - ▶ penetrate deeply and are primarily responsible for the acute radiation syndrome

Exposure Types

Medical Irradiation Source

- ▶ intentional during cancer radiation therapy
- ▶ no contamination hazard

Contamination

Internal

▶ inhalation or ingestion of radioactive substances
▶ treated in a similar manner to heavy-metal ingestions

External

▶ surface exposure to radioactive material
▶ treated by confining and removing the material

Acute Radiation Syndrome

General Principles

▶ results after a major portion of the body is irradiated by deeply penetrating radiation with a dose generally exceeding 1 Gy
▶ tissues with greater rates of cellular division are more radiosensitive
  ▶ the gastrointestinal and hematopoietic systems are most vulnerable
▶ massive exposure can affect any system due to cell death
▶ lethal doses after whole-body irradiation
  ▶ the LD_{50} without treatment is 3.5 Gy
  ▶ the LD_{50} with optimal treatment is 4.5 Gy
  ▶ doses over 10 Gy are uniformly fatal

Clinical Findings

Skin

▶ most common system affected
▶ areas of erythema that develop within 48 h will usually progress to ulceration or chronic radiodermatitis
  ▶ treatment is analogous to that for thermal burn and depends on the depth of injury

Hematopoietic

▶ pancytopenia due to bone marrow suppression follows a latent phase
  ▶ latent period 2–3 weeks with dose under 6 Gy
  ▶ symptomatic anemia
    ▶ treated with RBC transfusions

- ▶ thrombocytopenia causes petechiae and hemorrhage
  - ▹ present with doses exceeding 2–4 Gy after about 4 weeks
  - ▹ active bleeding or a platelet count below 20,000 mandates platelet infusion
- ▶ lymphopenia and neutropenia cause fever and infection susceptibility
  - ▹ absolute lymphocyte count (ALC) at 48 h correlates with prognosis
  - ▹ if infection can be prevented or controlled, with doses under 10 Gy the stem cells will eventually allow a return to normal
  - ▹ bone marrow transplantation is often considered with high radiation doses

Gastrointestinal (GI)

- ▶ nausea, vomiting, and anorexia lasts up to 48 h
  - ▶ radiation dose correlates with onset of these initial GI symptoms
    - ▹ under 0.5 Gy, over 6 h
    - ▹ under 2 Gy, 2–6 h
    - ▹ over 4 Gy, 30 min–2 h
    - ▹ under 10 Gy, under 30 min
- ▶ with doses over 10 Gy, after a latent period of 1 week, the GI mucosa becomes increasingly atrophic and then denuded
  - ▶ dehydration due to transudation of plasma into the GI tract, vomiting, and diarrhea
  - ▶ as bone marrow suppression ensues, the GI tract becomes a source of septicemia

Central Nervous System (CNS)

- ▶ headache, altered mental status, vertigo, sensorimotor symptoms
- ▶ occurs after massive exposure, and when following whole-body radiation is uniformly fatal
  - ▶ death expected within 48 h
  - ▶ potentially survivable if exposure is limited to head

Illness Categorization

- ▶ applies to brief exposure to whole-body penetration of gamma- or X-radiation (Table 36–1)

Treatment

General Principles

- ▶ irradiated but noncontaminated victims pose no risk to healthcare workers
- ▶ contaminated victims are unlikely to represent a significant risk of radiation exposure to healthcare workers after they are simply undressed

Table 36–1 Categorization of Illness Due to Irradiation

Degree	Exposure (Gy)	Clinical findings	Management
Mild	<2	• Asymptomatic or mild GI symptoms for ≈ 1 day • ALC (at 48 h) > 2000	• Can discharge if asymptomatic • Follow daily complete blood count/platelets
Moderate	2–4	• Moderate GI symptoms for ≈ 4 days • ALC (48 h) >1200	• Admit for gut decontamination, supportive care, and observation
Severe	4–10	• Severe GI symptoms for ≈ 7 days • ALC (at 48 h) <1200 • Symptomatic anemia • Opportunistic infections common	• Admit to protective isolation • Provide gut decontamination and intense supportive care which includes PRBC/platelet transfusions, antibiosis if febrile, and consider marrow transplant • About half will die
Fatal	>10	• GI/CNS symptoms within 30 min • ALC (at 48 h) negligible	• Admit for palliative measures • Death expected within 1 week

Internal Decontamination

▶ consider gastric lavage if within 2h of ingestion
▶ whole bowel irrigation

External Decontamination

▶ cleanse patients thoroughly
  ▶ first irrigate contaminated eyes, ears, and wounds profusely
  ▶ then use soap and water on intact skin
    ▸ gently scrub with a soft brush or sponge so as not to abrade the skin
    ▸ avoid hot water
  ▶ shampoo the hair several times and shave if the dose rate is not reduced to background levels
▶ utilize a survey meter to gauge adequate cleansing

Containment

▶ set up a radiation decontamination area and limit staff access in order to reduce contamination
  ▶ often the autopsy area of a hospital is converted to a decontamination area since it is typically remote, equipped with running water/floor drains, and has direct access to the outside
  ▶ staff should be declared noncontaminated by a radiation safety officer before being released
▶ floors, door handles, and light switches should be covered if time allows
▶ staff must use disposable protective clothing
▶ dispose of all waste properly
  ▶ ideally wash water should be collected and analyzed before release into sewage

Supportive Treatment

▶ adequate hydration to correct for GI losses
▶ symptomatic treatment with antiemetics and analgesics
▶ perform necessary operative procedures early to minimize risk of infection and bleeding due to the delayed hematopoietic effects of radiation
▶ reduce risk of opportunistic infection by utilizing protective isolation

37

Biologics

Bacterial Agents

Anthrax

▶ origin
  ▶ *Bacillus anthracis*
    ▹ very durable spore form
    ▹ occurs naturally in hoofed animals and is usually transmitted to humans by the cutaneous route
    ▹ responsible for "wool sorter's disease"
▶ clinical characteristics
  ▶ pulmonary
    ▹ incubation period 2–60 days after inhalation, the most likely route in a bioterrorism incident
    ▹ flu-like symptoms (fever, malaise, nonproductive cough) for about 3 days followed by abrupt ventilatory failure, shock, and death
    ▹ mediastinal lymphadenopathy and hemorrhagic medastinitis can cause widened mediastinum on chest radiograph (CXR)
    ▹ blood gram stain/culture may reveal gram-positive bacilli late in the disease
  ▶ cutaneous
    ▹ incubation period 1–7 days
    ▹ direct skin contact results in localized itching followed by papular and then vesicular rash, which later becomes a depressed black eschar
  ▶ gastrointestinal
    ▹ incubation period 1–7 days
    ▹ ingestion results in invasive gastroenteritis with septicemia and death
  ▶ mortality
    ▹ for pulmonary, over 90% if treated, 100% if untreated
    ▹ for cutaneous, 50% if untreated
▶ treatment
  ▶ begin antibiotics in the prodromal phase
    ▹ oral fluoroquinolones
    ▹ doxycycline

▶ secondary transmission
  ▶ occurs from direct contact with skin lesions, so maintain standard precautions
  ▶ airborne contact does not occur, so respiratory isolation is unnecessary

Plague

▶ called "back death"
▶ origin
  ▶ *Yersinia pestis*
    ▸ durable spore form
    ▸ naturally transmitted from infected rodents to humans by flea vector
▶ clinical characteristics
  ▶ pulmonary
    ▸ called pneumonic plague
    ▸ incubation period 2–3 days
    ▸ symptoms include fever, headache, cough, chest pain, hemoptysis
    ▸ sputum gram stain reveals gram-negative bacilli
    ▸ CXR consistent with pneumonia
  ▶ cutaneous
    ▸ purpuric lesions later become fluctuant buboes
    ▸ endotoxemia may cause septic shock and disseminated intravascular coagulation
  ▶ mortality
    ▸ for pulmonary, 95% if untreated
    ▸ for cutaneous, 50% if untreated
▶ treatment
  ▶ potentially treatable with intravenous antibiotics if begun during prodromal phase
    ▸ streptomycin
    ▸ doxycycline
    ▸ chloramphenicol
  ▶ post-exposure prophylaxis with an oral antibiotic for a one-week course is recommended
    ▸ doxycycline
    ▸ co-trimoxazole
▶ secondary transmission
  ▶ occurs from direct contact with skin lesions, so maintain standard precautions
  ▶ airborne contact occurs, so use respiratory precautions
    ▸ strict isolation for 48 h after treatment

Q fever

▶ organism characteristics
  ▶ rickettsial disease
    ▸ characteristics of both bacteria and viruses

- occurs naturally in hoofed animals and usually transmitted to humans by inhalation of dust contaminated by the feces of infected animals
- clinical characteristics
  - incubation period 10–40 days
  - flu-like symptoms and pleuritic chest pain for 2–10 days
  - mortality
    - under 1% even if untreated
- treatment
  - recovery occurs within 2 weeks without treatment
  - antibiotics shortens the duration of illness
    - doxycycline
- secondary transmission
  - airborne contact does not occur, so respiratory precautions are unnecessary

Viral Agents

Smallpox

- origin
  - the variola virus
    - probably not extinct as some believe
    - currently no herd immunity
    - transmitted by inhalation
- clinical characteristics
  - incubation period 7–17 days
  - flu-like symptoms for about 3 days followed by a rash
    - rash rapidly progresses from macules to papules to pustular vesicles
    - most prominent on the face and extremities (including palms/soles)
    - scabs over in 1–2 weeks
  - mortality
    - 30% if untreated
- treatment
  - antiviral agents may be effective
    - cidofovir IM
    - ribovirin PO
  - vaccinia-immune globulin (VIG) is effective in post-exposure prophylaxis when given within a week
- secondary transmission
  - occurs from direct contact with skin lesions, so maintain standard precautions
  - airborne contact occurs, so use respiratory precautions
    - quarantine contacts

Hemorrhagic Fevers

▶ origin
  ▶ types include Ebola, Lassa, Marburg, Rift Valley, Dengue, Argentinean, Yellow Fever
▶ clinical characteristics
  ▶ incubation period 1–3 weeks
  ▶ infectious gastroenteritis syndrome, petichiae/bleeding diathesis, followed by shock
  ▶ mortality
    ▸ approaches 90% for Ebola if untreated
▶ treatment
  ▶ potentially treatable with ribavirin
  ▶ vaccine exists for Yellow Fever
▶ secondary transmission
  ▶ occurs from direct contact with body fluids, so maintain standard precautions
    ▸ strict barrier precautions, especially if hemorrhage occurs
    ▸ quarantine contacts

Encephalitis

▶ origin
  ▶ Venezuelan Equine Encephalitis virus
  ▶ in nature, transmitted from equine species to man via mosquito vector
▶ clinical characteristics
  ▶ incubation period 2–14 days
  ▶ flu-like symptoms with meningismus for 3–5 days
  ▶ mortality
    ▸ if untreated, under 1%
▶ treatment
  ▶ potentially treatable with ribavirin
▶ secondary transmission
  ▶ airborne contact occurs, so use respiratory precautions

Toxins

Botulism

▶ origin
  ▶ *Clostridium botulinum*
    ▸ anaerobic gram-positive bacillus
    ▸ produces a potent neurotoxin
  ▶ naturally transmitted by ingestion of improperly canned foods

- ▶ clinical characteristics
  - ▶ onset about 24 h after ingestion and 48 h after inhalation
  - ▶ symptoms
    - ▹ generalized weakness
    - ▹ symmetric cranial neuropathies (ptosis, diplopia), blurred vision
    - ▹ descending flaccid paralysis, which persists for 2–3 months
    - ▹ eventual ventilatory failure
  - ▶ mortality approaches 60%
- ▶ treatment
  - ▶ botulinum antitoxin exists
- ▶ secondary transmission
  - ▶ does not occur

Ricin

- ▶ origin
  - ▶ toxin synthesized from the castor bean plant
  - ▶ naturally transmitted by ingestion of improperly canned foods
- ▶ clinical characteristics
  - ▶ onset about 18–24 h after ingestion
  - ▶ symptoms include weakness, fever, cough, and pulmonary edema
  - ▶ ventilatory failure, hypotension, and cardiovascular collapse within 12 h after symptoms begin
  - ▶ mortality high
- ▶ treatment
  - ▶ no available antitoxin exists
- ▶ secondary transmission
  - ▶ does not occur

Staphylococcus Enterotoxin B

- ▶ origin
  - ▶ toxin produced by *Staphylococcus*
  - ▶ normally ingested and causes "food poisoning"
- ▶ clinical characteristics
  - ▶ naturally transmitted by the ingestion of improperly kept foods
  - ▶ commonly referred to as "food poisoning"
    - ▹ abrupt, severe, and brief gastroenteritis syndrome with profuse, watery diarrhea for only 6–8 h
  - ▶ inhalation
    - ▹ pneumonitis within a few hours
    - ▹ fever for 2–5 days
    - ▹ persistent cough for weeks
    - ▹ high levels of exposure can lead to septic shock and death
    - ▹ CXR normal despite a pneumonia-like presentation
  - ▶ mortality is higher when the toxin inhaled, though most patients recover

▶ treatment
    ▶ antitoxin exists
▶ secondary transmission
    ▶ does not occur

38

Chemicals

Choking Agents

- ▶ agent characteristics
  - ▶ gases that rapidly dissipate
- ▶ examples
  - ▶ phosgene
    - ▸ odor like mown hay
  - ▶ chlorine
    - ▸ odor appreciated in swimming pools
- ▶ clinical characteristics
  - ▶ inhaled
    - ▸ immediately irritating to the respiratory tract
    - ▸ within hours, worsening coughing and bronchorrhea, which causes a "choking" sensation
  - ▶ cutaneous
    - ▸ irritating to the skin though not absorbed
- ▶ treatment
  - ▶ analgesia
  - ▶ eye irrigation
  - ▶ bronchodilators
- ▶ secondary transmission
  - ▶ occurs from direct contact, so maintain standard precautions
  - ▶ decontaminate the patient by removing all clothing and flushing the skin with copious amounts of water

Blister Agents

- ▶ agent characteristics
  - ▶ also called "vesicants"
  - ▶ these agents are rapidly absorbed in the skin
- ▶ examples (with military letter codes)
  - ▶ Mustard (H, HD, HN)
    - ▸ oily liquid with a garlic odor
  - ▶ Lewisite (L)
    - ▸ geraniums odor
  - ▶ Phosgene Oxime (CX)

- ▶ clinical characteristics
    - ▶ primarily cutaneous
        - ▹ within minutes causes erythroderma followed by skin blistering
    - ▶ respiratory irritant
- ▶ treatment
    - ▶ analgesia
    - ▶ standard burn care
- ▶ secondary transmission
    - ▶ occurs from direct contact, so maintain standard precautions
    - ▶ decontaminate the patient by removing all clothing and flushing the skin with copious amounts of water

Hemotoxins

- ▶ agent characteristics
    - ▶ can be vaporized and inhaled
    - ▶ odor of bitter almonds
    - ▶ fast-acting (seconds to minutes)
    - ▶ halt cellular respiration
- ▶ examples (with military letter codes)
    - ▶ hydrogen cyanide (AC)
    - ▶ cyanogen chloride (CK)
- ▶ clinical characteristics
    - ▶ vital signs
        - ▹ tachycardia and hypertension (early)
        - ▹ bradycardia and hypotension (late)
    - ▶ anxiety, headache, lightheadedness, vomiting
    - ▶ severe dyspnea despite red skin and lips
    - ▶ confusion, seizures, coma
    - ▶ rapidly progressive cardiorespiratory collapse and death
    - ▶ symptoms generally resolve when the source is no longer present
- ▶ treatment
    - ▶ use cyanide antidote kit
        - ▹ amyl nitrite pearls
        - ▹ sodium nitrite intravenously
        - ▹ sodium thiosulfate intravenously
    - ▶ hydroxocobalamin (vitamin B_{12})
    - ▶ hyperbaric oxygen
- ▶ secondary transmission
    - ▶ occurs from direct contact, so maintain standard precautions
    - ▶ decontaminate the patient by removing all clothing and flushing the skin with copious amounts of water

Neurotoxins

- agent characteristics
  - chemically are organophosphate compounds
  - can be vaporized and inhaled
  - colorless
  - may have slight fruity odor
  - fast acting (seconds to minutes)
  - halt cellular respiration
- examples (with military letter codes)
  - G agents
    - volatile and inhaled
    - types include Tabun (GA), Sarin (GB), and Soman (GD)
  - VX
    - evaporates slowly and persists longer in the environment
    - primarily affects by skin contact
- clinical characteristics
  - act in seconds to minutes to halt cellular respiration
  - effects nerve conduction by inhibition of cholinesterase
  - causes cholinergic toxidrome
    - miosis
    - "SLUDGE" syndrome (salivation, lacrimation, urination, defecation, GI cramps, emesis) and bronchorrhea
    - seizures
- treatment
  - control hypercholinergic signs
    - high-dose atropine
    - pralidoxime chloride (2-PAM)
    - protopam chloride
  - treat seizures
    - benzodiazepines
- secondary transmission
  - occurs from direct contact, so maintain standard precautions
  - decontaminate the patient by removing all clothing and flushing the skin with copious amounts of water

Part VI

USEFUL RESOURCES

39

Procedures

Airway

Chin Lift

▶ grasp mandible beneath patient's chin and pull forward to bring anterior
▶ in those requiring cervical immobilization, this procedure can be done
  without moving the neck

Jaw Thrust

▶ grasp the angles of the mandible bilaterally and push the mandible forward
  (Figure 39–1)
▶ use this technique while ventilating with a BVM device in order to make
  a tight seal

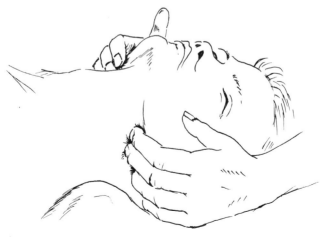

Figure 39–1

Oropharyngeal Airway

▶ select the proper size
  ▶ measure from the corner of the mouth to the external auditory canal
▶ open the mouth using the scissors technique
▶ using a tongue depressor to prevent pushing the tongue backward, slide in the airway

Nasopharyngeal Airway

▶ view each nares and nasopharynx and choose the side that seems the most patent
▶ select the proper size
▶ lubricate the airway and pass into the nasopharynx by gently pushing it straight in
▶ less likely to provoke gag reflex compared with an oropharyngeal airway

Bag-Valve-Mask (BVM) Ventilation

▶ the best results are achieved with a two-person effort when both are experienced
  ▶ one holds the mask in place with a tight seal
  ▶ the other squeezes the bag to provide adequate ventilation
  ▶ keep dentures in place to improve seal
▶ check effectiveness by auscultation and visually appreciating chest excursion
▶ expect insufflation of air into the stomach, which increases risk of regurgitation

Orotracheal Intubation

Equipment

▶ barrier precautions
▶ large-caliber, rigid suction device (e.g., Yankauer type)
▶ bag-valve-mask (BVM) and oxygen source

- ▶ oral airway
- ▶ 10-ml syringe
- ▶ pulse oximeter
- ▶ endotracheal (ET) tube size (mm)
    - ▶ for adult males use 7.5–8.5
    - ▶ for adult females use 7.0–8.0
    - ▶ for children
        - ▹ use the formula 4 + (age/4)
        - ▹ same caliber as width of patient's little fingernail (Figure 39–2)
    - ▶ check cuff of ET tube

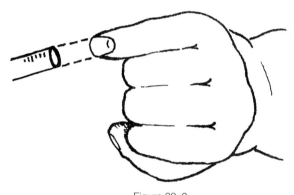

Figure 39–2

- ▶ stylet
- ▶ blade
    - ▶ in general, use what you are most adept at
    - ▶ curved blade (e.g., MacIntosh)
        - ▹ preferred for adults and especially short, thick-necked patients
        - ▹ wider blade is helpful in keeping tongue retracted
    - ▶ straight blade (e.g., Miller)
        - ▹ preferred for infants and small children
        - ▹ better for anterior larynx
        - ▹ better if larynx is fixed by scar tissue

Procedure

▶ align airway axis by putting patient in the "sniffing" position if there is no cervical spine injury (Figures 39–3A and 39–3B)

　▶ children, due to their relatively larger heads, are normally in the "sniffing" position when supine

　▶ this position may be facilitated in adults by placing a folded towel under the occiput

A

Airway Axis in Neutral Position

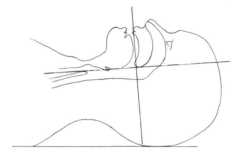

B

Airway Axis in "Sniffing" Position

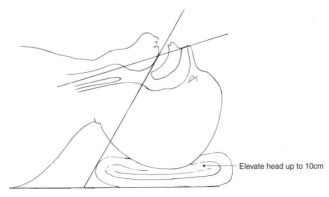

Elevate head up to 10cm

Figure 39–3A and B

▶ use a cross-finger ("scissors") technique to open mouth (Figure 39–4)
 ▶ with right hand, place thumb on lower teeth and 2nd and 3rd finger on upper teeth

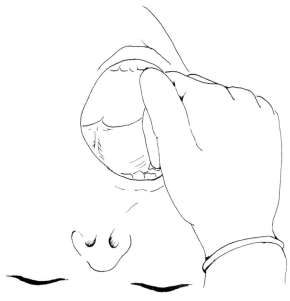

Figure 39–4

▶ introduce blade along right side of tongue, displacing the tongue to the left
 ▶ curved blade tip pushed into the vallecula lifts the epiglottis indirectly by moving the larynx (Figure 39–5A)
 ▶ straight blade tip lifts epiglottis directly (Figure 39–5B)

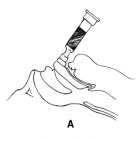

A

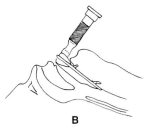

B

Figure 39–5A   Figure 39–5B

▶ apply upward traction (do not pivot the blade)
▶ visualize cords (Figure 39–6)

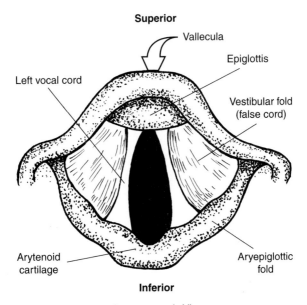

Superior

Vallecula

Epiglottis

Left vocal cord

Vestibular fold
(false cord)

Arytenoid
cartilage

Aryepiglottic
fold

Inferior

Laryngoscopic View

Figure 39–6

▶ place the ET tube through vocal cords
  ▶ pass the cuff 1—2 cm beyond the vocal cords
▶ inflate cuff just enough to seal off any air leak (about 5–7 ml of air)
▶ check for bilateral breath sounds and chest excursion
  ▶ auscultate both axillae and also over the stomach
▶ confirm adequate pulse oximetry readings
▶ secure ET tube
  ▶ 21 cm at teeth for women and 23 cm for men
  ▶ 3 times ET tube diameter (in cm) approximates where to tape at the
    teeth in children
▶ confirm tube position
  ▶ colorimetric capnometry device
  ▶ piston device
  ▶ chest radiograph (CXR)

Complications

- ▶ damage to teeth
- ▶ laceration of lips or oral mucosa
- ▶ esophageal intubation
- ▶ vomiting and aspiration

Nasotracheal Intubation

Advantages

- ▶ for patients with impaired neck or jaw motion
- ▶ cervical spine motion unnecessary for intubation
- ▶ avoids paralyzing or excessive sedation of patient
- ▶ facilitates surgery of oral cavity
- ▶ avoids dental injuries

Contraindications

- ▶ apnea
- ▶ severe maxillofacial or nasal trauma
- ▶ coagulopathy or anticoagulant use
- ▶ avoid in patient with elevated ICP unless pharmacologic agents used to blunt rise of ICP

Equipment

- ▶ alpha-agonist/anesthetic preparation
  - ▶ phenylephrine with either lidocaine or cetacaine
  - ▶ topical cocaine
- ▶ viscous lidocaine for lubrication
- ▶ ET tube
- ▶ 10-ml syringe
- ▶ BVM and oxygen source
- ▶ pulse oximeter
- ▶ suction

Procedure

- ▶ administer 100% oxygen by mask for 5 min
- ▶ apply alpha-agonist/anesthetic deeply into the nasopharynx using cotton-tipped applicators
  - ▶ wait 2 min until full vascoconstrictor/anesthesia effect achieved
- ▶ head position
  - ▶ "sniffing" position optimal if there is no cervical spine injury
  - ▶ neutral position with cervical immobilization if cervical spine injury is possible

▶ ET tube selection
- ▶ 6.5–7.5 for women
- ▶ 7.0–8.0 for men
- ▶ Endotrol tubes allow flexion of distal tip to direct tube into larynx

▶ lubricate the tube and the nostril

▶ introduce the tube with bevel edge toward the nasal septum (Figure 39–7A)

▶ once in the pharynx, curvature of the tube should face inferiorly (Figure 39–7B)

▶ advance the tube to hypopharynx

▶ listen for breath sounds (Figure 39–7C)

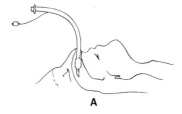

A

Figure 39–7A

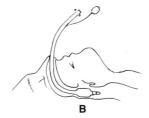

B

Figure 39–7B

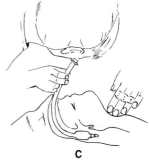

C

Figure 39–7C

- ▶ place second hand over larynx
  - ▶ apply posterior pressure to facilitate passage of tube through the vocal cords
  - ▶ palpate the paratracheal area for misdirection of ET tube
- ▶ pass the tube firmly but not forcibly at onset of inhalation
- ▶ if the tube passes posteriorly into esophagus
  - ▶ pull back on the tube until breath sounds are heard
  - ▶ apply pressure to larynx
  - ▶ extend neck (if cervical spine uninjured)
  - ▶ reinsert at onset of inhalation
- ▶ if the tube passes laterally to side of larynx
  - ▶ pull back slightly on the tube
  - ▶ rotate the tube toward center
- ▶ if the tip of the tube is on the vocal cords but cannot pass due to laryngospasm
  - ▶ squirt 25–50 mg of lidocaine down the ET tube to anesthetize the vocal cords
  - ▶ reinsert at onset of inhalation
- ▶ if the tube is in correct position
  - ▶ patient will cough and not be able to phonate
  - ▶ good bilateral breath sounds will be heard with BVM ventilation
  - ▶ good air movement through ET tube
    - ▶ condensation seen within tube during exhalation
- ▶ secure the tube in place
  - ▶ usually 28 cm from the external nares in males
  - ▶ usually 26 cm from the external nares in females
- ▶ confirm tube position
  - ▶ colorimetric capnometry device
  - ▶ piston device
  - ▶ CXR

Complications

- ▶ epistaxis
- ▶ turbinate fracture
- ▶ retropharyngeal laceration
- ▶ esophageal intubation

Laryngeal Mask Airway

General Principles

- ▶ specially designed mask placed into the hypopharynx
- ▶ used as an alternative when ET intubation is unsuccessful and effective BVM is difficult or impossible
- ▶ aspiration remains a possibility
  - ▶ if gag reflex is present, apply a topical anesthetic or sedate the patient

Procedure (Figure 39–8A and B)

- ▶ lubricate mask
- ▶ insert with the opening facing patient's tongue
- ▶ push the mask into the hypopharynx with index finger
  - ▶ resistance correlates with correct position at upper esophageal sphincter
- ▶ inflate cuff

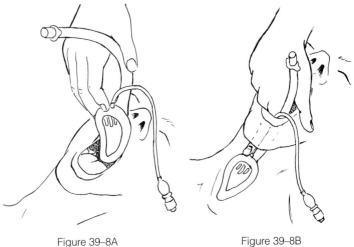

Figure 39–8A   Figure 39–8B

Cricothyrotomy

Contraindications

- ▶ age under 5–10 years old (depending on child's size)
  - ▶ age cut-off controversial
- ▶ larynx/cricoid cartilage injury or tracheal transection
- ▶ tracheal transection
- ▶ expanding hematoma over cricothyroid membrane
- ▶ preexisting laryngeal pathology

Equipment

- ▶ scalpel with #11 blade
- ▶ Trousseau dilator
- ▶ tracheal hook
- ▶ small, curved hemostat
- ▶ tracheostomy tube size 6–8 in adults or ET tube
- ▶ suction

▶ 10-ml syringe
▶ good lighting

Procedure

▶ 100% oxygen
▶ prepare the neck with betadine
▶ hyperextend head if cervical spine cleared
▶ grasp the thyroid cartilage with thumb and long finger of the nondominant hand and locate the cricothyroid membrane with the index finger (Figure 39–9)
▶ incise the skin and cricothyroid membrane with the scalpel through one stab incision (Figure 39–10)
   ▶ avoid too deep an incision, which could injure the esophagus
▶ make a transverse incision through the membrane in each direction while keeping the scalpel in place (Figure 39–11)
▶ insert a tracheal hook to retract larynx upward (Figure 39–12)
▶ remove the scalpel
▶ insert a Trousseau dilator or curved hemostat to dilate the opening (optional) (Figure 39–13)
▶ place a tracheostomy or ET tube (Figure 39–14)

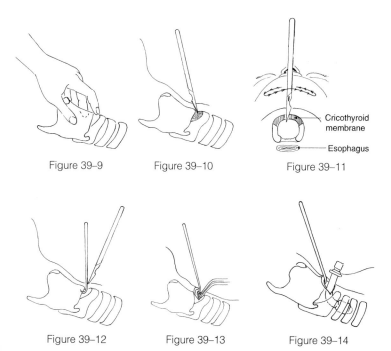

Figure 39–9   Figure 39–10   Cricothyroid membrane — Esophagus — Figure 39–11

Figure 39–12   Figure 39–13   Figure 39–14

Alternative Procedure

▶ midline vertical incision 3–4 cm long (Figure 39–15)
   ▶ allows for better identification of cricothyroid membrane in patients with difficult landmarks
▶ follow with transverse incision through cricothyroid membrane
▶ insert a tracheal hook to retract larynx upward
▶ remove the scalpel
▶ insert a Trousseau dilator (optional)
▶ place a tracheostomy or ET tube

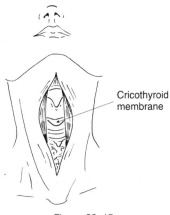

Cricothyroid membrane

Figure 39–15

Complications

▶ esophageal perforation
▶ hemorrhage
▶ subcutaneous emphysema
▶ vocal cord injury
▶ prolonged procedure time

Tracheostomy

Indications

▶ patient for which cricothyrotomy would be technically difficult
   ▶ pediatric cases

- laryngeal fracture
- tracheal transection
- expanding hematoma over cricothyroid membrane
- laryngeal foreign body

Contraindications

- expanding hematoma over tracheotomy site

Equipment

- same as for cricothyrotomy with two additional clamps

Procedure

- 100% oxygen
- hyperextend neck if cervical spine fracture is excluded
- prepare neck with betadine
- midline vertical skin incision from the cricoid cartilage to the suprasternal notch (Figure 39–16)
    - continue incision deep until the pretracheal fascia is reached
- retract wound edges
- use blunt dissection to separate the thyroid isthmus from the trachea
- place two clamps on the isthmus and divide it (Figure 39–17)

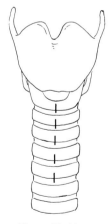

Figure 39–16

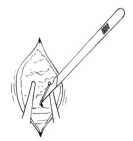

Figure 39–17

▶ place a tracheostomy hook between the first and second tracheal rings to provide stabilization and upward traction (Figure 39–18)
▶ make a vertical incision through the 3rd and 4th tracheal rings
▶ insert the tube (Figure 39–19)
  ▶ tracheal tube size 6, 7, or 8
  ▶ ET tube size 6.0
▶ remove the obturator from the tracheal tube and inflate the cuff

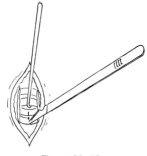

Figure 39–18

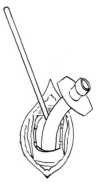

Figure 39–19

Complications

▶ hemorrhage
▶ mediastinal emphysema
▶ false passage

Percutaneous Transtracheal Jet Insufflation

General Principles

▶ temporizing measure for patients who need ventilation but cannot be immediately intubated
▶ carbon dioxide retention remains a problem
▶ aspiration is not prevented
▶ procedure of choice in children under 5 years old when ET intubation is unsuccessful
  ▶ surgical airway is difficult in this age group

Indications

▶ failure to achieve ET intubation in a timely fashion

Contraindications

▶ total obstruction of airway above the vocal cords
▶ tracheal transection
▶ damage to cricoid cartilage or larynx

Equipment

▶ ideally use oxygen directly from an ordinary oxygen wall outlet or standard oxygen cylinder (50 PSI), but practically may only be able to use a flow regulator turned up to the maximum liter flow
  ▶ liter flow regulators (15—17 L/min) do not provide sufficient flow
▶ standard oxygen tubing
▶ 14-gauge angiocath or similar cannula manufactured specifically for percutaneous ventilation
▶ commercial valve apparatus or three-way plastic stopcock

Procedure

▶ if a commercial valve apparatus is unavailable, create a valve
  ▶ place the three-way plastic stopcock in the oxygen tubing
  ▶ cut a side hole near the distal end of a length of standard oxygen tubing
▶ attach the oxygen to the wall source
▶ prepare the neck with betadine
▶ puncture the cricothyroid membrane at a 45° angle caudally with 14-gauge angiocath attached to a syringe (Figure 39–20)
  ▶ advance with negative pressure applied to syringe
  ▶ gush of air into syringe signifies entry into larynx
  ▶ remove needle
▶ secure the catheter to the skin using a suture
▶ attach to oxygen tubing

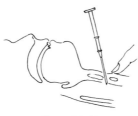

Figure 39–20

▶ begin jet ventilation (Figure 39–21)
   ▶ provide oxygen at no greater then 50 PSI (adults) or 30 PSI (children) by watching the pressure monitor (when available)
   ▶ allow the oxygen jet to insufflate lungs for 1 s
   ▶ allow exhalation for 3 s

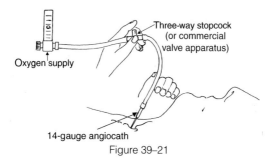

Figure 39–21

Complications

▶ esophageal puncture
▶ barotrauma
   ▶ subcutaneous and mediastinal emphysema
▶ progressive hypercapnia, which decreases cerebral perfusion

Retrograde Guidewire Intubation

Indications

▶ failure to achieve ET intubation in a timely fashion
▶ severe orofacial trauma distorting the anatomy
▶ bloody field making endotracheal intubation difficult

Contraindications

▶ coagulopathy
▶ expanding hematoma over cricothyroid membrane
▶ inability to open mouth for guidewire retrieval

Equipment

▶ Cook Retrograde Intubation Set
   ▶ 110 cm guidewire with a J tip
   ▶ guidewire-introducer needle
   ▶ 11 French black 70-cm TFE catheter
▶ long forceps (e.g., Magill type) to grasp guidewire
▶ ET tube (at least 4 mm ID)

Procedure

▶ provide supplemental oxygen to the patient throughout the procedure
▶ anesthetize and apply betadine to skin over the cricothyroid membrane
▶ puncture the lower half of the cricothyroid membrane with the needle with bevel facing cephalad
▶ aspirate air to assure placement in the lumen
▶ angle needle 30–45° cephalad
▶ introduce the guidewire through the needle until the tip is visible in the patient's mouth
▶ grasp and retrieve the guidewire from the oropharynx with Magill forceps
▶ remove the needle from the cricothyroid site over the guidewire
▶ secure the cricothyroid end of the guidewire with a clamp (Cook kit has a black positioning mark) (Figure 39–22A)
▶ introduce the catheter antegrade over the guidewire and, while pulling the guidewire taught, advance the catheter until resistance felt and tenting is noted at the cricothyroid access site (Figure 39–22B)
  ▷ if unsure that the correct position has been obtained, consider confirming with direct laryngoscopy
▶ now can either advance the ET tube over the catheter into the trachea or remove the clamp and pull the guidewire through the cricothyroid site while simultaneously advancing the catheter into the trachea (Figure 39–22C)
  ▷ intubating with a catheter only allows ventilation through the catheter
  ▷ be aware that the ET tube can "hang up" at the veleculla and may require gentle twisting to overcome resistance
▶ pull the catheter from the ET tube and confirm its correct placement (Figure 39–22D)
  ▷ colorimetric capnometry device
  ▷ piston device
  ▷ CXR

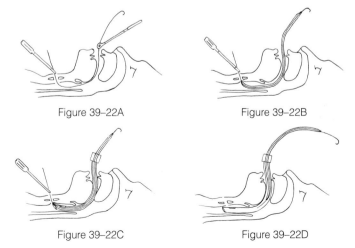

Figure 39–22A   Figure 39–22B

Figure 39–22C   Figure 39–22D

Complications

▶ subcutaneous and mediastinal emphysema
▶ vocal cord injury
▶ hemorrhage
▶ esophageal puncture
▶ infection

Digital Intubation

Indications

▶ conventional methods failed
▶ upper airway obscured by blood or secretions
▶ short-necked individuals
▶ ET equipment is lacking or not functioning

Procedure

▶ patient must be deeply sedated or paralyzed
▶ place a bite block between upper and lower molars
▶ place a stylet in the ET tube and curl into a "J" formation
▶ palpate the tip of the epiglottis with the middle finger of the nondominant hand (Figure 39–23)
▶ use tactile sensation to guide the ET tube anteriorly through the vocal cords (Figure 39–24)

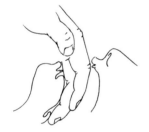

Figure 39–23

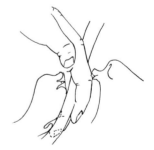

Figure 39–24

Typical Initial Ventilator Settings

Minute Volume

▶ V_T is 10–15 ml/kg
▶ RR is 12–14/min

F_iO_2

▶ 100%
▶ titrate down to maintain S_pO_2 over 95%

Positive End-Expiratory Pressure (PEEP)

▶ 5 cm H_2O

Inspiratory Time

▶ 33%
▶ correlates to I:E ratio of 1:2

Pause Time

▶ 0%

Volume Control

▶ no sigh

Waveform

▶ square

Pressure Limits

▶ start at 50 cm H_2O
▶ adjust to 10–15 cm H_2O above observed peak inspiratory pressure

Trigger Sensitivity

▶ -1 to -3 cm H_2O

Vascular Access

General Principles

▶ for subclavian and internal jugular cannulation, place the patient in the Trendelenburg position (head down at least 15°) to distend the neck veins and prevent air embolism
▶ after vein cannulation, cover the catheter at all times to prevent air embolism
▶ prepare and drape the area using aseptic sterile technique

Seldinger Technique

▶ basic equipment
  ▶ guidewire with a J tip
  ▶ guidewire-introducer needle
  ▶ #11 blade scalpel
  ▶ catheter (with indwelling dilator)
  ▶ lidocaine and local anesthesia needle
  ▶ 5–10 ml syringe
  ▶ suture to secure catheter
▶ determine the point of insertion and apply betadine
▶ anesthetize the skin and subcutaneous tissues in awake patients
▶ keep 1/2 ml of lidocaine in the syringe and switch to the guidewire-introducer needle to evacuate any skin plug after passing through the skin
▶ cannulate the vessel (Figure 39–25A)
  ▶ confirmed when able to freely aspirate venous blood
▶ thread guidewire through the guidewire-introducer needle until resistance is met or only 3 cm of wire is left outside the needle (Figure 39–25B)
  ▶ if resistance is felt before the guidewire enters vessel, remove it, re-confirm vessel cannulation, and rethread the guidewire
▶ remove the needle (Figure 39–25C)
▶ make a small stab incision adjacent to the guidewire using the scalpel tip (Figure 39–25D)
▶ pass the catheter (with indwelling dilator) over guidewire (Figure 39–25E)
▶ grasp the proximal end of the guidewire through the proximal end of the catheter
▶ advance the catheter over the guidewire through the skin and into the vessel using a twisting motion (Figure 39–25F)
▶ remove the guidewire (Figure 39–25G)
▶ remove the dilator
▶ confirm free aspiration of venous blood from catheter
▶ connect the catheter to IV tubing
▶ secure the catheter with sutures and apply a dressing

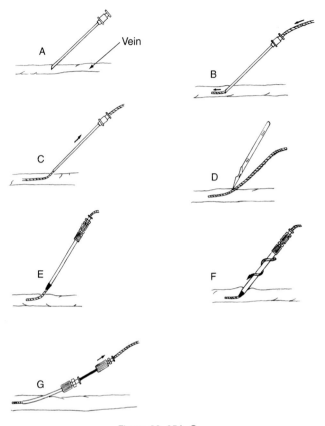

Figure 39–25A–G

Complications

► pneumothorax
► air embolism
► infection
► thoracic duct laceration
► hematoma
► arterial perforation
► catheter malposition

Internal Jugular Landmarks

Traditional Anterior Approach

▶ turn the head toward the contralateral side of venous cannulation (after the cervical spine is cleared)
▶ palpate and locate the carotid artery to prevent inadvertent puncture
▶ insert the needle at apex of the triangle formed by two heads of stern-ocleidomastoid muscle (Figure 39–26A) at a 30° posterior angle with the frontal plane and direct toward the ipsilateral nipple (Figure 39–26B)
▶ the vein should be entered within 2 cm of needle advancement

Middle (Central) Approach

▶ turn the head toward the contralateral side of venous cannulation (after the cervical spine is cleared)
▶ palpate and locate the carotid artery to prevent inadvertent puncture
▶ insert the needle in the middle of the triangle formed by the two heads of sternocleidomastoid muscle at a 30° posterior angle with the frontal plane and direct parallel to the sagital plane
▶ the vein should be entered within 2 cm of needle advancement

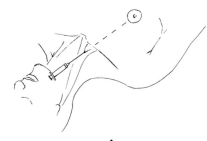

Figure 39–26A

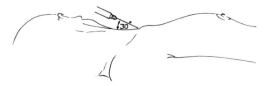

Figure 39–26B

Direct Anterior Approach

▶ keep the head in neutral position or turned minimally (only 5°) toward the contralateral side (after the cervical spine is cleared)
▶ palpate and locate the carotid artery to prevent inadvertent puncture
▶ insert the needle at the apex of the triangle formed by the two heads of the sternocleidomastoid muscle and direct toward the ipsilateral nipple at a 60° angle to the skin
▶ the vein should be entered within 1.5 cm of needle advancement

Posterior Approach

▶ insert the needle at the posterior border of the sternocleidomastoid muscle just cephalad to the crossing of the external jugular and direct toward the suprasternal notch (Figure 39–27)
▶ the vein should be entered within 5 cm of needle advancement

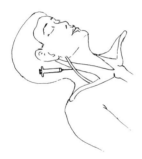

Figure 39–27

Subclavian Landmarks

Infraclavicular Approach

▶ insert the needle 1 cm inferior to the clavicle at the junction of the medial and middle thirds

▶ direct the needle under the clavicle toward the operator's left index finger placed in the suprasternal notch (Figure 39–28)
  ▶ start with the bevel upward (cephalad) and, once the vein is entered, rotate the bevel downward (caudad)
  ▶ the vein should be entered within 4 cm of needle advancement

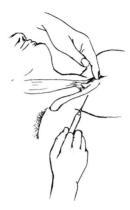

Figure 39–28

Supraclavicular Approach

▶ insert the needle 1 cm lateral to the clavicular head of sternocleidomastoid (SCM) and 1 cm above the superior border of the clavicle (Figure 39–29)

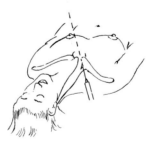

Figure 39–29

▶ direct the needle 10–15° above the horizontal plane bisecting the angle formed by the junction of the clavicle and the SCM angle, aiming just caudal to contralateral nipple (in males)

    ▶ the vein should be entered within 3 cm of needle advancement

▶ the right side is preferred

    ▶ the right subclavian has a straighter course in relation to the innominate and superior vena cava than the left subclavian

    ▶ thoracic duct is on the left

Femoral Landmarks

Procedure

▶ while palpating the femoral artery with the nondominant index and middle finger, insert the needle cephalad at a 45° angle 1–2 cm inferior to the inguinal crease and 0.5–1.0 cm medial to the artery (Figure 39–30)

▶ the vein is located midway between the pubic tubercle and anterior superior iliac spine

    ▶ use these landmarks when attempting the procedure in the pulseless patient

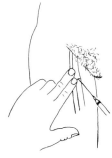

Figure 39–30

Saphenous Cut-Down (Ankle)

Procedure

▶ make a 2–3 cm incision two finger breadths above the medial malleolus transversely from the anterior border of the tibia to the posterior border of the medial malleolus (Figure 39–31A)

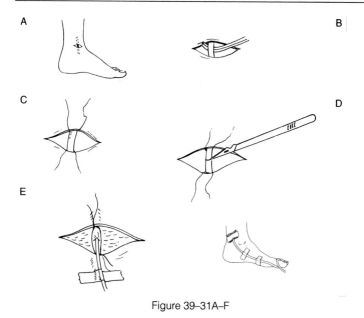

Figure 39–31A–F

▶ using a curved hemostat to bluntly dissect, isolate the saphenous vein and pass two ligatures under the vein (Figure 39–31B)
▶ ligate the distal aspect of the vein, leaving the suture ends long to provide traction (Figure 39–31C)
▶ using a #11 blade scalpel, make a transverse incision through one-half of the width of the vein and gently dilate with the tip of a closed hemostat (Figure 39–31D)
▶ insert the cannula (beveled IV extension tubing or 14-gauge angiocath) about 4 cm into the vein (Figure 39–31E)
▶ tie the proximal ligature snugly around the catheterized vein
▶ secure the IV tubing by taping to the skin and wrapping it once around the great toe (Figure 39–31F)
▶ close the skin with a suture and apply a sterile dressing

Saphenous Cut-Down (Groin)

Procedure

▶ make a transverse skin incision from where the scrotum or labial fold meets the medial aspect of the thigh to 6 cm laterally (Figure 39–32)

▶ bluntly dissect and isolate the saphenous vein, which is superficial and medial to the femoral artery and vein

   ▶ lies at the point where the transverse incision meets a line drawn directly inferior from the lateral edge of the hair of the mons pubis

▶ pass two ligatures under the vein

▶ using a #11 blade scalpel, make a transverse incision through one-half of the width of the vein

▶ insert the cannula (beveled IV extension tubing or 14-gauge angiocath) into the vein

▶ tie off both the proximal ligature around the catheterized vein and the distal ligature

▶ secure the IV tubing by taping to the skin

▶ close the skin with a suture

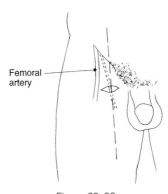

Femoral
artery

Figure 39–32

Intraosseous

Needles

▶ intraosseus (IO) needle (e.g., Dieckmann Modification, Cook Critical Care)
▶ short 18-gauge spinal needle with stylet

Procedure (Figure 39–33)

▶ insertion site prepared with betadine and anesthetized
  ▶ usually in the midline of the flat surface of the anterior tibia (if uninjured) 2 cm below the tibial tuberosity
  ▶ alternatively, can use the distal anterior femur
▶ direct needle at 60° away from the epiphyseal plate
▶ entry into the marrow is signified by sudden decrease in resistance
▶ remove the stylet and aspirate for bone marrow, which confirms placement in the medullary cavity
▶ infuse fluid
▶ tape in place

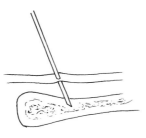

Figure 39–33

Complications

▶ needle forced completely through bone
▶ incomplete bone penetration
▶ fluid extravasation from previous puncture sites after multiple attempts
▶ osteomyelitis

Needle Thoracostomy

Equipment

▶ long, large-bore over-the-needle catheter

▶ 5–10-ml syringe
▶ flutter valve
  ▶ commercial device or use fingertip of a sterile glove to create one

Procedure

▶ place the catheter in the second intercostal space in the midclavicular line whenever a tension pneumothorax is suspected
  ▶ often done bilaterally in patients with pulseless electrical activity, which could be due to tension pneumothorax
▶ if placement is met by a sudden rush of air, pneumothorax is confirmed
▶ if the patient's hemodynamic status improves suddenly, tension pneumothorax is confirmed
▶ in viable patients, follow needle thoracostomy with a tube thoracostomy on the same side

Tube Thoracostomy

Equipment

▶ chest tube size
  ▶ for hemothorax in adults
    ▶ use large tube (36–40 Fr) to prevent blood from coagulating within the tube
  ▶ for a simple pneumothorax in adults
    ▶ use a smaller caliber (22–24 Fr)
  ▶ for hemothorax in children and infants use quadruple the estimated endotracheal tube size
    ▶ equivalent to 16 + age
▶ scalpel with #10 blade
▶ large curved clamp
▶ large straight clamp
▶ scissors
▶ 2–0 silk sutures

Procedure

▶ position the patient with the head of the bed elevated 30–60° (if possible) and the ipsilateral arm above the head
▶ prepare the area with betadine and anesthetize the skin and deeper structures with lidocaine
  ▶ intercostal nerve blocks above and below tube sites provide excellent anesthesia
  ▶ local anesthetic injected into parietal pleura makes the most painful part of procedure more tolerable
▶ cut the proximal end of the chest tube transversely and clamp

▶ make a 2–4 cm incision along the 5th or 6th rib just anterior from the mid axillary line (Figure 39–34)
▶ insert a curved clamp or scissors and tunnel upward
▶ enter the thorax in the 4th or 5th intercostal space between the lateral border of the pectoralis major and the medial border of the latissimus dorsi
▶ the pleural cavity is entered by puncturing through the intercostal muscles and parietal pleura superiorly over the rib to avoid the neurovascular bundle below each rib (Figure 39–34B)
  ▸ strong force is required but must be controlled to prevent an iatrogenic pulmonary injury
  ▸ trocar devices are not used since they are associated with serious pulmonary injuries in patients with pleural adhesions, which occur in up to 25% of the population

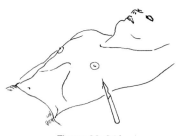

Figure 39–34A

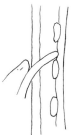

Figure 39–34B

▶ insert a gloved finger into thoracic cavity and perform a digital examination (Figure 39–34C)
  ▸ confirm correct location of underlying structures
  ▸ feel for adhesions
  ▸ break up hematomas
▶ using a finger as a guide or with a curved clamp on the end of the chest tube, insert the chest tube past its last hole into the thoracic cavity (Figure 39–34D)

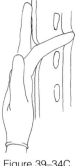

Figure 39–34C

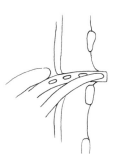

Figure 39–34D

▶ the tube should be gently directed as far posteriorly as possible in the pleural space
▶ attach the chest tube to a suction device
▶ secure the tube to the skin, placing a suture through the skin and wrapping the long ends around the chest tube multiple times in opposite directions and tying a knot (Figure 39–34E)
▶ cover the site with Vaseline gauze and bandage
▶ after the procedure, confirm lung reexpansion and adequate evacuation of a hemothorax with CXR

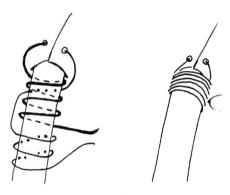

Figure 39–34E

Complications

▶ infection
▶ bleeding
  ▶ intercostal vessel laceration
  ▶ pulmonary vessel injury
  ▶ local incision hematoma
▶ injury to abdominal organs
  ▶ spleen
  ▶ liver
▶ incorrect tube placement
  ▶ subcutaneous placement
  ▶ extraparietal placement
  ▶ kinked tube

Autotransfusion

▶ place 100 ml of citrate solution in a collecting bag
▶ after blood fills up the bag, detach from the chest tube, connect to blood tubing, and infuse
▶ 4 h limit to the use of blood that is draining from thorax

Pericardiocentesis

Equipment

▶ local anesthesia with needle and syringe
▶ betadine prep solution
▶ 50-ml syringe
▶ 18-gauge spinal needle
▶ alligator clips (optional)
▶ ECG monitor (optional)

Subxiphoid Approach (Figure 39–35)

▶ position the patient supine and, if possible, sitting at a 45° angle, which brings the heart closer to the chest wall
▶ prepare the area with betadine and drape in a sterile manner
▶ attach an 18-gauge spinal needle to a 60-ml syringe
▶ if there is cardiac activity, attach an ECG monitor V lead to the needle (optional)
▶ insert the needle in the angle between the xiphoid process and the left costal arch and direct the needle toward the left shoulder at a 30° angle to the skin
▶ continuously aspirate for blood
▶ watch the cardiac monitor for change or ventricular ectopy when the needle touches the epicardium

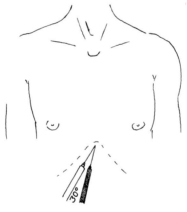

Figure 39–35

Parasternal Intercostal Approach

▶ same as subxiphoid approach except that the needle is inserted perpendicular to the skin at the 5th or 6th intercostal space just to the left of the sternum

Complications

▶ high false negative rate due to clotted blood in pericardium
▶ laceration of myocardium or coronary vessels
▶ arrhythmias
▶ pneumothorax

Thoracotomy

Equipment

▶ scalpel with #20 blade
▶ Mayo's scissors, curved
▶ rib spreaders
▶ vascular clamps
▶ needle holder
▶ 10-inch tissue forceps
▶ suture scissors
▶ 10-inch Debakey tangential occlusion clamp
▶ 2–0 silk sutures
▶ prepare the area with iodophore solution

Procedure

▶ prepare the area with betadine and drape the chest
▶ incise the skin, subcutaneous tissues, and superficial musculature along
  the 5th intercostal space from just to the right of the sternum then across
  the sternum and along the left 5th interspace to the posterior axillary line
  laterally (Figure 39–36A)
  ▶ approximated by an incision just below the left nipple in males or the
    inframammary crease in women while elevating breast tissue
▶ while momentarily pausing mechanical ventilation, identify and puncture
  the intercostal muscles at the anterior axillary line with curved Mayo's
  scissors
▶ using the Mayo's scissors, cut the intercostal muscles superiorly and then
  inferiorly using the 2nd and 3rd finger of the left hand to separate the
  pleura of the lungs from the chest wall while incising the intercostal muscles (Figure 39–36B)
▶ insert a rib spreader with the ratchet bar downward and open up the chest
  cavity (Figure 39–36C)
▶ move the lung superiorly and identify the pericardial sac
▶ perform a pericardiotomy by incising and cutting the pericardial sac lon-
  gitudinally anterior to the phrenic nerve (Figure 39–36D)
▶ evacuate pericardial blood, control bleeding, and repair any cardiac injury
  (Figure 39–36E)
▶ if indicated, begin open heart massage by compressing the ventricles between two hands or the sternum

- ▶ cross-clamp the aorta using a noncrushing vascular clamp
  - ▶ the aorta is located by sweeping the hand along the posterior thoracic wall just above the diaphragm and separated from the esophagus if possible
  - ▶ the aorta is the first structure anterior to the vertebral bodies
- ▶ cross-clamp affected pulmonary hilum to control significant pulmonary hemorrhage

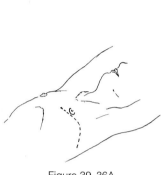

Figure 39–36A

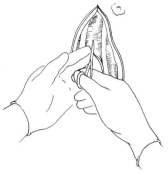

Figure 39–36B

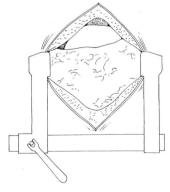

Figure 39–36C

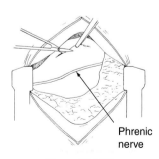

Phrenic nerve

Figure 39–36D

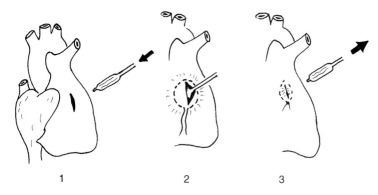

1. Urinary catheter passed through myocardial rent.

2. Urinary catheter inflated and slight tension applied to stop hemorrhage; purse-string suture placed with care not to penetrate catheter balloon.

3. Catheter deflated and removed; purse-string suture tightened and tied.

Figure 39–36E

Diagnostic Peritoneal Lavage

General Preparation

▶ place a urinary catheter and a gastric tube to decompress the bladder and stomach
▶ prepare the area with betadine and drape the abdomen
▶ anesthetize the skin at the incision puncture site down to the linea alba, using lidocaine with epinephrine for hemostasis

Equipment

▶ Seldinger-type DPL kit

Closed Technique/Infraumbilical Approach

▶ insert an 18-gauge needle attached to a 10-ml syringe 1 cm inferior to umbilicus at 60° to the skin directed caudal toward the pelvis
▶ carefully puncture into the peritoneal cavity by feeling two "pops"
  ▶ first when through linea alba
  ▶ second when through peritoneum

▶ advance 1/2 cm into the peritoneal cavity and aspirate for blood
▶ insert the guidewire and catheter using the same Seldinger technique as for vascular access (see p. 438)
▶ aspirate for blood

Open Technique/Supraumbilical Approach

▶ procedure
  ▶ requires an assistant to retract
  ▶ make a 2–3 cm vertical incision with the inferior aspect 1–2 cm above the umbilicus
  ▶ bluntly dissect to the linea alba using army–navy retractors
  ▶ incise the linea alba with the scalpel and carefully dissect down to the peritoneum
  ▶ gently elevate the peritoneum with two hemostats and incise the peritoneum (5 mm) under direct visualization (Figure 39–37A)
  ▶ insert the catheter, directing it toward the pelvis (Figure 39–37B)
  ▶ aspirate for blood
  ▶ place a purse string suture around the catheter with absorbable suture

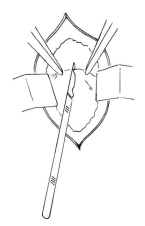
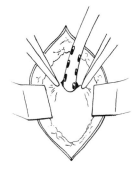

Figure 39–37A   Figure 39–37B

Lavage Procedure

▶ infuse 1 liter of warm, isotonic, sterile saline into the peritoneal cavity (10–15 ml/kg in children)
▶ gently agitate the abdomen to distribute the fluid and allow it to mix with any intraperitoneal blood
▶ toward the end of the infusion when about 50 ml is left, place the IV bag on the floor to collect the fluid (with no fluid left in the bag, the siphon effect is gone)

▶ if fluid does not return, may try the following methods to promote fluid return
  ▷ place the patient alternately in Trendelenburg and reverse Trendelenburg
  ▷ advance/withdraw the catheter until flow resumes
  ▷ infuse a second liter of fluid if still unsuccessful, and then repeat the above
▶ remove the catheter after fluid is obtained
▶ if the open technique was used, close the linea alba with 2-0 silk and close skin incision with 4-0 nylon
▶ cover the puncture/incision site with a sterile dressing
▶ send fluid for analysis

Complications

▶ bowel perforation causing peritonitis
▶ wound infection at the puncture/incision site
▶ bleeding within rectus sheath
▶ infusion of fluid into abdominal wall
▶ bladder penetration
▶ lack of fluid return (nondiagnostic study)
▶ laceration of mesenteric vessels (false positive study)

Burr Holes

Equipment

▶ hand drill, perforator, and burr bits
▶ Frazier suction catheter and self-retaining retractors
▶ scalpel with #11 blade and periosteal elevator
▶ bone currette
▶ rongeur
▶ dural hook

Location Sequence

▶ first burr hole site
  ▷ over or adjacent to any obvious fracture site on the side of a blown pupil
  ▷ if unsuccessful, proceed to second site
▶ second burr hole site
  ▷ location
    ▹ in temporal bone on the side of a blown pupil
    ▹ two finger breadths superior to the zygomatic arch
    ▹ two finger breadths posterior to frontal process of the zygoma
  ▷ evacuates middle fossa epidural hematoma (secondary to laceration of middle meningeal artery)
    ▹ where 70% of epidural hematomas are located
  ▷ if unsuccessful, proceed to third site

▶ third burr hole site
  ▶ two finger breadths superior to pinna of ear
  ▶ two finger breadths posterior to external auditory meatus
  ▶ on the side of a blown pupil

Procedure

▶ elevate head of bed to 15–20° (if possible)
▶ shave, prepare the area with betadine, and incise the scalp and periosteum
▶ clean off the bone with a periosteal elevator or the blunt end of a scalpel
▶ drill perforating hole first
  ▶ use hand drill with chisel point bit to perforate the skull (Figure 39–38)
  ▶ drill perpendicular to the skull
  ▶ clean off bone fragments and check depth of penetration periodically
  ▶ when the bit has penetrated the skull, there will be a change in turning resistance
▶ after penetration of the inner table of the skull, switch the perforator bit to the burr bit on the drill
▶ continue drilling until there is a thin rim of bone left under the burr bit
▶ scoop the remaining rim of bone out with a bone currette
▶ enlarge the hole if necessary with a rongeur
▶ check for epidural blood
  ▶ clots should be suctioned
  ▶ nonclotted blood implies continued bleeding

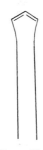

Figure 39–38

▶ if there is no epidural blood, open the dura
  ▶ insert a dural hook through outer layer of dura
  ▶ pull the dura upward and incise with #11 blade scalpel
  ▶ carefully suction out blood/blood clots
    ▶ overzealous suctioning can injure unprotected brain beneath the clot

Complications

▶ inadvertent plunge into brain with perforator or burr bit
▶ bleeding
▶ infection
▶ injury to vessels and sinuses from poor placement of burr hole

Laceration Repair

Gluing

General Principles

▶ 2-octyl cyanoacrylate (Dermabond) is commonly used
▶ appropriate in skin-only lacerations over nontension areas
▶ impractical when suturing of deeper structures is necessary
▶ do not use on or very near mucous membranes or in areas with dense hair (e.g., scalp)
▶ avoid dripping the adhesive into the eye or a mucous membrane

Technique

▶ local anesthesia is sometimes necessary for adequate cleansing and debridement
▶ dry the wound well afterward
▶ approximate the wound edges manually
▶ gently brush the adhesive over the wound edges using the applicator tip
▶ apply carefully so that a drop does not run
▶ polymerization occurs in seconds
▶ repeat brushings until at least 3 layers of adhesive have been applied

Aftercare

▶ do not apply antibiotic ointments as they dissolve the adhesive
▶ wound may get wet during daily shower but otherwise keep dry
▶ avoid rubbing or scratching the adhesive
▶ cover with bandage and change bandage daily
    ▶ do not place tape directly over the adhesive
    ▶ do not expose the wound to direct sunlight for a prolonged period
▶ adhesive sloughs in 1 week

Sutures

General Principles

▶ choose suture material according to the following guide:

Location	Skin	Deep	Removal (days)
Scalp	3.0 or 4.0 NAb	3.0 Ab if needed	7–10
Face	6.0 NAb	5.0 Ab	3–5
Inner lip	5.0 Ab	5.0 Ab	Dissolve
Outer lip	6.0 silk or 6.0 Ab	5.0 Ab	5 (silk) or Dissolve
Neck	5.0 NAb	5.0 Ab	5–7
Torso	4.0 NAb	4.0 Ab if needed	7–10
Extremity	4.0 NAb	4.0 Ab if needed	10–14
Hand or foot	5.0 NAb	Never necessary	10–14

NAb = nonabsorbable suture such as dermalon or prolene
Ab = absorbable suture such as dexon or vicryl

▶ maximum allowable time from occurrence to closure of laceration
  ▶ 8 h for torso and extremity wounds
  ▶ 24 h for facial wounds
▶ for wounds that present too late for primary closure
  ▶ may perform delayed closure 3–4 days after injury
  ▶ dress wound with sterile wet dry dressings changed daily

Wound Preparation

▶ apply betadine to skin surrounding the wound
▶ perform local anesthesia
  ▶ maximum dose of plain lidocaine = 4 mg/kg
  ▶ maximum dose of lidocaine with epinephrine = 7 mg/kg
▶ debride particulate matter from wound
▶ perform jet irrigation with 0.9NS using 18-gauge angiocath attached to 20-ml syringe for optimal force
▶ avoid instilling products within the wound that retard wound healing
  ▶ hydrogen peroxide
  ▶ betadine scrub

Suturing

▶ gently *evert* the edges of all wounds when suturing (Figure 39–39)
▶ minimize local tissue trauma during repair
▶ layered closure
  ▶ mandatory on deep facial laceration
  ▶ optimal in areas of high tension on wounds
  ▶ necessary for deep lacerations with large amount of dead space
  ▶ inappropriate in hand or foot lacerations

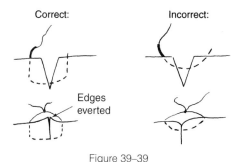

Figure 39–39

Aftercare Instructions (see p. 522)

▶ daily application of antibiotic ointment (bacitracin) prevents wound crusting but does not reduce wound infection rates
▶ leave the initial dressing in place for 24 h
▶ thereafter, wash gently with soap and water daily and reapply antibiotic ointment and dressing
▶ apply steristrips after suture removal when sutures are removed early (face) or are over high-tension areas (joints)
▶ prophylactic antibiotics for high-risk lacerations (5-day course)
  ▶ tendon, muscle, or fascia involvement
    ▶ dicloxicillin or cephalexin
  ▶ deep intraoral lacerations that are sutured
    ▶ penicillin or clindamycin
  ▶ deep human or animal bites
    ▶ amoxicillin/clavulonic acid or combination cephalexin/penicillin
▶ use sunscreen containing para-aminobenzoic acid during exposure of the wound to sun for the first 6 months post injury to prevent darkening of scar

Special Lacerations

Facial Laceration

- ▶ thoroughly irrigate facial wounds
- ▶ suture up to 24 h after the injury for improved cosmesis
- ▶ place buried deep sutures in deep facial lacerations to minimize scar formation
- ▶ vermilion border lacerations require meticulous reapproximation
  - ▶ align the vermilion border and place a single suture or mark the border prior to infiltration of local anesthesia
  - ▶ use field block when possible
  - ▶ layer closure is important if the wound extends into subcutaneous tissue or muscle
- ▶ deep tongue lacerations require double-layer repair
- ▶ periorbital
  - ▶ lid margin lacerations should be repaired by an ophthalmologist
  - ▶ suspect lacrimal duct injury with medial canthus lacerations
  - ▶ do not shave or debride eyebrow lacerations
- ▶ consult a plastic surgeon when
  - ▶ complex lacerations
  - ▶ extensive debridement required
  - ▶ avulsed skin (over 1 cm^2)
  - ▶ tissue loss of lip

Hand Lacerations

- ▶ to determine the presence of tendon and joint injuries, put the fingers through a full range of motion while inspecting the wound
- ▶ a finger tourniquet facilitates exploration and repair
  - ▶ technique
    - ▶ apply a sterile glove to the hand
    - ▶ cut finger tip of the glove and roll back to the base of the finger
    - ▶ creates both a sterile field and a tourniquet
  - ▶ remove within 20 min of application
  - ▶ excessive tourniquet pressure may cause tissue damage
- ▶ nail bed injuries
  - ▶ repair with 5-0 absorbable sutures
  - ▶ for nail avulsions, place a small section of the nail or Telfa back in nail matrix to preserve function of nail matrix

► simple subungual hematoma where the nail is firmly adherent
  ► do not need to remove nail to search for nailbed laceration
  ► drain subungual hematoma when present under the majority of the nail surface for pain control
    ► drill using an 18-gauge needle or electric cautery

Ear Lacerations

► for wounds that involve the cartilage of the pinna
  ► reapproximate cartilage using 4-0 or 5-0 absorbable sutures at major pinna landmarks
    ► incorporate perichondrium into arc of the skin sutures
    ► apply minimum tension
  ► place a well-molded dressing to the pinna that supports architectural integrity
    ► cover the laceration with bacitracin ointment and xeroform
    ► pack the crevice of the auricle with mineral-oil–soaked cotton balls
    ► apply a bulky dressing supported by head wrap

Nerve Blocks

Indications

► when used in the setting of lacerations
  ► prevent distortion of tissues from infiltration of local anesthetic
  ► allow repair large or multiple lacerations where multiple injections or large doses of local anesthetic would otherwise be required

Procedure

► identify the site of desired nerve block (see below)
► prepare the site of injection with betadine
► use 25–30-gauge needle for hand/foot/face
► use 23-gauge needle for other blocks
► insert needle and aspirate for blood to prevent intravascular injection of anesthetic
► inject anesthetic agent
► half 1% lidocaine and half 0.5% bupivacaine can be used when prolonged anesthesia is desired
► anesthetic with epinephrine can be used for all injections except those in acral areas (e.g., ears, nose, fingers, penis, toes)

Facial

Supraorbital and Supratrochlear Nerve (Figure 39–40A)

▶ locate by palpating the supraorbital ridge until the notch is identified
  ▶ where the supraorbital nerve traverses
▶ supratrochlear nerve exits just medial to supraorbital nerve
▶ inject 2–3 ml of anesthetic in the area of the notch and at a site 0.5–1.0 cm medial to the notch
▶ an alternative technique is to locally infiltrate anesthetic agent along both supraorbital ridges
  ▶ blocks all branches of supraorbital and supratrochlear nerves bilaterally

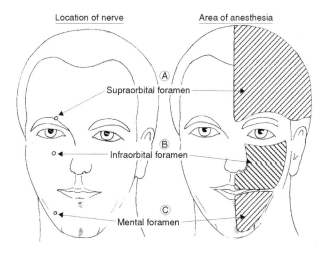

Figure 39–40

Infraorbital Nerve (Figure 39–40B)

▶ intraoral approach
  ▶ anesthetize the mucous membrane at the site of injection by placing a few drops of lidocaine on the mucous membrane just
  ▶ insert the needle at the buccogingival fold just medial to the canine tooth of the maxilla
  ▶ place a finger externally at the inferior orbital rim
  ▶ avoid needle entry into the orbit
  ▶ advance the needle toward the infraorbital foramen
    ▶ do not enter the foramen
    ▶ injection in area of the foramen will provide sufficient anesthesia
  ▶ aspirate, then inject 1–2 ml of anesthetic

▶ extraoral approach
  ▷ palpate a notch in the infraorbital rim
  ▷ insert the needle perpendicular to the skin 0.5 cm inferior to the notch in the area of the infraorbital foramen
  ▷ aspirate, then inject 1–2 ml of anesthetic

Mental Nerve (Figure 39–40C)

▶ intraoral approach
  ▷ anesthetize the mucous membrane at site of injection
  ▷ insert the needle at the level of the inferior canine and direct toward the mental foramen, which lies directly below the level of the second premolar
  ▷ aspirate, then inject 2 ml of anesthetic
▶ extraoral approach
  ▷ locate the area of the mental foramen
  ▷ insert the needle perpendicular to the skin
  ▷ advance to the bone
  ▷ aspirate, then inject 3 ml of anesthetic

Auricular Area (Figure 39–41)

▶ infiltrate 5–10 ml of local anesthetic along the entire base of the ear in circumferential fashion

Intercostal Nerve Blocks (Figure 39–42)

▶ perform block midway between the posterior axillary line and the midaxillary line or just lateral to the lateral border of the erector spinae muscles
▶ insert the needle perpendicular to the skin at the lower portion of the rib
▶ advance the needle until it strikes the rib

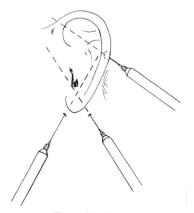

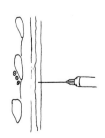

Figure 39–41   Figure 39–42

► carefully "walk" the needle down inferiorly until it slips off the inferior margin of the rib
► advance the needle 3 mm
► inject 2–5 ml of anesthetic (half 1% lidocaine, half 0.5% bupivacaine)
► repeat on the adjacent ribs superiorly and inferiorly to provide anesthesia for affected rib(s)

Upper Extremity

Thumb (Figure 39–43)

► insert the needle at the midline of proximal, palmar thumb crease
► advance through soft tissue and direct the needle to both the radial and ulnar aspects of the thumb
► deposit 1–2 ml of anesthetic on each side
► in addition, raise a wheel along dorsal aspect of the proximal thumb

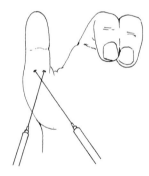 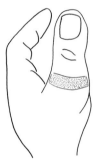

Figure 39–43

Fingers (Figure 39–44)

► many techniques are available but the one described below is recommended
  ► insert the needle perpendicular to the skin on the palmar aspect at the midline of the digit at the level of the MCP joint
  ► advance through soft tissue and direct the needle to both the radial and ulnar aspects of metacarpal head without withdrawing the needle
► deposit 1–2 ml of anesthetic on each side

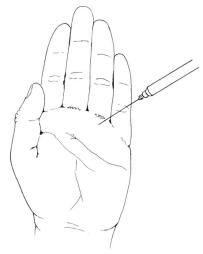

Figure 39–44

Wrist Block

▶ hand sensation distribution depicted in Figure 39–45

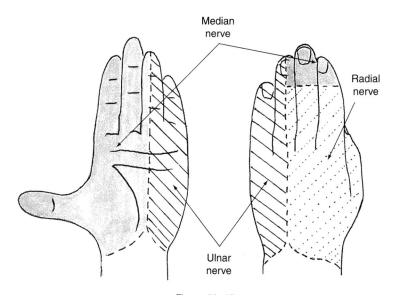

Figure 39–45

▶ radial nerve block (Figure 39–46)
  ▶ inject anesthetic subcutaneously in a band extending from the volar aspect of the radial styloid extending to the dorsal aspect of the wrist to block the branches of the radial nerve

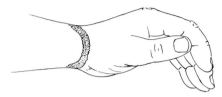

Figure 39–46

▶ median nerve block (Figure 39–47)
  ▶ locate the palmaris longus tendon by opposing the thumb and 5th finger and palpating at the wrist (absent in 10–15%)
  ▶ locate the flexor carpi radialis (FCR) by flexing the wrist with radial deviation
  ▶ insert the needle perpendicular to the skin between the palmaris longus and FCR tendons at the proximal aspect of the proximal skin crease
  ▶ advance the needle through the flexor retinaculum (resistance felt)
  ▶ advance an additional 5 mm
  ▶ if paresthesias are elicited, inject 2 ml of anesthetic agent
  ▶ if no paresthesias are elicited, inject 5 ml of anesthetic agent
▶ ulnar nerve block (Figure 39–48)
  ▶ locate the flexor carpi ulnaris (FCU) tendon by palpating the pisiform while flexing the wrist
  ▶ insert the needle perpendicular to the skin on the radial side of the FCU at the level of the proximal skin crease

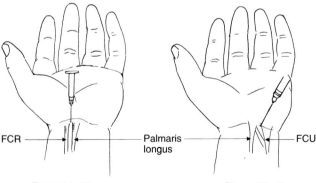

Figure 39–47   Figure 39–48

- ▶ direct needle under the FCU but not through flexor retinaculum
- ▶ inject 2 ml of anesthetic to block the volar branches
- ▶ block the dorsal branches of the nerve by thorough subcutaneous infiltration of anesthetic (5–10 ml) from lateral border of the FCU to the dorsal midline (Figure 39–49)

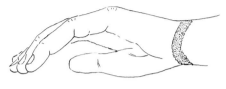

Figure 39–49

Anesthesia of Plantar Aspect of Foot

▶ perform both sural and posterior tibial nerve blocks (Figure 39–50)

Sural Nerve Block

- ▶ introduce the needle just lateral to the Achilles tendon, 1 cm superior to the lateral malleolus, directed 1 cm above the distal fibula
- ▶ infiltrate a band of 3–5 ml of anesthetic between the Achilles tendon and the lateral malleolus

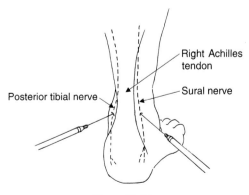

Figure 39–50

Posterior Tibial Nerve Block

▶ palpate the posterior tibial artery
▶ the posterior tibial nerve is adjacent to the artery and lies lateral and deep to the artery
▶ insert the needle perpendicular to the skin medial to the Achilles tendon at the level of the upper border of the medial malleolus
▶ direct the needle lateral to the artery and advance until it touches the tibia
▶ if paresthesias are elicited with medial lateral motion of the needle, inject 5 ml of anesthetic
▶ if no paresthesias are elicited, inject 10 ml of anesthetic while in deep space and while withdrawing the needle

Compartment Pressure Measurement

Needle-Manometer Technique

▶ materials
  ▶ 18-gauge needle
  ▶ 20-ml syringe
  ▶ three-way stopcock
  ▶ IV extension tubing (2)
  ▶ normal saline
▶ setup
  ▶ place the needle on the first IV extension tubing
  ▶ attach opposite end of the IV extension tubing to the three-way stopcock
  ▶ attach the syringe to the stopcock
  ▶ attach the second IV extension tubing to the stopcock and then to a BP manometer
▶ technique
  ▶ close the stopcock to the manometer
  ▶ aspirate sterile normal saline halfway up the first extension tubing
  ▶ close the first extension tubing
  ▶ remove the syringe from the stopcock and place 20 ml of air in the syringe
  ▶ place the syringe back on the stopcock
  ▶ insert the needle into the compartment using sterile technique
  ▶ turn the stopcock to create an open system between three attachments
  ▶ push down the syringe plunger to increase pressure in the system
  ▶ as the air/fluid meniscus begins to move, read the pressure on the manometer (this is the tissue pressure)
    ▶ the pressure normally is under 20 mm Hg

Splinting Techniques

Hairpin/Distal Phalanx Splinting (Figure 39–51)

▶ DIP in full extension
▶ splint distal to PIP

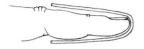

Figure 39–51

Dynamic Splint (Figure 39–52)

▶ after placing a thin layer of padding in between, "buddy tape" the affected digit to the normal adjacent digit to provide stability

Volar Finger Splint (Figure 39–53)

▶ aluminum splint placed along the volar aspect of the affected finger, extending to the distal forearm
▶ joint position
  ▶ DIP at 10° flexion
  ▶ PIP at 15° flexion
  ▶ MCP at 70° flexion
▶ may wrap the splint around the end of the finger and have volar and dorsal splint to provide better protection

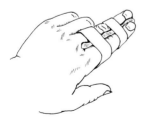
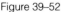
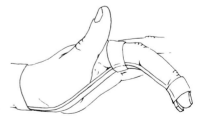

Figure 39–52   Figure 39–53

Volar Short Arm Splint (Figure 39–54)

▶ plaster strip placed along the volar aspect of the forearm, wrist, and hand
▶ PIP and DIP flexed at 15–30°
▶ MCP flexed at 70°

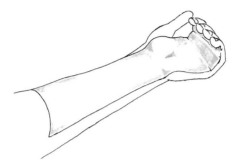

Figure 39–54

Thumb Spica Splint (Figure 39–55)

▶ wide plaster strip placed along the radial aspect of the forearm, extending to the hand and immobilizing the thumb
▶ thumb should be in same position as when holding a can of soda
▶ wrist and thumb should be immobile

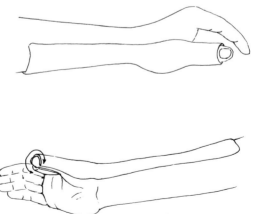

Figure 39–55

Long Arm Splint (Figure 39–56)

▶ plaster strip placed along the ulnar aspect of the forearm from the wrist, extending to the proximal posterior humerus

▶ use a sling to support the splint

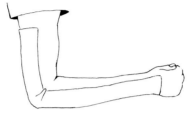

Figure 39–56

Coaptation Splint (Figure 39–57)

▶ plaster strip placed on the superior aspect of the shoulder, extending along the lateral aspect of the humerus under 90° flexed elbow and up along medial aspect of humerus to axilla

▶ use splint to support forearm

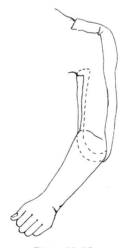

Figure 39–57

Kenny Howard Shoulder Harness

▶ immobilizes the shoulder

Sling and Swathe (Figure 39–58)

► immobilizes elbow and shoulder

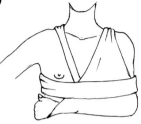

Figure 39–58

Clavicular Strap (Figure 39–59)

► "figure of 8" method stabilizes the clavicle
► tighten to maintain good reduction of fracture fragments

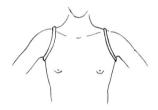 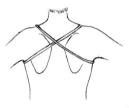

Figure 39–59

Short Leg Posterior Splint (Figure 39–60)

► plaster strip placed along the posterior leg distal to the knee, extending to the plantar aspect of the foot
► ankle should be at 90° flexion

Jones Dressing

► stabilizes the knee or ankle
► place several layers of padding over the affected joint
► follow with an elastic compression dressing

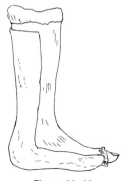

Figure 39–60

40

Radiograph Interpretation

Cervical Spine

Lateral View

General Principles

▶ ensure visualization of all cervical vertebrae as well as the atlanto-occipital and C7–T1 articulations (Figure 40–1)
  ▶ techniques to improve the ability to demonstrate the C7–T1 level
    ▻ increase penetration
    ▻ pull the shoulders down
    ▻ obtain "swimmer's" view
    ▻ trauma obliques
    ▻ CT (when the above techniques fail)
▶ proceed according to the following "ABCs" mnemonic (alignments, bones, cartilage)

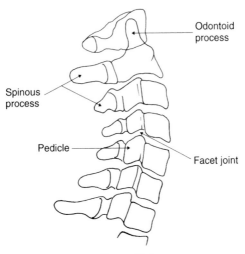

Figure 40–1

Alignments (Figure 40–2)

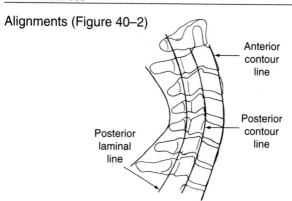

Figure 40–2

- ▶ anterior contour line
  - ▶ anterior margin of vertebral bodies should match within 1 mm
  - ▶ pseudosubluxation up to 3 mm is often seen in children at C2–C3 and C3–C4 levels
- ▶ posterior contour line
  - ▶ posterior margin of vertebral bodies
- ▶ spinolaminal line
  - ▶ bases of spinous processes
- ▶ posterior aspect of spinous processes
- ▶ posterior laminal line (Figure 40–3)
  - ▶ C1 and C3 should line up within 2 mm of the base of the C2 spinous process

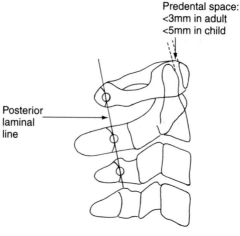

Figure 40–3

▶ the predental space between posterior aspect of C1 and anterior aspect of the odontoid (Figure 40–3) should be
  ▸ under 3 mm in adult
  ▸ under 5 mm in child
▶ vertical basion–dens distance under 12 mm
  ▸ distance from tip of dens to base of skull

Bony Integrity

▶ vertebral bodies
▶ facet joints
▶ posterior spinous processes
▶ odontoid peg

Cartilage (Intervertebral Disks)

▶ uniform height

Soft Tissue (Figure 40–4)

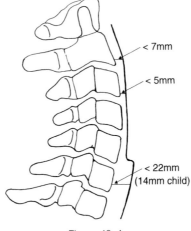

< 7mm

< 5mm

< 22mm
(14mm child)

Figure 40–4

▶ swelling, especially in the prevertebral space
▶ normal configuration
▶ prevertebral space should run parallel to the anterior vertebrae from C2 to C4
▶ standard widths for adults
  ▸ in front of C2, under 7 mm
  ▸ in front of C3–C4, under 5 mm
  ▸ in front of C6, under 22 mm

- standard widths for children
    - in front of C3–C4, under 2/3 of width of C2 body
    - in front of C6, under 14 mm
- check for local bulges
- swelling occurs in approximately 50% of bony injuries
- investigate for ligamentous injuries if soft tissue swelling is present without bony injury

AP View

- inspect spinous processes
    - should lie in a straight line (Figure 40–5)
    - malalignment may indicate a unilateral facet dislocation (Figure 40–6)
    - single spinous process out of alignment may indicate a fracture
- check interspinous process distance
    - distance between the spinous processes should be equal
    - no single space should be 50% wider than the one immediately above or below
        - unless the neck is held in flexion from spasm
    - abnormal widening of an interspinous space is indicative of an anterior cervical dislocation (Figure 40–7)
    - malalignment occurs with fractures and bilateral facet dislocations
- check pedicles
    - appear as upright ovals
    - look for fractures through these structures
- look at intervertebral disk spaces
    - should be equal
- check the vertebral bodies for fractures
- inspect the upper chest for rib fractures and pneumothoraces

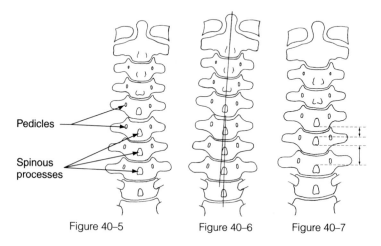

Pedicles

Spinous processes

Figure 40–5   Figure 40–6   Figure 40–7

Odontoid (Open Mouth) View

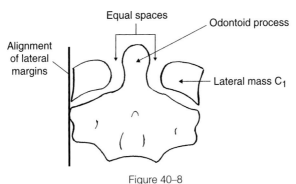

Figure 40–8

▶ check alignment (Figure 40–8)
  ▶ lateral margins of C1 should align with the lateral margins of C2
  ▶ space on each side of the odontoid should be equal
    ▸ slight rotation of the neck may cause these spaces to appear as unequal
    ▸ lateral margins of C1 and C2 should remain normally aligned if unequal spaces are due to rotation
▶ inspect the odontoid and the rest of C2 for fractures
  ▶ overlying shadows may cause artifact (called Mach effect) due to superimposition of
    ▸ arch of C1
    ▸ incisor teeth
    ▸ occiput
    ▸ soft tissues at the nape of the neck
▶ submental (or closed-mouth) view for uncooperative patients

Oblique Views

▶ general principles
  ▶ trauma oblique views are performed with the neck immobilized
    ▸ order when the three-view series is suspicious of fracture or locked facets
▶ check for "shingles on the roof" appearance of overlapping laminae (Figure 40–9)
  ▶ disruption suggestive of facet dislocation
▶ lamina appears as an intact ellipse posteriorly
  ▶ scrutinize for fractures
▶ interlaminar distance should be equal
  ▶ increased distance suggestive of subluxation

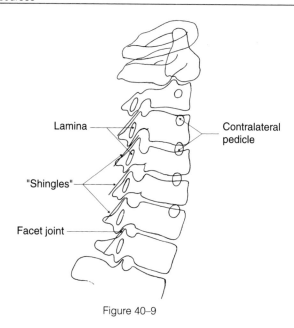

Figure 40–9

Flexion–Extension Views

► general principles
  ► perform if plain radiographs are normal but there is a high suspicion of ligamentous injury
    ► focal posterior midline cervical spine tenderness
    ► severe cervical pain
  ► patient must be sober, cooperative, and neurologically intact
  ► patient moves neck independently for positioning and stops if increased pain, paresthesias, or neurologic signs develop
► check for interruption of contour lines or widening of interspinous spaces on lateral view

Thoracic Spine

Lateral View

► use the mnemonic "ABC"
  ► alignment
  ► bones
  ► cartilage
► visualize all thoracic vertebrae
  ► swimmer's view is needed for upper thoracic vertebrae

▶ check the alignment of the vertebral bodies
  ▶ anterior margins line up within 1 mm
  ▶ posterior margins line up within 1 mm
  ▶ disruption of posterior line demonstrates encroachment of bony fragments on spinal canal
▶ inspect bones for fractures
  ▶ vertebral bodies are the same height both anteriorly and posteriorly
  ▶ posterior margin of each vertebral body is slightly concave
  ▶ check the posterior elements
▶ cartilage—check intravertebral disk spaces, which should be equal

AP View

▶ visualize all 12 vertebrae and evaluate in terms of (Figure 40–10)
  ▶ symmetry
  ▶ height
  ▶ contour
  ▶ cortices
▶ spinous processes
  ▶ alignment
  ▶ interspinous distance between vertebrae above and below
  ▶ breaks in the cortex indicate fracture
▶ pedicles
  ▶ check for continuity of the oval cortex of the pedicles
    ▶ break in the cortex indicates fracture of the pedicle
  ▶ abnormal widening of the interpedicle distance of a vertebra may indicate disruption of posterior elements
▶ paraspinal line should be closely applied to the vertebral bodies
  ▶ widening indicates hematoma resulting from a fracture (Figure 40–11)
▶ inspect
  ▶ posterior portions of ribs
  ▶ transverse processes
  ▶ costovertebral junctions

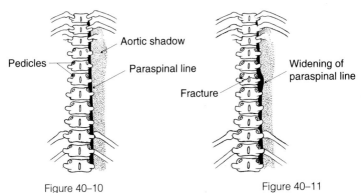

Pedicles

Aortic shadow

Paraspinal line

Fracture

Widening of paraspinal line

Figure 40–10

Figure 40–11

Lumbar Spine

Lateral View (Figure 40–12)

▶ visualize L1–L5 in addition to T11 and T12
▶ use the mnemonic "ABC"
  ▶ alignment
  ▶ bones
  ▶ cartilage
▶ check the alignment of the vertebral bodies
  ▶ anterior margins line up within 1 mm
  ▶ posterior margins line up within 1 mm
  ▶ disruption of posterior line demonstrates encroachment of bony fragments on spinal canal
▶ bones
  ▶ vertebral bodies are the same height both anteriorly and posteriorly
  ▶ posterior margin of each vertebral body is slightly concave
  ▶ check the posterior elements
▶ cartilage
  ▶ intervertebral disk spaces should be equal

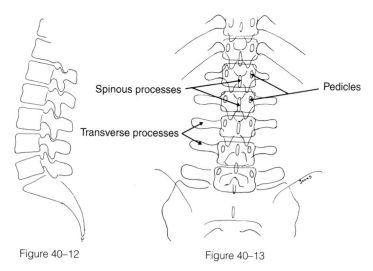

Spinous processes

Pedicles

Transverse processes

Figure 40–12

Figure 40–13

AP View (Figure 40–13)

▶ visualize all five vertebrae—evaluate in terms of
  ▶ symmetry
  ▶ height
  ▶ contour
  ▶ cortices

- ▶ spinous process
  - ▶ check alignment
  - ▶ check interspinous distance between vertebrae above and below
  - ▶ break in the cortex indicates fracture
- ▶ pedicles
  - ▶ check for continuity of oval cortex
    - ▹ break in the cortex indicates fracture
  - ▶ the distance between the pedicles of each vertebra becomes gradually wider from L1 to L5
    - ▹ abnormal widening may indicate disruption of posterior elements
- ▶ scrutinize the vertebral bodies and transverse processes for fractures
- ▶ check the lower ribs and sacroiliac areas for fractures
- ▶ localized ileus may be associated with lumbar spine trauma

Chest

AP or PA View

- ▶ trachea
  - ▶ midline location
- ▶ mediastinum
  - ▶ supine AP gives false impression of widening
    - ▹ under 8 cm is normal
  - ▶ upright PA better estimates mediastinal width
    - ▹ under 6 cm is normal
    - ▹ 6–10 cm is equivocal
    - ▹ over 10 cm is abnormal
  - ▶ aortic knob
  - ▶ nasogastric tube displacement
  - ▶ pneumomediastinum due to
    - ▹ pneumothorax
    - ▹ tracheal/bronchial injury
    - ▹ esophageal disruption
  - ▶ heart size and shape
- ▶ thoracic spine
  - ▶ fracture
  - ▶ displacement
- ▶ lung fields
  - ▶ pneumothorax
  - ▶ hemothorax
  - ▶ pulmonary contusion
- ▶ costophrenic angles
  - ▶ should be sharp in upright patient
    - ▹ blunting indicates fluid
- ▶ hemidiaphragm
  - ▶ distinct
  - ▶ appropriately curved
  - ▶ right slightly higher than left
  - ▶ look for free intraperitoneal air

▶ ribs
  ▶ fractures
  ▶ displacement
  ▶ upper rib fractures (first three)
    ▹ due to major force
    ▹ associated with vascular injury
  ▶ lower rib fractures (last three)
    ▹ associated with splenic, hepatic, and renal injuries
    ▹ not well visualized
    ▹ rib radiographs better demonstrate fractures
▶ soft tissue
  ▶ subcutaneous emphysema, which suggests pneumothorax
  ▶ foreign body

Lateral View

▶ sternal fracture
▶ thoracic spine fracture
▶ hemothorax
▶ pulmonary contusion
▶ pneumomediastinum

Pelvis

AP Pelvis (Figure 40–14)

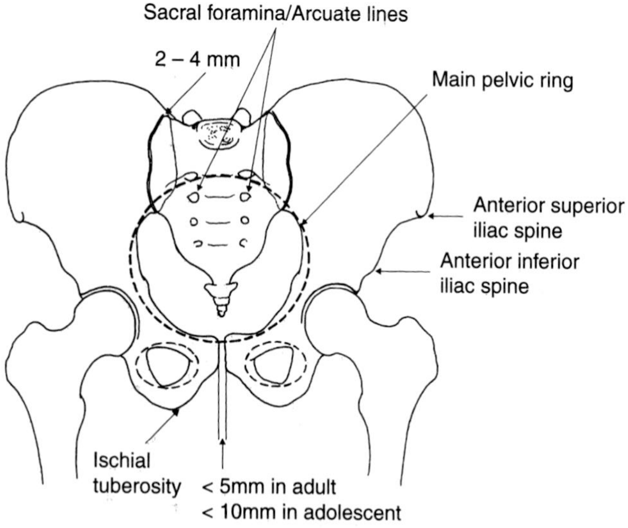

Figure 40–14

▶ look for symmetry of the hemipelves
▶ scrutinize the three pelvic rings for fractures
  ▶ main pelvic ring
  ▶ two smaller rings formed by pubic and ischial bones
▶ sacroiliac joints
  ▶ normal width is 2–4 mm
  ▶ widths should be equivalent bilaterally
  ▶ scrutinize the inferior aspect of the joint for displacement
  ▶ fracture of the 5th lumbar transverse process often accompanies a sacroiliac joint disruption
▶ pubic symphysis
  ▶ superior surfaces of pubic rami should align
    ▹ offset over 2 mm indicates disruption
  ▶ normal width of joint
    ▹ under 5 mm in adult
    ▹ up to 10 mm in adolescent
▶ sacral foramina
  ▶ fractures are difficult to detect due to overlying gas and stool
  ▶ arcuate lines should be complete and symmetric
  ▶ disruption of the arcuate lines indicates a sacral fracture
▶ acetabulum
  ▶ compare each side for symmetry
  ▶ check for fractures/abnormalities
    ▹ often difficult to detect fractures
    ▹ obtain Judet and inlet/outlet views or CT when there is any clinical suspicion
▶ hip
  ▶ check the femoral head, femoral neck, and intertrochanteric region for fractures
  ▶ osteopenic bones in older patients hide fractures
    ▹ bone scan, MRI, or CT may be needed to diagnose fracture
▶ sites for avulsion fractures (see Figure 16–1, p. 217)
  ▶ anterior superior iliac spine (rectus femoris)
  ▶ anterior inferior iliac spine (sartorius)
  ▶ ischial tuberosity (adductor magnus)
▶ fractures
  ▶ a break at one point in a ring assumes a second break in the ring is present
  ▶ a widened sacroiliac joint or pubic symphysis represents a break of the main ring

Additional Views

▶ Judet
  ▶ 45° internal and external oblique
  ▶ better demonstrates acetabular fractures
▶ inlet
  ▶ 25–40° caudad angulation
  ▶ better demonstrates the pelvic rim

▶ outlet
  ▶ 35° cephalad angulation
  ▶ better demonstrates the posterior acetabular rim and inferior pubic rami
▶ CT
  ▶ demonstrates fractures and associated retroperitoneal hematomas

Face

Standard Views (Figure 40–15)

 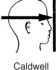 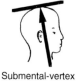 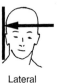

Waters'   Caldwell   Submental-vertex   Lateral

Figure 40–15

Waters' View

▶ most useful view in facial series
▶ demonstrates greatest number of fractures
▶ structures identified (Figure 40–16)
  ▶ zygoma and zygomatic arches
  ▶ orbital rim
  ▶ arch of nasal bone
  ▶ nasal septum
  ▶ maxillary and frontal sinuses where blood appears as an air–fluid level
    when the patient is upright or diffuse haziness when the patient is supine

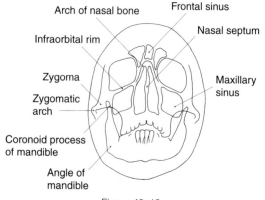

Figure 40–16

► reading system using the three lines of McGrigor (Figure 40–17)
  ► line A
    ▹ trace through the zygomatic–frontal suture across the superior orbital margin and frontal sinus and continue to the other side
    ▹ search for fractures, widening of the zygomatic–frontal suture, and fluid in the frontal sinus
  ► line B
    ▹ trace through the superior border of the zygomatic arch, across the body of the zygoma, continue through the inferior margin of the orbit and along the contour of the nose, and continue to the other side
    ▹ search for fracture of the zygomatic arch (disruption of the "elephant's trunk"—Figure 40–18), fracture through the inferior rim of orbit, presence of teardrop in the roof of the maxillary antrum representing herniating orbital contents in a blow-out fracture, depression/asymmetry of the nasal contour

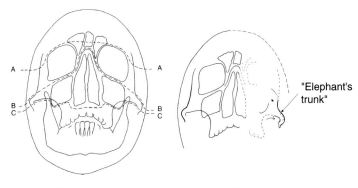

Figure 40–17   Figure 40–18

  ► line C
    ▹ trace along the inferior margin of the zygomatic arch, down the maxillary antrum, along the inferior margin of the antrum and across the maxilla, including the roots of the teeth, and continue to the other side
    ▹ search for fractures of the zygoma and maxillary antrum, and a fluid level in the maxillary antrum

Lateral View

► best view to demonstrate fractures of frontal sinus
  ► scrutinize the anterior and posterior walls
  ► fracture of the posterior wall serves as a portal for CSF infection
► difficult to interpret because of superimposition of bilateral structures

► scrutinize the anterior and posterior walls of maxilla for fractures
► check for air–fluid levels in sinuses
  ► sphenoid
  ► maxillary
  ► frontal
  ► ethmoid

Caldwell's View (Figure 40–19)

► best demonstrates fracture of the superior/lateral orbital rim
► check the orbital rim for fractures
► check for air–fluid levels in the sinuses
  ► frontal
  ► ethmoid sinuses

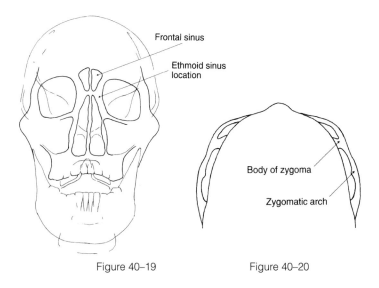

Figure 40–19   Figure 40–20

Submental–Vertex View (Figure 40–20)

► best view to identify zygomatic arch fracture
► obtain when significant pain, tenderness or deformity are present over the zygomatic arches
► check the zygomatic arches for fracture and depression

Common Fractures

Orbital Floor ("Blow-Out") Fracture

▶ mechanism
  ▶ increased intraorbital pressure causes a fracture of the orbital floor or less commonly the medial orbital wall, which are the weakest parts of the orbit
  ▶ orbital contents may herniate downwards through the orbital floor
▶ radiographic appearance on Waters' view (Figure 40–21)
  ▶ soft tissue "teardrop sign" in the roof of the maxillary sinus
  ▶ orbital emphysema
  ▶ fluid in maxillary sinus
  ▶ fractures of inferior or medial orbit are difficult to visualize

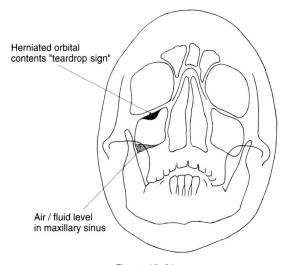

Herniated orbital contents "teardrop sign"

Air / fluid level in maxillary sinus

Figure 40–21

Tripod Fracture

▶ three-part fracture (Figure 40–22)
  ▶ widening of zygomatico-frontal suture
  ▶ widening of zygomatico-temporal suture
  ▶ fracture through the body of the zygoma or through the anterolateral wall of the maxillary sinus

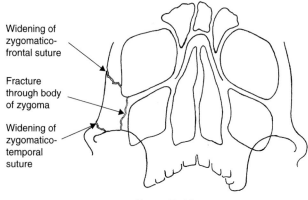

Widening of
zygomatico-
frontal suture

Fracture
through body
of zygoma

Widening of
zygomatico-
temporal
suture

Figure 40–22

Hand

PA/Oblique Views

▶ search carefully for fractures/dislocations
  ▶ distance between the carpometacarpal joints should be 1–2 mm
  ▶ scrutinize all joint lines for subtle fractures

Lateral View

▶ search for fractures/dislocations
▶ look for the degree of anterior angulation in metacarpal fractures

Common Fractures/Dislocations

Bennett's Fracture (see Figure 19–13, p.254)

▶ oblique avulsion fracture of the base of the articular surface of the 1st
  metarcarpal bone with radial subluxation of the carpometacarpal joint

Boxer Fracture (see Figure 19–18, p. 258)

▶ fracture of the neck of the 5th metacarpal
▶ most common metacarpal fracture

Gamekeeper's Thumb (see Figure 19–15, p. 256)

▶ rupture of ulnar collateral ligament of the 1st MCP joint
▶ associated with avulsion fracture of the ulnar surface of the 1st proximal
  phalanx
▶ stress views aid in diagnosis

Mallet Finger (see Figure 19–3, p. 250)

▶ intraarticular avulsion fracture of the dorsal surface of the distal phalanx causing loss of full extension at DIP joint

Rolando's Fracture (see Figure 19–14, p. 255)

▶ comminuted intraarticular fracture of the base of the 1st metacarpal

Wrist

PA View (Figure 40–23)

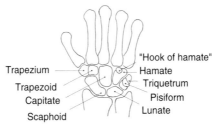

Trapezium
Trapezoid
Capitate
Scaphoid

"Hook of hamate"
Hamate
Triquetrum
Pisiform
Lunate

Figure 40–23

▶ check the alignment of the carpal bones in two rows
  ▶ look for the three carpal arcs (Figure 40–24)
    ▹ arc 1 = proximal articular margins of proximal row of carpus (scaphoid, lunate, triquetrum)
    ▹ arc 2 = distal articular margins of proximal row
    ▹ arc 3 = proximal articular margins of capitate and hamate
▶ joint spaces between the carpal bones should be 1–2 mm and uniform (Figure 40–24)
  ▶ widening suggests intercarpal subluxation
  ▶ confirm normal radial length (8–18 mm), radial inclination (14–30°)

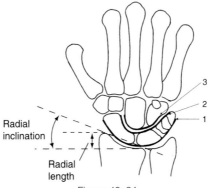

Radial
inclination

3
2
1

Radial
length

Figure 40–24

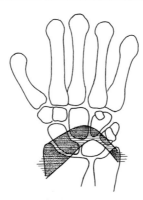

Figure 40–25

▶ carefully search for fractures and dislocations
 ▶ 90% of carpal fractures involve scaphoid
  ▹ 10% of scaphoid fractures missed on initial radiographs
  ▹ if highly suspicious of the scaphoid fracture but the initial radiograph is negative, obtain a special scaphoid view of wrist, which increases sensitivity
 ▶ most injuries of the carpus occur within the zone of vulnerability (Figure 40–25)
 ▶ check for fractures of the distal radius and ulna
▶ check for disruption of the radioulnar joint
 ▶ head of the ulna is usually 1–2 mm shorter than the radius
 ▶ head of the ulna either touches or slightly overlaps the radius at the distal radioulnar joint

Lateral View

▶ check the bone alignment
 ▶ radius, lunate and capitate articulate with each other and lie in a straight line (Figure 40–26)
 ▶ check for lunate dislocation (Figure 40–27)
  ▹ lunate dislocates anteriorly
  ▹ concavity of the lunate is empty
  ▹ radius and capitate remain in straight line
 ▶ check for perilunate dislocation (Figure 40–28)
  ▹ whole of carpus (except for lunate) is displaced posteriorly
  ▹ concavity of lunate is empty
  ▹ radius and lunate remain in a straight line
  ▹ capitate lies posteriorly
  ▹ check for accompanying scaphoid fracture

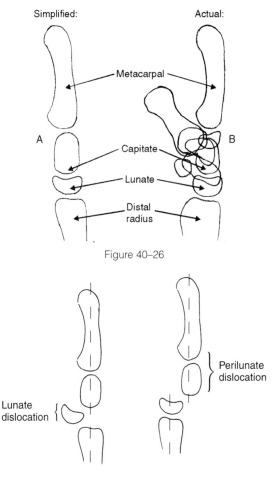

Figure 40–26

Figure 40–27   Figure 40–28

▶ check for normal volar tilt of radius (2–24°)
▶ carefully search for fractures and dislocations

Elbow

AP View

▶ trace the cortices for fractures

▶ capitellum articulates with the radial head
  ▶ check the radiocapitellar line (Figure 40–29)
    ▹ a line drawn along the center of the shaft of the proximal radius should pass through the capitellum in adults
    ▹ if the line does not pass through the capitellum, a dislocation of the radial head is suspected
▶ trochlea articulates with ulna

Lateral View

▶ examine the cortices for fractures
▶ check for anterior or posterior dislocation of the elbow
▶ check the radiocapitellar line (Figure 40–30)
  ▶ a line drawn along the center of the shaft of the proximal radius should pass
    ▹ through the capitellum in adults
    ▹ through the capitellum ossification center in children
  ▶ if the line does not pass through the capitellum, a dislocation of the radial head is suspected
  ▶ the rule is always valid on a true lateral
  ▶ Monteggia fracture/dislocation (see Figure 21–14, p. 278)
    ▹ dislocation of radial head
    ▹ fracture of proximal third of ulna

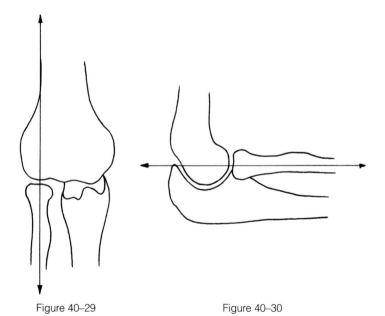

Figure 40–29   Figure 40–30

► check the anterior humeral line
  ► on a true lateral film, a line traced along the anterior cortex of the humerus should pass through the middle third of the capitellum (Figure 40–31)
  ► if less than a third of the capitellum lies anterior, check carefully for a supracondylar fracture (Figure 40–32)
  ► less reliable in young children who have only partial ossification of the capitellum

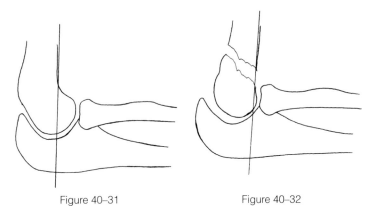

Figure 40–31   Figure 40–32

► check the two fat pads
  ► normal findings (Figure 40–33)
    ▸ situated anterior and posterior to the distal humerus
    ▸ anterior fat pad is visible on a normal true lateral radiograph
    ▸ in contact with the joint capsule
    ▸ seen as a black streak in surrounding gray soft tissues
  ► abnormal findings (Figure 40–34)
    ▸ joint effusion due to fracture displaces fat pads away from bone
    ▸ visible posterior fat pad is always indicative of an effusion since it should be hidden in the olecranon fossa
    ▸ bulging anterior fat pad is also indicative of an effusion
    ▸ absence of visible fat pad does not exclude a fracture

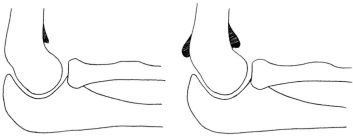

Figure 40–33   Figure 40–34

▶ with fat pad displacement but no obvious fracture, search carefully for the following fractures:
  ▶ radial head
  ▶ supracondylar (especially in children)
▶ with fat pad displacement and no visible fracture
  ▶ treat as radial head fracture and immobilize in a sling
  ▶ recheck in 10 days
▶ for children, check the location of ossification centers (Figure 40–35)
  ▶ the mnemonic "CRITOL" is used to recall the usual order in which ossification centers appear radiographically
    ▹ C = capitellum (1 year old)
    ▹ R = radial head (3–6 years old)
    ▹ I = medial (internal) epicondyle (5–7 years old)
    ▹ T = trochlea (9–10 years old)
    ▹ O = olecranon (9–10 years old)
    ▹ L = lateral (external) epicondyle (9–13 years old)

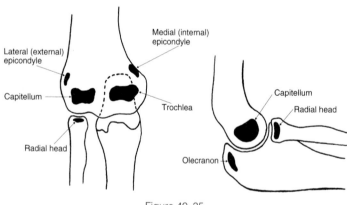

Figure 40–35

▶ check for avulsion of the medial epicondyle
  ▹ common injury due to insertion of forearm flexors
  ▹ if trochlea is ossified, should see medial epicondyle
  ▹ if medial epicondyle not visible in normal position, suspect avulsion fracture and search joint for displaced fragment
  ▹ obtain comparison views to better demonstrate abnormalities

Knee

AP View

▶ check for fractures/dislocations
  ▶ most are obvious
  ▶ scrutinize the patella, which is visualized through the head of the femur, for fractures
    ▹ check location
    ▹ high riding patella is associated with infrapatellar rupture of quadriceps tendon
  ▶ avulsion fractures of the tibial spine or femoral condyles may indicate ligamentous injury
▶ tibial plateau fractures may be difficult to visualize
  ▶ a vertical line drawn at the most lateral margin of the femur should have no more than 5 mm of adjacent tibia outside of it (Figure 40–36)
    ▹ when this rule is violated, check closely for tibial plateau fracture
    ▹ look for areas of increased bone density

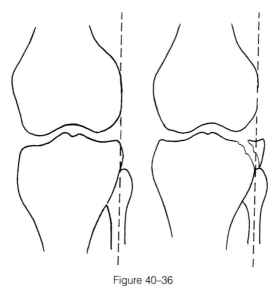

Figure 40–36

Lateral View

▶ check for fractures/dislocations
▶ search for joint effusion
  ▶ distension of suprapatellar bursa displacing patella away from femur

Sunrise View

▶ angled beam with knee flexed (Figure 40–37)
▶ obtain when suspect patellar fracture
  ▶ especially useful for nondisplaced vertical patellar fractures

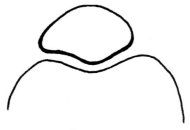

Figure 40–37

Ankle

AP View

▶ mortise joint space should be uniform
▶ check integrity of the talar dome
▶ search for fractures in the distal tibia and fibula
  ▶ if fracture is seen on one side of the joint, scrutinize the opposite side for fracture or signs of ligament rupture
  ▶ if the following injuries are present obtain radiograph of entire tibia and fibula to check for fracture of proximal fibula (Maisonneuve fracture)
    ▷ fracture of posterior lip of the distal tibia
    ▷ widening of the medial joint
    ▷ displaced fracture of the medial malleolus without fracture of the lateral malleolus or distal fibula
▶ check the base of the 5th metatarsal for an avulsion fracture

Ankle Mortise View

▶ AP view taken with 15° of internal rotation (Figure 40–38)
▶ check joint space around the talus for symmetry/disruption
▶ search for fractures of the distal tibia and fibula

Lateral View

▶ scrutinize the distal fibula for fractures through the overlying tibia
▶ check the tibial surface (especially the posterior aspect) for fractures

► check the base of 5th metatarsal for an avulsion fracture
► check other tarsal bones visualized for fractures

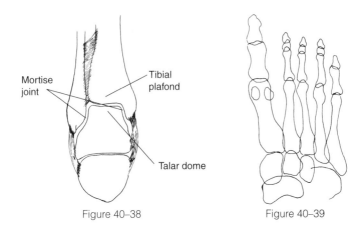

Figure 40–38   Figure 40–39

Foot

AP and Oblique Views

► scrutinize the cortical margins on all of the bones for fractures
► normal alignments of AP view (Figure 40–39)
  ► lateral margin of 1st metatarsal and lateral margin of medial cuneiform
  ► medial margin of base of 2nd metatarsal and medial margin of medial cuneiform
► normal alignments of oblique view
  ► medial margin of the base of the 3rd metatarsal and medial margin of the lateral cuneiform
  ► lateral margin of base of the 3rd metatarsal and lateral margin of the lateral cuneiform
  ► medial border of the 4th metatarsal and medial border of the cuboid bone (may be 2–3 mm offset)
► check for
  ► Lisfranc injury is a tarsometatarsal dislocation and is appreciated by one or more of the following findings
    ► fracture base of the 2nd metatarsal
    ► diastasis of the 1st and 2nd metatarsals
    ► diastasis of the middle and medial cuneiforms

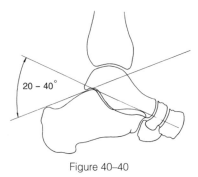

Figure 40–40

- ▶ stress fracture most commonly seen in 2nd and 3rd metatarsal
- ▶ Jones fracture
  - ▹ transverse fracture at the base of the 5th metatarsal 1.5–2 cm distal to the tarsal–metatarsal joint
- ▶ avulsion fracture base of the 5th metatarsal after inversion injury

Lateral Foot

- ▶ scrutinize the cortical margins of all bones for fractures
- ▶ check the base of the 5th metatarsal for fracture
- ▶ check the calcaneus for fractures
  - ▶ measure Boehler's angle (Figure 40–40)
    - ▹ normal angle (20–40°) does not exclude fracture
    - ▹ angle is reduced with compression fracture of calcaneus
  - ▶ additional views
    - ▹ axial view demonstrates the medial and lateral surfaces (Figure 40–41)
  - ▶ calcaneal fractures are associated with lumbar compression fractures

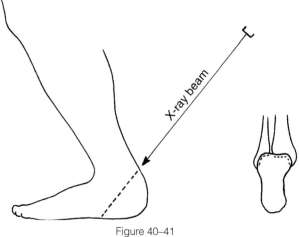

Figure 40–41

41

Radiographic Anatomy

▶ this chapter consists of illustrations depicting special radiographic studies often obtained in the setting of trauma

Angiography

Facial (Figure 41–1)

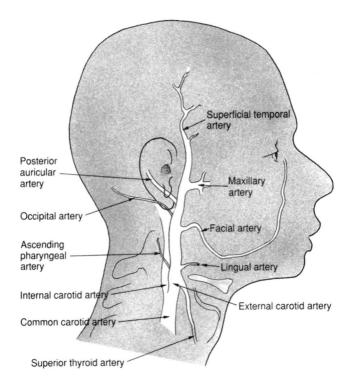

Figure 41–1

Thoracic Aorta

▶ anterior–posterior (Figure 41–2)

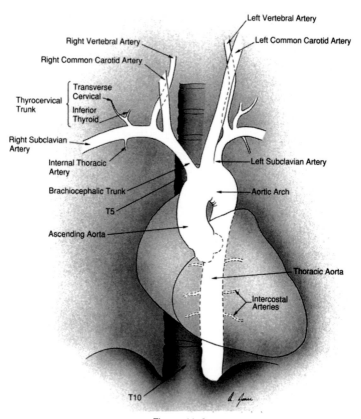

Figure 41–2

▶ lateral (Figure 41–3)

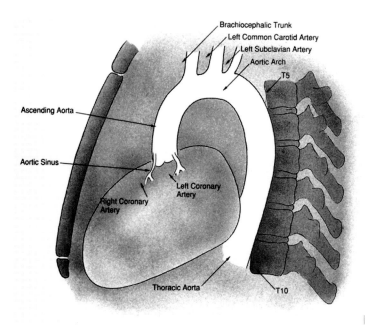

Figure 41–3

Extremity

▶ upper (Figures 41–4 and 41–5)

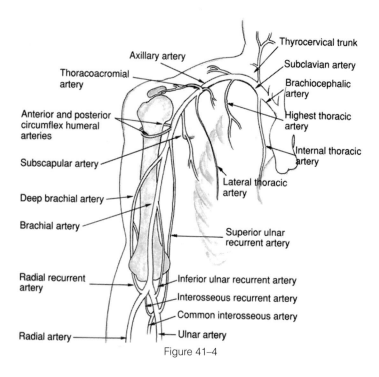

Figure 41–4

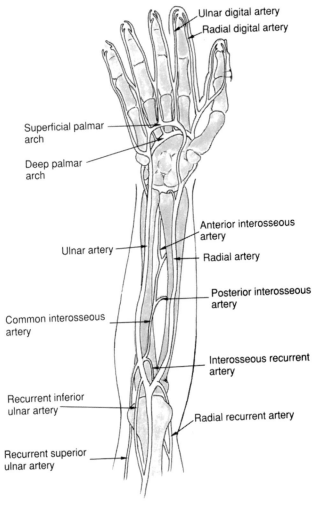

Figure 41–5

► lower (Figures 41–6 and 41–7)

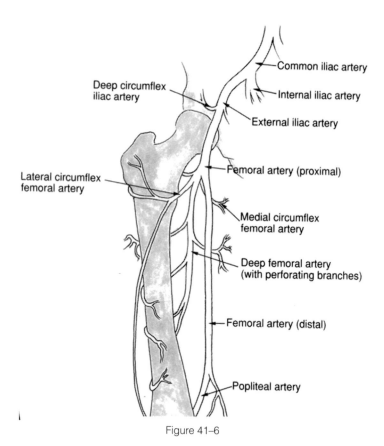

Figure 41–6

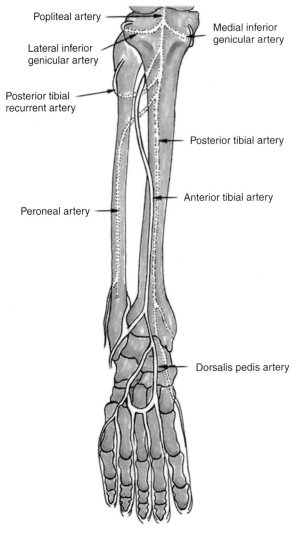

Popliteal artery

Medial inferior genicular artery

Lateral inferior genicular artery

Posterior tibial recurrent artery

Posterior tibial artery

Anterior tibial artery

Peroneal artery

Dorsalis pedis artery

Figure 41–7

IVP (Figure 41–8)

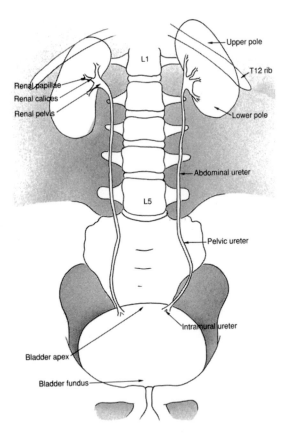

Figure 41–8

Computer Tomography (CT)

Head (Figures 41–9 to 41–15)

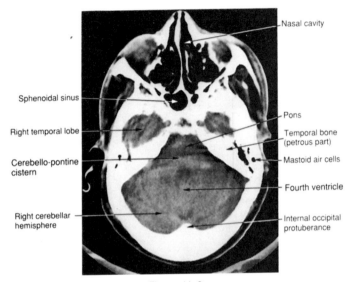

Nasal cavity

Sphenoidal sinus

Right temporal lobe

Cerebello-pontine cistern

Right cerebellar hemisphere

Pons

Temporal bone (petrous part)

Mastoid air cells

Fourth ventricle

Internal occipital protuberance

Figure 41–9

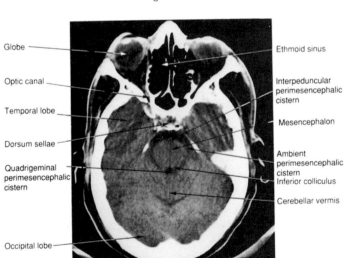

Globe

Optic canal

Temporal lobe

Dorsum sellae

Quadrigeminal perimesencephalic cistern

Occipital lobe

Ethmoid sinus

Interpeduncular perimesencephalic cistern

Mesencephalon

Ambient perimesencephalic cistern

Inferior colliculus

Cerebellar vermis

Figure 41–10

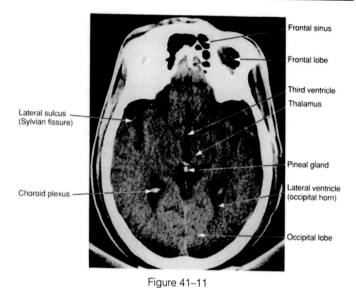

Frontal sinus

Frontal lobe

Third ventricle

Thalamus

Lateral sulcus
(Sylvian fissure)

Pineal gland

Lateral ventricle
(occipital horn)

Choroid plexus

Occipital lobe

Figure 41–11

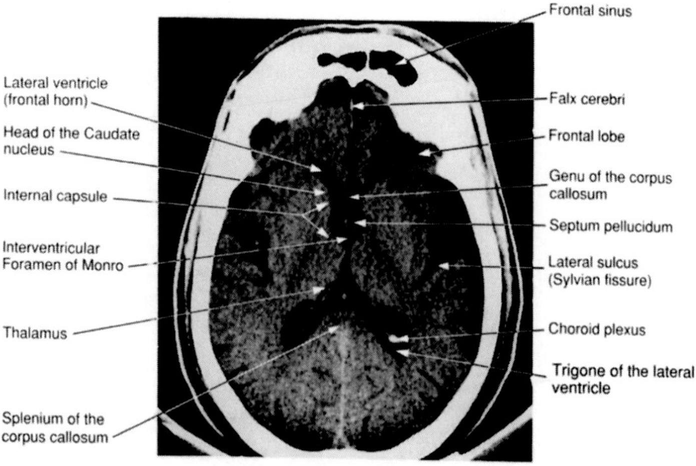

Frontal sinus

Lateral ventricle
(frontal horn)

Falx cerebri

Head of the Caudate
nucleus

Frontal lobe

Genu of the corpus
callosum

Internal capsule

Septum pellucidum

Interventricular
Foramen of Monro

Lateral sulcus
(Sylvian fissure)

Thalamus

Choroid plexus

Trigone of the lateral
ventricle

Splenium of the
corpus callosum

Figure 41–12

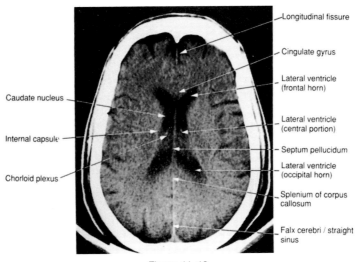

Longitudinal fissure

Cingulate gyrus

Lateral ventricle (frontal horn)

Caudate nucleus

Lateral ventricle (central portion)

Internal capsule

Septum pellucidum

Choroid plexus

Lateral ventricle (occipital horn)

Splenium of corpus callosum

Falx cerebri / straight sinus

Figure 41–13

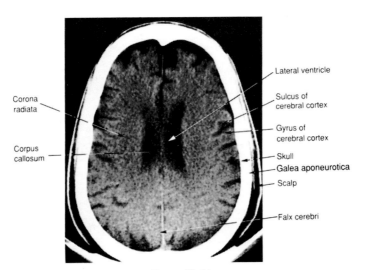

Corona radiata

Lateral ventricle

Sulcus of cerebral cortex

Gyrus of cerebral cortex

Corpus callosum

Skull

Galea aponeurotica

Scalp

Falx cerebri

Figure 41–14

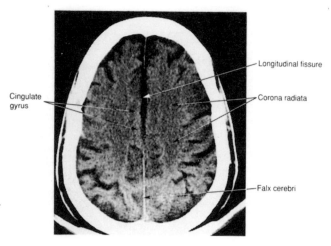

Figure 41–15

Abdomen (Figures 41–16 to 41–21)

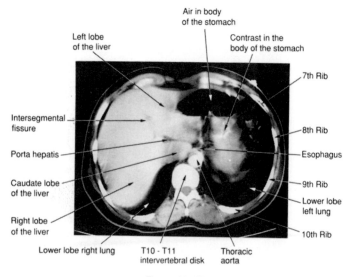

Figure 41–16

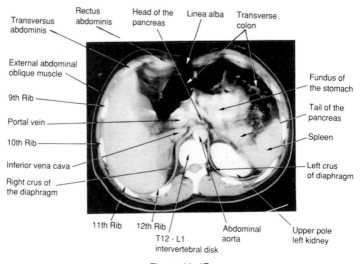

Transversus abdominis
Rectus abdominis
Head of the pancreas
Linea alba
Transverse colon
External abdominal oblique muscle
9th Rib
Portal vein
10th Rib
Inferior vena cava
Right crus of the diaphragm
Fundus of the stomach
Tail of the pancreas
Spleen
Left crus of diaphragm
11th Rib
12th Rib
T12 - L1 intervertebral disk
Abdominal aorta
Upper pole left kidney

Figure 41–17

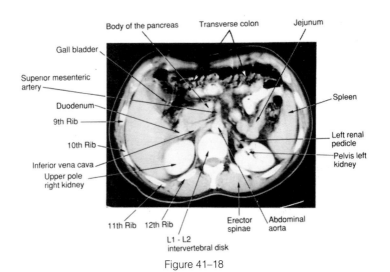

Body of the pancreas
Transverse colon
Jejunum
Gall bladder
Superior mesenteric artery
Duodenum
9th Rib
10th Rib
Inferior vena cava
Upper pole right kidney
Spleen
Left renal pedicle
Pelvis left kidney
11th Rib
12th Rib
L1 - L2 intervertebral disk
Erector spinae
Abdominal aorta

Figure 41–18

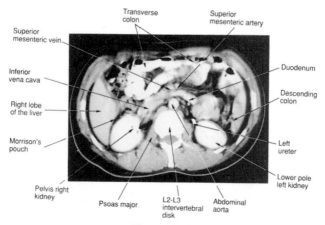

Figure 41-19

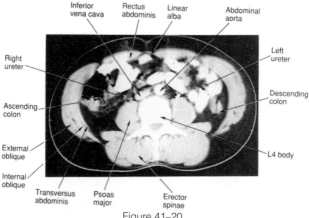

Figure 41-20

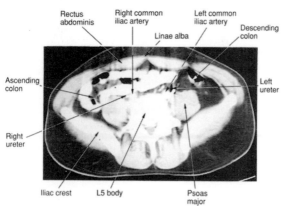

Figure 41-21

Male Pelvis (Figures 41–22 and 41–23)

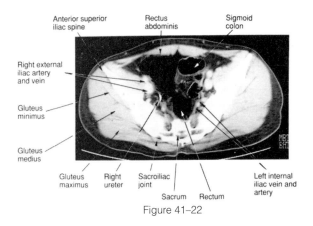

Figure 41–22

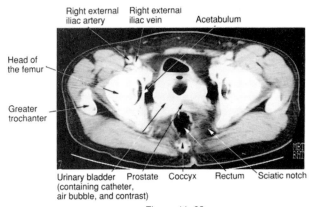

Figure 41–23

Cervical Spine (Figures 41–24 to 41–26)

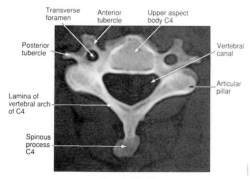

Transverse foramen · Anterior tubercle · Upper aspect body C4 · Vertebral canal · Posterior tubercle · Articular pillar · Lamina of vertebral arch of C4 · Spinous process C4

Figure 41–24

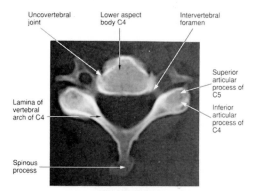

Uncovertebral joint · Lower aspect body C4 · Intervertebral foramen · Superior articular process of C5 · Lamina of vertebral arch of C4 · Inferior articular process of C4 · Spinous process

Figure 41–25

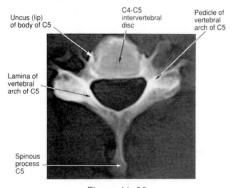

Uncus (lip) of body of C5 · C4-C5 intervertebral disc · Pedicle of vertebral arch of C5 · Lamina of vertebral arch of C5 · Spinous process C5

Figure 41–26

42

Organ Procurement

General Principles

▶ 40% of sudden death victims are suitable donors and organ donation occurs in the minority
  ▶ two-thirds due to head trauma
  ▶ other common causes include ruptured cerebral aneurysm, overdose, and anoxic brain injury

Considerations

▶ make contact with regional organ procurement organization when brain death is expected
  ▶ comply with institutional policy and the Uniform Anatomical Gift Act
  ▶ nursing supervisor is usually responsible
▶ common exclusion criteria
  ▶ death from overwhelming infection
  ▶ serious communicable disease
  ▶ long-standing medical problem that jeopardizes organ function
  ▶ certain types of cancer
▶ role of treating physician
  ▶ continue advanced medical care and optimize organ function prior to procurement
    ▶ maintain normal blood pressure and renal function
    ▶ treat cardiac arrhythmias
    ▶ prevent hypothermia
  ▶ explain the definition of brain death and answer all questions
  ▶ provide emotional support to the family
▶ expect the regional organ procurement organization to supervise the following process
  ▶ explain the concept of organ donation and obtain consent
  ▶ test for communicable diseases
  ▶ arrange short- and long-term follow-up with the family

Brain Death

Definition

▶ two licensed physicians concur on the following criteria
  ▶ presence of clinical or neuroradiographic evidence of a nonreversible brain insult
  ▶ absence of medical conditions that can mimic brain death
    ▶ these include hypoglycemia, hypoxia, hypothermia, and oversedation

Clinical Criteria

▶ the presence of all of the following sustained for several hours denotes brain death
▶ coma
  ▶ GCS of 3
▶ absence of brain stem signs
  ▶ no pupillary reaction
  ▶ no extraoccular movement
    ▶ can use cold calorics to test
  ▶ no corneal reflex
  ▶ no gag or cough reflex
▶ apnea, which can be tested in the following manner
  ▶ begin when the patient is well-oxygenated, normocarbic, and has a SBP greater than 90 mm Hg
  ▶ obtain baseline arterial blood gas (ABG) and remove the patient from the ventilator
  ▶ terminate the procedure (inconclusive) if SBP drops below 90 mm Hg or cardiac arrhythmia is provoked by hypoxia
  ▶ at 8 minutes, obtain second ABG and return the patient to the ventilator
  ▶ positive test implies no respiratory muscle movement for 8 minutes and pCO_2 increased to greater than 60 mm Hg

Confirmatory Testing

▶ recommended when clinical criteria are unreliable or inconclusive
▶ options
  ▶ electroencephalogram (EEG) without brain waves for 30 minutes
  ▶ cerebral angiography or transtemporal doppler ultrasonography demonstrate no cerebral blood flow

43

Infection Prophylaxis

Tetanus

General Principles

▶ all traumatic wounds are "tetanus prone," though the degree of risk varies
▶ most victims of tetanus are unable to recall the wound

Treatment

Prior tetanus immunization	TT	TIG
Unknown	Yes	Yes
Incomplete	Yes	Yes
>5 years ago	Yes	No
<5 years ago	No	No

TIG = tetanus immune globulin   TT = tetanus toxoid

Doses

Tetanus/Diphtheria Toxoid

▶ tetanus component
  ▶ 0.5 ml IM is standard dose
▶ diphtheria component
  ▶ standard dose for infant diphtheria immunization is denoted with an upper-case "D"
  ▶ diphtheria booster is 1/4–1/10 strength of "D" and is denoted by a lower-case "d"
▶ dose
  ▶ if under 6 years, diphtheria–pertussis–tetanus (DPT) is recommended
    ▹ exclude pertussis whenever contraindicated
  ▶ if 6 years or older, diphtheria–tetanus (dT) is recommended

Tetanus Immune Globulin (TIG)

▶ 250 U IM for children
▶ 500 U IM for adults
▶ use separate sites for tetanus toxoid and TIG injection

Rabies

Animal Factors

High Risk

▶ bats
  ▶ largest threat in the United States
  ▶ if a bat is found in the same room as the patient and it is unsure whether a bite has occurred (e.g., nonverbal child or sleeping adult), then treat as high risk
▶ coyotes
▶ foxes
▶ raccoons
▶ skunks
▶ woodchucks

Intermediate Risk

▶ domesticated dogs, cats, and ferrets
▶ livestock

No Risk

▶ rodents
  ▶ mice and rats
  ▶ squirrels and chipmunks
  ▶ hamsters, guinea pigs, and gerbils
▶ lagomorphs
  ▶ rabbits and hares

Treatment

General Principles

▶ initiate treatment in all high-risk animal bites
  ▶ clean the wound with a virucidal agent (e.g., povidone iodine)
  ▶ give both rabies immune globulin and vaccine
▶ ruling out the possibility of rabies obviates the need for continuing treatment
  ▶ observe domesticated animals for 10 days, and if they remain healthy discontinue treatment
  ▶ kill and test wild animals
    ▸ send the animal's head (refrigerated) to the appropriate local laboratory for fluorescent rabies antibody testing
    ▸ discontinue treatment if negative
▶ for domesticated animal bites when the animal is unknown

> ▶ handle on a case-by-case basis and use the public health department as a resource
>> ▷ in areas where domesticated animal rabies is endemic, initiate treatment if the animal appeared unhealthy or the bite was unprovoked
>> ▷ in areas where domestic animals are immunized, treatment is generally unnecessary unless the local public health authority recommends otherwise

Human Rabies Immune Globulin (HRIG)

▶ offers passive antibody protection for several weeks
▶ 20 IU/kg
▶ inject half the dose IM into the gluteus and infiltrate the area of the bite with the rest

Vaccine

▶ comparable products
> ▷ Human Diploid Cell Vaccine (HDCV)
> ▷ Rabies Vaccine Adsorbed (RVA)
> ▷ Purified Chick Embryo Cell Vaccine (PCEC)
▶ offer active antibody protection within 10 days and last for over 2 years
▶ 1 ml IM immediately and on days 3, 7, 14, and 28 following for a total of 5 doses
▶ do not use same syringe as for HRIG

Antibiotic Use

General Principles

▶ much variation among institutions and practitioners
▶ institutional sensitivity reports guide choices
▶ 5-day course commonly recommended for prophylaxis
▶ at greater than 48 h after injury, if there is no clinical evidence of infection, prophylactic antibiosis unnecessary

Lacerations

▶ use first-generation cephalosporins (or equivalent coverage) for injuries involving
> ▷ tendon or sheath
> ▷ cartilage
> ▷ joint capsule
> ▷ fascia
> ▷ neurovascular structures
> ▷ lacerations caused by pressure injection

▶ consider ciprofloxacin (or equivalent coverage) when the wound is significantly contaminated by
  ▶ raw meat
  ▶ sea or lake water

Puncture Wounds

▶ foot punctures from a nail through gym shoes have a high incidence of pseudomonal infections
  ▶ use ciprofloxacin in adults
  ▶ use ampicillin/clavulanate in children

Bites

▶ thorough cleansing is essential
▶ human
  ▶ need coverage for skin organisms, *Eiknella corrodens,* and oral anaerobes
  ▶ clenched-fist injuries
    ▷ highly prone to infection
    ▷ radiograph necessary to rule out retained tooth fragment
  ▶ acceptable antibiotic regimes
    ▷ ampicillin/sulbactam or cefazolin/penicillin intravenously (IV) for in-patients
    ▷ amoxicillin/clavulanate by mouth (PO) for out-patients
    ▷ erythromycin if penicillin-allergic
▶ dog or cat
  ▶ provide coverage for *Pasturella multocida*
    ▷ causes infection within 24 h
    ▷ cat bites (and scratches) are far more prone to infection than dog bites
    ▷ some use an initial intravenous dose for cat bites
    ▷ some do not prophylax dog bites
  ▶ ampicillin/sulbactam IV
  ▶ amoxicillin/clavulanate PO
  ▶ use doxycycline if penicillin-allergic

Penetrating Injuries

General Principles

▶ low-velocity missiles never become "hot" enough to be considered sterile
▶ penetration results in inoculation of tissue with debris and bacteria from nonsterile clothes and skin

Neck or Thoracic Cavity

▶ use first-generation cephalosporins (or equivalent coverage)

Esophageal Penetration

▶ use broad-spectrum coverage when suspected or confirmed

Abdominal Cavity or Pelvis

▶ use second- or third-generation cephalosporins
▶ use clindamycin/aminoglycoside if penicillin-allergic

Blunt Injuries

Open Fractures

▶ use first-generation cephalosporins (or equivalent coverage)

Maxillofacial Fractures

▶ use penicillin or clindamycin for mandibular fractures with intraoral communication
  ▶ typically angle or body fractures
▶ use first-generation cephalosporins (or equivalent coverage) for orbital
floor or other sinus fractures

Hollow Viscus Rupture

▶ use second- or third-generation cephalosporins (or equivalent coverage)

Antibiotics Unnecessary

▶ basilar skull fractures
▶ noninfected burns
▶ hemothorax or pneumothorax from blunt trauma

44

Aftercare Instructions

Instructions in English and Spanish appear on the two pages following.

English

Wound Care

▶ keep your wound clean and dry
▶ return in 2 days for a wound check
▶ keep the wound covered to prevent it from getting dirty
▶ if the wound becomes dirty, wash it with soap and water, and dry it well with a towel
▶ return immediately if your wound turns red, hot, or swollen, if it shows pus or red streaks, or if you feel more pain
▶ return in __ days to remove the stitches

Sprains/Contusions/Fractures

▶ fill a plastic bag with ice and place it over the injured area for 20 minutes every 6 hours for 2 days
▶ keep the injured area elevated for less swelling
▶ if you have an elastic bandage, loosen it if it is too tight or rewrap it if it is too loose
  ▶ loosen the bandage if you notice swelling, numbness, tingling, or change in color (pale or blue)
▶ keep the splint on until you see the specialist—don't walk on your splint; use crutches if necessary
  ▶ don't get the splint wet and don't scratch underneath the dressing because you may cause a skin infection

Head Injury

▶ avoid strenuous activities for 24 hours
▶ keep the patient in bed if he/she has a headache or other symptoms develop
▶ take 2 Tylenol tablets every 4 hours for the headache
▶ apply ice packs over the injured area for 30 minutes every 6 hours
▶ wake the patient up every 2 hours to see if his/her mental state is okay
▶ return immediately if any of the following occurs
  ▶ repeated vomiting, nausea, or fever
  ▶ dilated pupil (if the pupils are not the same size)
  ▶ constantly sleeping, unconscious, or seizures
  ▶ problems with his/her balance, paralysis or trouble wakening, problems using his/her arms or legs or numbness of the skin
  ▶ mental confusion, disorientation, dizziness
  ▶ irregular breathing or trouble breathing

Español

Cuidado de Heridas

- ▶ mantenga la herida limpia y seca
- ▶ regrese en 2 dias para revisarle la herida
- ▶ mantenga la herida cubierta si tiene que trabajar en un ambiente sucio
- ▶ si se le ensucia la herida, lávela con agua y jabón, secandola bien con una toalla
- ▶ regrese pronto si su herida se pone roja, caliente, hinchada, muestra pus o rayas rojas o si siente más dolor
- ▶ regrese en __ dias para quitarle las puntadas

Torceduras/Contusiones/Fracturas

- ▶ llene una bolsa de plástico con hielo y póngala sobre el área por 20 minutos cada 6 horas por 2 dias
- ▶ mantenga la área lastimada elevada para disminuir la hinchazón
- ▶ si tiene una venda elástica vuelva a envolverla si está muy apretada o muy suelta
  - ▶ afloje la venda si usted nota hinchazón, entumecimiento, o sensación de hormigueo o cambio de color (pálido o azul)
- ▶ mantenga el yeso puesto hasta que vea al especialista—no camine con la pierna entablillada, use muletas si es necesario
  - ▶ no moje el yeso o trate de rascarse debajo del vendaje porque puede infectarse la piel

Golpes en la Cabeza

- ▶ evite el juego o trabajo fuerte por 24 horas
- ▶ mantenga al paciente en cama si el dolor de cabeza continua o si presentan otros síntomas
- ▶ administre 2 tabletas de Tylenol para el dolor de cabeza cada 4 horas
- ▶ aplique compresas de hielo sobre el area que se golpeó, por 30 minutos cada 6 horas
- ▶ despierte al paciente cada 2 horas para ver si su estado mental esta bien
- ▶ regrese inmediatamente si le ocurre lo siguiente
  - ▶ vómitos repetidos, nausea o fiebre
  - ▶ pupilas de los ojos dilatadas (si las pupilas de los ojos no son del mismo tamaño)
  - ▶ sueño constante, inconciente, convulsiones
  - ▶ problemas con el balance, parálisis o problemas con el uso normal de los brazos y piernas o adormecimiento de la piel
  - ▶ confusión mental, desorientación, mareos
  - ▶ respiración irregular o dificultad al respirar

45

Drug Formulary

General Principles

Purpose

▶ this formulary includes drugs that are commonly used in the emergency management of trauma patients
▶ it is not an exhaustive formulary and drugs infrequently used may not be included

Caveats

▶ only a partial list of pertinent or common prescribing information is listed
▶ indications listed are exclusively those that relate to trauma
  ▶ e.g., epinephrine indications include cardiac arrest and adjunct to local anesthesia but not anaphylaxis or asthma
▶ the practitioner must consult a definitive pharmacologic reference when unfamiliar or inexperienced in treating certain medical conditions or prescribing certain medications
▶ it is implied (and therefore not repetitively written) that a known allergy to the same class of medications is a contraindication to a drug's use
▶ this formulary is to be used for general guidance and in no way replaces sound clinical judgment
  ▶ clinicians should routinely refer to specific prescribing information for all medications they order
▶ always consult a definitive pharmacologic reference in patients with impaired renal or hepatic function as it may be necessary to reduce the dose or lengthen the dosing interval
▶ IO doses are the same as IV doses and IV use implies that IO use is acceptable

Pregnancy Categories

▶ A
  ▶ no risk documented by studies

► B
  ► no risk documented though not adequately studied
► C
  ► adverse effects documented in animals and not humans; benefits often outweigh risks; consulting an obstetrician is recommended
► D
  ► evidence of risk to human fetus documented, so relatively contraindicated; benefits may outweigh risks in certain situations; obstetrical consultation necessary
► X
  ► evidence of fetal abnormalities documented; absolutely contraindicated

Abbreviations

General Principles

► the following abbreviations are used commonly in prescription writing and are found throughout this text

Dosing Frequency

► BID, twice daily
► d, day
► h, hour
► HS, at bedtime
► min, minute
► mo, month
► prn, as needed
► q, every
► QID, four times daily
► s, second
► TID, three times daily
► yr, year

Route

► ET, by endotracheal tube
► IM, intramuscularly
► IO, intraosseously
► IV, intravenously
► PO, by mouth
► PR, rectally
► SC, subcutaneously
► SL, sublingually

Amounts

- ▶ g, grams
- ▶ gtt, drops
- ▶ max, maximum
- ▶ mcg, micrograms
- ▶ mEq, milliequivalents
- ▶ mg, milligrams
- ▶ ml, milliliters
- ▶ MU, milliunits; MIU, milliunits using the International System
- ▶ U, units; IU, units using the International System

Form

- ▶ div, divided
- ▶ susp, suspension
- ▶ tabs, tablets
- ▶ caps, capsules
- ▶ amps, ampules
- ▶ elix, elixir
- ▶ liq, liquid
- ▶ supp, suppositories
- ▶ oint, ointment
- ▶ sln, solution
- ▶ inj, injection
- ▶ ophth, ophthalmic preparation

Other

- ▶ sig, signature or dosing information
- ▶ NSAID, non-steroidal anti-inflammatory
- ▶ avg, average

Drugs

Acetaminophen (Anacin-3, Datril, Tempra, Tylenol)

- ▶ class
  - ▶ analgesic, nonopioid, antipyretic
- ▶ indication
  - ▶ relief of mild pain and fever
- ▶ precautions/contraindications
  - ▶ pregnancy category B
  - ▶ avoid when there is hepatic insufficiency or history of chronic alcohol abuse

- ▶ dosage/route
  - ▶ children: 10–15 mg/kg PO q 4–6 h prn
  - ▶ adults: 650–1,000 mg PO q 4–6 h prn; not to exceed 4 g/d acutely
- ▶ how supplied
  - ▶ tabs 160 mg, 325 mg, 500 mg, 650 mg
  - ▶ chewable tabs 80 mg, 120 mg, 160 mg
  - ▶ caps 325/500 mg
  - ▶ supp 120 mg, 325 mg, 650 mg
  - ▶ elix 120 or 160 or 320 mg/5 ml
  - ▶ liq 160 mg/5 ml, 500 mg/15 ml

Acetaminophen/Codeine (Tylenlol #2, #3 or #4)

- ▶ class
  - ▶ analgesic, opioid
- ▶ indication
  - ▶ relief of moderate pain
- ▶ precautions/contraindications
  - ▶ pregnancy category C (D near term)
  - ▶ avoid when there is hepatic insufficiency
  - ▶ adverse effects include CNS depression, hypotension, vomiting, and respiratory depression
- ▶ dosage/route
  - ▶ children: 10–15 mg/kg (of acetaminophen) PO q 4–6 h prn pain
  - ▶ adults: 1–2 tabs PO q 4–6 h prn pain
- ▶ how supplied
  - ▶ elix 120/12 mg/5 ml
  - ▶ tabs #2 = 300/15 mg, #3 = 300/30 mg, #4 = 300/60 mg

Acetominophen/Hydrocodone (Vicodin, Lortab)

- ▶ class
  - ▶ analgesic, opioid
- ▶ indication
  - ▶ relief of moderate to severe pain
- ▶ precautions/contraindications
  - ▶ pregnancy risk category C (D near term)
  - ▶ avoid when hepatic insufficiency
  - ▶ adverse effects include CNS depression, hypotension, vomiting, and respiratory depression
- ▶ dosage/route
  - ▶ children: 10–15 mg (of acetominophen) PO q 4–6 h prn pain
  - ▶ adults: 1–2 tabs PO q 4–6 h prn
- ▶ how supplied
  - ▶ elix 2.5/167 mg/5 ml
  - ▶ tabs 5/500 mg, 7.5/500 mg

Acetaminophen/Oxycodone (Percocet)

▶ class
  ▶ analgesic, opioid
▶ indication
  ▶ relief of moderate to severe pain
▶ precautions/contraindications
  ▶ pregnancy category C (D near term)
  ▶ avoid when hepatic insufficiency
  ▶ adverse effects include CNS depression, hypotension, vomiting, and respiratory depression
▶ dosage/route
  ▶ children: safe use not established
  ▶ adults: 1–2 tabs PO q 4–6 h prn
▶ how supplied
  ▶ requires triplicate prescription (C-II restriction)
  ▶ tabs acetaminophen 325 mg/oxycodone 5 mg

Acetazolamide (Ak-zol, Diamox)

▶ class
  ▶ carbonic anhydrase inhibitor
▶ indication
  ▶ eye trauma associated with intraocular pressure (IOP) over 20 mm Hg (e.g., retrobulbar hemorrhage, complication of hyphema)
▶ precautions/contraindications
  ▶ pregnancy risk category C
  ▶ do not use when there is electrolyte imbalance, hepatic dysfunction, or renal insufficiency
  ▶ use cautiously in patients with respiratory problems since they may cause acidosis
▶ dosage/route
  ▶ children: 5 mg/kg PO/IV/IM q 4–6 h
  ▶ adults: 250 mg PO/IV/IM q 4–6 h
▶ how supplied
  ▶ tabs 125 mg, 250 mg
  ▶ caps 500 mg (extended release)
  ▶ inj 500 mg

Adenosine (Adenocard)

▶ class
  ▶ antiarrhythmic
▶ indications
  ▶ first-line drug for narrow-complex supraventricular tachycardia (SVT)
  ▶ can be used diagnostically for tachyarrhythmias of unknown type

- ▶ pharmacodynamics/kinetics
  - ▶ pregnancy risk category C
  - ▶ natural nucleoside that slows atrial–ventricular (AV) nodal conduction
    - ▹ transient heart block or asystole is expected
  - ▶ antagonized by methylxanthines (e.g., theophylline), so higher dose may be necessary
  - ▶ potentiated by dipyridamole—smaller dose may be necessary
  - ▶ transient chest pain and irritability are common side effects
- ▶ precautions/contraindications
  - ▶ patients with underlying second- or third-degree heart block or sick sinus syndrome may become hemodynamically unstable after the SVT is terminated
    - ▹ a pacemaker must be readily available
  - ▶ possible bronchoconstriction in asthmatics
- ▶ dosage/route
  - ▶ always given rapid IV push followed by immediate NS flush
  - ▶ stop if SVT is terminated or if atrial fibrillation or atrial flutter are diagnosed
  - ▶ children: 0.1–0.2 mg/kg initially; repeat within 1–2 min increasing in increments of 0.05 mg/kg; stop when maximum dose of 0.25 mg/kg is achieved
  - ▶ adults: 6-mg IV rapid bolus injection—if SVT is not terminated within 1–2 min, increase dose to 12 mg; then repeat 12 mg prn
- ▶ how supplied
  - ▶ inj 3 mg/ml

Alfentanil (Alfenta)

- ▶ class
  - ▶ analgesic, opioid
- ▶ indication
  - ▶ anesthesia induction
- ▶ pharmacodynamics/kinetics
  - ▶ duration under 30 min
  - ▶ can cause skeletal muscle rigidity and difficult ventilation because of rigid chest wall
  - ▶ hypoventilation reversed with naloxone; repeat doses of naloxone may be required
  - ▶ bradycardia treated with atropine
- ▶ precautions/contraindications
  - ▶ pregnancy risk category C
  - ▶ adverse effects include "tight chest syndrome," respiratory depression, bradycardia, dysrhythmia, bronchospasm, and vomiting
- ▶ dosage/route
  - ▶ doses based on ideal body weight, for patients up to 20% above ideal weight
  - ▶ children under 12 yr: safe use not established
  - ▶ children over 12 yr and adults: 8–20 mcg/kg for induction, then 3–5 mcg/kg incrementally

▶ how supplied
  ▶ inj 500 mcg/ml

Amikacin (Amikin)

▶ class
  ▶ antibiotic, aminoglycoside
▶ precautions/contraindications
  ▶ pregnancy risk category D
  ▶ adverse effects include reversible nephrotoxicity and possibly irreversible ototoxicity
  ▶ use cautiously when there are prior hearing problems, neuromuscular disease, renal insufficiency or concomitant loop diuretics
▶ dosage/route—IV/IM
  ▶ children and adults: 15 mg/kg/d IV/IM div q 8–12 h; IV preferable over 30–60 min
  ▶ in those with impaired renal function, dosing interval (h) = creatinine (mg/dL) times 9
  ▶ lower dose as necessary based on peak/trough levels measured after the third dose; peak should be 15–30 mcg/ml and trough, 5–10 mcg/ml
▶ how supplied
  ▶ inj 50 or 250 mg/ml

Amiodarone (Cordarone)

▶ class
  ▶ antiarrhythmic, class III
▶ indication
  ▶ ventricular and supraventricular arrhythmias
▶ pharmacodynamics/kinetics
  ▶ duration 3 weeks–3 months
▶ precautions/contraindications
  ▶ pregnancy risk category D
  ▶ do not use when heart block
  ▶ adverse effects include hypotension, pneumonitis, and hepatic failure
  ▶ arrhythmias
▶ dosage/route
  ▶ adults: when VF/pulseless VT give 300 mg IVP, otherwise give 150 mg over 10 min (and repeat if necessary) followed by 1 mg/min for the next 6 h followed by 0.5 mg/min; total daily dose is 2.2 g
  ▶ children: 5 mg/kg IV
▶ how supplied
  ▶ inj 50 mg/mL

Amoxicillin (Amoxil, Polymox, Trimox, Wymox)

▶ class
  ▶ aminopenicillin antibiotic

► precautions/contraindications
  ► pregnancy risk category B
  ► causes rash in patients with mononucleosis
► dosage/route
  ► children: 20–40 mg/kg/d PO div TID
  ► adults: 250–500 mg PO TID
► how supplied
  ► susp 125 mg/5 ml or 250 mg/5 ml
  ► caps 250 mg, 500 mg
  ► chewable tabs 125 mg, 250 mg

Amoxicillin/Clavulanic Acid (Augmentin)

► class
  ► antibiotic, aminopenicillin with beta-lactamase inhibitor
► precautions/contraindications
  ► pregnancy risk category B
  ► causes rash in patients with mononucleosis
► dosage/route
  ► based on amoxicillin
  ► children: 20–40 mg/kg/d PO div TID
  ► adults: 250–500 mg PO TID
► how supplied
  ► tabs 250/125 mg, 500/125 mg, 875/125mg
  ► chewable tabs 250/62.5 mg, 125/31.25 mg, 200/31.25 mg, 400/62.5 mg
  ► susp 250/62.5 mg/5 ml, 125/31.25 mg/5 ml, 200/28.5 mg/5 ml, 400/57 mg/5 ml

Ampicillin (Amcil, Omnipen, Polycillin, Principen, Totacillin)

► class
  ► antibiotic, aminopenicillin
► precautions/contraindications
  ► pregnancy risk category B
  ► causes rash in patients with mononucleosis
► dosage/route
  ► children: 50–100 mg/kg/d div PO QID or 100–200 mg/kg IV/IM q 6 h
  ► adults: 250–500 mg PO QID or 500 mg–4 g IV/IM q 6 h
► how supplied
  ► elix and susp 125 mg/5 ml, 250 mg/5 ml, 500 mg/5 ml
  ► caps 250 mg, 500 mg

Ampicillin/Sulbactam (Unasyn)

► class
  ► antibiotic, aminopenicillin with beta-lactamase inhibitor

▶ precautions/contraindications
- ▶ pregnancy risk category B
- ▶ causes rash in patients with mononucleosis

▶ dosage/route
- ▶ based on ampicillin
- ▶ children: IM or IV 100–200 mg/kg/d div q 6 h
- ▶ adults: IM or IV 1.5–3 g every 6 h

▶ how supplied
- ▶ 1.5 g (1 g ampicillin/500 mg sulbactam)
- ▶ 3 g (2 g ampicillin/1 g sulbactam)

Aspirin (ASA, Ascriptin, Bayer, Bufferin, Ecotrin, Empirin)

▶ class
- ▶ analgesic, NSAID, antipyretic

▶ indication
- ▶ relief of mild pain, fever, inflammation

▶ precautions/contraindications
- ▶ pregnancy risk category D
- ▶ do not use in children with viral infection as Reye's syndrome may develop
- ▶ anticoagulant effects may worsen bleeding after trauma
- ▶ avoid use with other NSAIDs

▶ dosage/route
- ▶ children: 15 mg/kg PO q 4–6 h prn pain
- ▶ adults: 325–650-mg tabs PO or PR q 4–6 h prn pain

▶ how supplied
- ▶ enteric-coated tabs available
- ▶ tabs 81 mg, 325 mg, 500 mg, 650 mg
- ▶ caps 325 mg, 500 mg
- ▶ supp 60 mg, 125 mg, 325 mg, 650 mg, 1200 mg

Aspirin/Codeine (Empirin with Codeine)

▶ class
- ▶ analgesic, opioid

▶ indication
- ▶ relief of moderate pain

▶ precautions/contraindications
- ▶ pregnancy risk category D
- ▶ do not use in children with viral infection as Reye's syndrome may develop
- ▶ anticoagulant effects may worsen bleeding after trauma
- ▶ adverse effects include CNS depression, hypotension, vomiting, and respiratory depression

▶ dosage/route
- ▶ children: safe use not established
- ▶ adults: 1–2 tabs PO q 4–6 h prn pain

- how supplied
  - tabs 325/30 mg

Atracurium (Tracrium)

- class
  - paralytic, nondepolarizing
- indication
  - paralysis for intubation, mechanical ventilation, procedures
- pharmacodynamics/kinetics
  - onset max effect in 3–5 min
  - duration 20–35 min
- precautions/contraindications
  - pregnancy risk category C
  - do not use when neuromuscular disease or myasthenia gravis
- adverse effects
  - histamine release is common at doses over 0.5 mg/kg
- dosage/route
  - children under 1 mo: safe use not established
  - children 1 mo–2 yr: 0.3–0.4 mg/kg initially and for maintenance
  - children over 2 yr and adults: 0.4 mg/kg initially and for maintenance 0.08 to 0.1 mg/kg q 30–45 min
- how supplied
  - inj 10 mg/ml

Atropine (Isopto)

- class
  - antiarrhythmic, anticholinergic, vagolytic
- indications
  - symptomatic bradycardia
  - preinduction for vagolysis and decreasing secretions
- pharmacodynamics/kinetics
  - onset max effect in 2–3 min
  - causes tachycardia
- precautions/contraindications
  - pregnancy risk category C
  - may precipitate narrow-angle glaucoma
- dosage/route
  - children: 0.01–0.02 mg/kg IV/IM/ET q 5 min to max 1 mg
  - adults: 0.5–1 mg IV/IM/ET q 5 min to max 2 mg; ET dose is 2.5 times IV dose
  - use single, lower dose for preinduction
- how supplied
  - inj variable concentrations

Azithromycin (Zithromax)

▶ class
  ▶ antibiotic, macrolide
▶ pharmacodynamics/kinetics
  ▶ half-life is 68 h
  ▶ rapidly absorbed from GI tract
▶ precautions/contraindications
  ▶ pregnancy risk category B
  ▶ avoid when hepatic dysfunction
  ▶ interacts with oratadine and may precipitate arrhythmias
▶ dosage/route
  ▶ children: safe use not established
  ▶ adults: 500 mg PO on day 1, then 250 mg PO q d for 4 days
  ▶ take on an empty stomach
▶ how supplied
  ▶ caps 250 mg

Aztreonam (Azactam)

▶ class
  ▶ antibiotic, monobactam
▶ precautions/contraindications
  ▶ pregnancy risk category B
  ▶ adverse effects include seizures, confusion, and hypotension
  ▶ dose adjustment with renal insufficiency
▶ dosage/route
  ▶ children: 90–120 mg/kg/d div q 6–8 h
  ▶ adults: 500 mg–2 g q 6–8 h; max 8 g/d
▶ how supplied
  ▶ inj 500 mg, 1 g, 2 g vials

Bacitracin (Aktracin, Baciguent)

▶ class
  ▶ antibiotic, polypeptide
▶ precautions/contraindications
  ▶ pregnancy risk category C
  ▶ do not use in the external ear canal if the tympanic membrane is perforated
▶ dosage/route
  ▶ children and adults: apply ophthalmic to eyes or topical ointment to skin wounds BID–QID
▶ how supplied
  ▶ oint 500 U/g

Betaxolol (Betoptic, Kerlone)

- ► class
  - ► topical beta-blocker
- ► indication
  - ► reduces increased IOP due to hyphema or other ocular injury
- ► pharmacodynamics/kinetics
  - ► thought to lower IOP by reducing aqueous humor production
- ► precautions/contraindications
  - ► pregnancy risk category C
  - ► do not use when second- or third-degree AV block or CHF present
- ► dosage/route
  - ► adults: one gtt in affected eye BID
- ► how supplied
  - ► ophth sln 0.5% in 2.5, 5, 10 and 15 ml dropper bottles

Brimondine (Alphagan)

- ► class
  - ► topical alpha-2-adrenergic agonist
- ► indication
  - ► eye trauma associated with IOP over 20 mm Hg
- ► pharmacodynamics/kinetics
  - ► onset 1–4, 2 h
  - ► duration 12 h
- ► precautions/contraindications
  - ► pregnancy risk category B
  - ► avoid when concurrent monoamine oxidase (MAO) inhibitor use
  - ► adverse effects include hypotension
- ► dosage/route
  - ► children: safe use not established
  - ► adults: 1 gtt in effected eye
- ► how supplied
  - ► ophth 0.2% sln

Bupivacaine (Marcaine, Sensorcaine)

- ► class
  - ► local anesthetic, amide
- ► indication
  - ► long-acting local anesthesia
  - ► regional nerve block
- ► pharmacodynamics/kinetics
  - ► pregnancy risk category C
  - ► duration of sensory block 6–8 h, motor block 1–2 h
  - ► often given in combination with lidocaine, which has faster onset of anesthesia, and with epinephrine, which prolongs the duration

▶ precautions/contraindications
  ▹ adverse effects include seizures, hypotension, bradycardia
▶ dosage/route
  ▹ children under 12 years: safe use not established
  ▹ children over 12 years and adults: inject locally in wound, maximal dose is 2.5 mg/kg (plain), 3 mg/kg (with epinephrine)
▶ how supplied
  ▹ inj 0.25% or 0.5%, with or without epinephrine (1:200,000)

Calcium Chloride

▶ class
  ▹ cardiotonic
▶ indications
  ▹ cardiac resuscitation and suspected hypocalcemia (e.g., arrest after massive blood transfusion) or hyperkalemia (e.g., arrest in patient with renal failure)
  ▹ do not use routinely in cardiac arrest since can cause cardiac syncope
▶ precautions/contraindications
  ▹ pregnancy risk category C
  ▹ do not use when there is digitalis toxicity or ventricular fibrillation (unless hypocalcemia is highly suspect)
  ▹ IM or SC administration or IV extravasation causes severe skin necrosis
  ▹ adverse effects include hypotension, bradycardia, and arrhythmias
▶ dosage/route
  ▹ do not mix with sodium bicarbonate
  ▹ children: 10–20 mg/kg slow IV push; may repeat every 10 min if necessary
  ▹ adults: 500 mg–1 g slow IV push over 5–10 min
▶ how supplied
  ▹ inj 10% (100 mg/ml) sln

Cefaclor (Ceclor)

▶ class
  ▹ antibiotic, cephalosporin (second-generation)
▶ precautions/contraindications
  ▹ pregnancy risk category B
  ▹ caution with penicillin allergy
  ▹ excreted in breast milk
▶ dosage/route
  ▹ children: 40 mg/kg PO div TID
  ▹ adults: 250–500 mg PO TID or 375–500 mg PO BID with extended release
▶ how supplied
  ▹ susp 125 mg/5 ml, 250 mg/5 ml, 375 mg/5 ml
  ▹ caps 250 mg, 500 mg
  ▹ tabs (extended release) 375 mg, 500 mg

Cefadroxil (Duricef)

- ▶ class
  - ▶ antibiotic, cephalosporin (first-generation)
- ▶ precautions/contraindications
  - ▶ pregnancy risk category B
  - ▶ caution with penicillin allergy
  - ▶ excreted in breast milk
- ▶ dosage/route
  - ▶ children: 30 mg/kg PO div BID
  - ▶ adults: 1–2 g PO q d or div BID
- ▶ how supplied
  - ▶ susp 125 or 250 or 500 mg/5 ml
  - ▶ caps 500 mg
  - ▶ tabs 1 g

Cefamandole (Mandol)

- ▶ class
  - ▶ antibiotic, cephalosporin (second-generation)
- ▶ precautions/contraindications
  - ▶ pregnancy risk category B
  - ▶ caution with penicillin allergy
  - ▶ excreted in breast milk
- ▶ dosage/route
  - ▶ children: 50–150 mg/kg/d IV/IM div q 4–8 h
  - ▶ adults: 500 mg–1 g IV/IM q 4–8 h IV/IM
- ▶ how supplied
  - ▶ inj 500 mg, 1 g, 2 g

Cefazolin (Ancef, Kefzol, Zolicef)

- ▶ class
  - ▶ antibiotic, cephalosporin (first-generation)
- ▶ precautions/contraindications
  - ▶ pregnancy risk category B
  - ▶ caution with penicillin allergy
  - ▶ excreted in breast milk
- ▶ dosage/route
  - ▶ children under 1 mo: safe use not established
  - ▶ children over 1 mo: 50–100 mg/kg/d div every 6–8 h
  - ▶ adults: 250 mg–1 g IV/IM q 6–8 h
- ▶ how supplied
  - ▶ inj 250, 500 mg, 1 g

Cefepime (Maxipime)

▶ class
  ▶ antibiotic, cephalosporin (fourth-generation)
▶ precautions/contraindications
  ▶ pregnancy risk category B
  ▶ caution with penicillin allergy
▶ dosage/route
  ▶ children over 12 years and adults: 0.5–2 g IV q 12 h
▶ how supplied
  ▶ inj 500 mg, 1 g, 2 g

Cefixime (Suprax)

▶ class
  ▶ antibiotic, cephalosporin (third-generation)
▶ precautions/contraindications
  ▶ pregnancy risk category B
  ▶ caution with penicillin allergy
▶ dosage/route
  ▶ children under 6 mo: safe use not established
  ▶ children over 6 mo: 8 mg/kg PO q d or div BID; max 400 mg
  ▶ adults: 400 mg PO q d or div BID
▶ how supplied
  ▶ susp 100 mg/5 ml
  ▶ tabs 200 mg, 400 mg

Cefmetazole (Zefazone)

▶ class
  ▶ antibiotic, cephalosporin (second-generation)
▶ precautions/contraindications
  ▶ pregnancy risk category B
  ▶ adverse effects include possible disulfiram-like reaction
  ▶ caution with penicillin allergy
▶ dosage/route
  ▶ children: safe use not established
  ▶ adults: 2 g IV q 6–12 h
▶ how supplied
  ▶ inj 1 g, 2 g

Cefonocid (Monocid)

▶ class
  ▶ antibiotic, cephalosporin (second-generation)

▶ precautions/contraindications
  ▶ pregnancy risk category B
  ▶ caution with penicillin allergy
▶ dosage/route
  ▶ children: safe use not established
  ▶ adults: 500 mg–2 g IV/IM q d
▶ how supplied
  ▶ inj 500 mg, 1 g

Cefoperazone (Cefobid)

▶ class
  ▶ antibiotic, cephalosporin (third-generation)
▶ precautions/contraindications
  ▶ pregnancy risk category B
  ▶ caution with penicillin allergy
▶ dosage/route
  ▶ children: safe use not established
  ▶ adults: 2–4 g IV/IM q 12 h
▶ how supplied
  ▶ inj 1 g, 2 g

Cefotaxime (Claforan)

▶ class
  ▶ antibiotic, cephalosporin (third-generation)
▶ precautions/contraindications
  ▶ pregnancy risk category B
  ▶ caution with penicillin allergy
▶ dosage/route
  ▶ children under 50 kg: 50–200 mg/kg/d IV/IM div q 4–6 h
  ▶ children over 50 kg and adults: 1–2 g IV/IM q 6–12 h; max 12g/d
▶ how supplied
  ▶ inj 1 g, 2 g

Cefotetan (Cefotan)

▶ class
  ▶ antibiotic, cephalosporin (second-generation)
▶ precautions/contraindications
  ▶ pregnancy risk category B
  ▶ caution with penicillin allergy
▶ dosage/route
  ▶ children: safe use not established
  ▶ adults: 1–2 g IV/IM q 12 h
▶ how supplied
  ▶ inj 1 g, 2 g

Cefoxitin (Mefoxin)

▶ class
  ▶ antibiotic, cephalosporin (second-generation)
▶ precautions/contraindications
  ▶ pregnancy risk category B
  ▶ caution with penicillin allergy
▶ dosage/route
  ▶ IM injection is painful
  ▶ children (over 3 mo): 80–160 mg/kg/d IV/IM div q 4–6 h
  ▶ adults: 1–2 g IV/IM q 6–8 h; max 12 g/d
▶ how supplied
  ▶ inj 1 g, 2 g

Cefpodoxime (Vantin)

▶ class
  ▶ antibiotic, cephalosporin (second-generation)
▶ precautions/contraindications
  ▶ pregnancy risk category B
  ▶ caution with penicillin allergy
▶ dosage/route
  ▶ children under 6 mo: safe use not established
  ▶ children over 6 mo: 5 mg/kg/dose IV/IM q 12 h, not to exceed 200 mg
  ▶ adults: 100–400 mg PO BID
▶ how supplied
  ▶ susp 50 or 100 mg/5 ml
  ▶ tabs 100 mg, 200 mg

Cefprozil (Cefzil)

▶ class
  ▶ antibiotic, cephalosporin (second-generation)
▶ precautions/contraindications
  ▶ pregnancy risk category B
  ▶ caution with penicillin allergy
▶ dosage/route
  ▶ children: 15 mg/kg/d PO div BID
  ▶ adults: 250–500 mg PO BID or q d
▶ how supplied
  ▶ susp 125 or 250 mg/5 ml
  ▶ tabs 250 mg, 500 mg

Ceftazadime (Fortaz, Tazicef, Tazidime)

▶ class
  ▶ antibiotic, cephalosporin (third-generation)

► precautions/contraindications
  ► pregnancy risk category B
  ► caution with penicillin allergy
► dosage/route
  ► children: 30–50 mg/kg/dose IV/IM q 8 h
  ► adults: 500 mg–2 g IV/IM q 8–12 h, max 6 g/d
► how supplied
  ► inj 500 mg, 1 g, 2 g

Ceftizoxime (Cefizox)

► class
  ► antibiotic, cephalosporin (third-generation)
► precautions/contraindications
  ► pregnancy risk category B
  ► caution with penicillin allergy
► dosage/route
  ► children under 6 mo: safe use not established
  ► children over 6 mo: 50 mg/kg IV/IM q 6–8 h
  ► adults: 500 mg–2 g IV/IM q 8–12 h

Ceftriaxone (Rocephin)

► class
  ► antibiotic, cephalosporin (third-generation)
► pharmacodynamics/kinetics
  ► duration: half-life averages 7 h
► precautions/contraindications
  ► pregnancy risk category B
  ► adverse effects include "pseudocholelithiasis" (sludge in gallbladder)
  ► caution with penicillin allergy
► dosage/route
  ► children: 50–75 mg/kg/d IV/IM div q 12 h, max 2 g/d
  ► adults: 1–2 g IV/IM q d or div q 12 h, max 4 g/d

Cefuroxime (Ceftin, Kefurox, Zinacef)

► class
  ► antibiotic, cephalosporin (second-generation)
► precautions/contraindications
  ► pregnancy risk category B
  ► caution with penicillin allergy
► dosage/route
  ► children under 3 mo: safe use not established
  ► children over 3 mo: 50–150 mg/kg/d IV/IM div q 6–8 h or 125 mg PO BID (under 10 kg)/250 mg PO BID (over 10 kg)
  ► adults: 750 mg–1.5 g IV/IM q 8 h or 250–500 mg PO BID

▶ how supplied
  ▶ tabs 125 mg, 250 mg, 500 mg
  ▶ susp 125 mg/5 ml
  ▶ inj 750 mg, 1.5 g

Celecoxib (Celebrex)

▶ class
  ▶ analgesic, NSAID
▶ indications
  ▶ osteoarthritis
▶ precautions/contraindications
  ▶ pregnancy risk category C (D in third trimester)
  ▶ avoid when peptic ulcer disease or renal insufficiency
  ▶ hepatic insufficiency
  ▶ sulfa allergy
▶ dosage/route
  ▶ adults: 200 mg/d q d or BID
▶ how supplied
  ▶ caps 100 mg, 200 mg

Cephalexin (Keflex, Keftab)

▶ class
  ▶ antibiotic, cephalosporin (first-generation)
▶ precautions/contraindications
  ▶ pregnancy risk category B
  ▶ caution with penicillin allergy
▶ dosage/route
  ▶ children: 25–100 mg/kg/d div PO QID
  ▶ adults: 250 mg–1 g PO QID
▶ how supplied
  ▶ tabs 250 mg, 500 mg, 1 g
  ▶ caps 250 mg, 500 mg
  ▶ susp 125 or 250 mg/5 ml

Cephradine (Anspor, Velosef)

▶ class
  ▶ antibiotic, cephalosporin (first-generation)
▶ precautions/contraindications
  ▶ pregnancy risk category B
  ▶ caution with penicillin allergy
▶ dosage/route
  ▶ children under 1 yr: safe use not established

- children over 1 yr: 25–100 mg/kg/d div PO QID or 12.5–25 mg/kg IV/IM q 6 h
- adults: 250–500 mg–1 g PO QID or IV/IM q 6 h
▶ how supplied
  - caps 250 mg, 500 mg
  - susp 125 or 250 mg/5 ml

Chloral Hydrate (Aquachloral, Noctec, Novochlorhydrate)

▶ class
  - sedative, nonspecific
▶ indication
  - short-term sedative/hypnotic for diagnostic and therapeutic procedures
▶ pharmacodynamics/kinetics
  - onset 30–60 min
  - duration half-life 8–10 h
▶ precautions/contraindications
  - pregnancy risk category C, caution in patients with hepatic disease/dysfunction or renal dysfunction
▶ dosage/route
  - administer at least 30 min before procedure
  - children: sedation, 5–15 mg/kg PO or PR; hypnosis, 25–75 mg/kg PO or PR
  - adults: sedation, 250 mg PO or PR; hypnosis, 500–1000 mg PO or PR
▶ how supplied
  - caps 250 mg, 500 mg
  - syrup 250 or 500 mg/5 ml
  - supp 325 mg, 500 mg, 650 mg

Chlorpromazine (Chlorazine, Ormazine, Promapar, Promaz, Sonazine, Thorazine, Thor-Prom)

▶ class
  - antipsychotic, antiemetic, phenothiazine
▶ indication
  - sedation, management of acute psychosis
▶ pharmacodynamics/kinetics
  - onset within 20 min, PO
  - duration 4–6 h, PO
▶ precautions/contraindications
  - pregnancy risk category C
  - adverse effects include orthostatic hypotension and dystonic reactions (treated with diphenhydramine or benztropine)
  - avoid when cardiac disease, seizure disorder, or neuroleptic malignant syndrome
▶ dosage/route
  - children over 6 mo: 0.25–0.5 mg/kg IV/IM q 6–8 h; repeat dose in 20 min if necessary
  - adults: 25–100 mg IV/IM; repeat dose in 20 min if necessary

▶ how supplied
  ▷ inj 25 mg/ml

Ciprofloxacin (Cipro)

▶ class
  ▷ antibiotic, quinolone
▶ important pharmacodynamics/kinetics
  ▷ antacids reduce absorption by up to 98% so do not co-administer within 2 h; may increase theophylline and warfarin levels.
▶ precautions/contraindications
  ▷ pregnancy risk category C,
  ▷ patients with a history of seizure disorder or CNS conditions that can increase risk for seizure; adjust dose w/renal impairment.
▶ dosage/route
  ▷ children (under 18 years old): contraindicated
  ▷ adults: 250–750 mg PO BID or 400 mg IV q 12 h
▶ how supplied
  ▷ tabs 250 mg, 500 mg, 750 mg
  ▷ inj 200 mg, 400 mg

Clarithromycin (Biaxin)

▶ class
  ▷ antibiotic, macrolide
▶ pharmacodynamics/kinetics
  ▷ increases theophylline and carbamazepine levels
▶ precautions/contraindications
  ▷ pregnancy risk category C
  ▷ concomitant use of loratadine or terfenidine since ventricular arrhythmias have occurred with other macrolides
  ▷ may increase PT and INR in patients taking warfarin
▶ dosage/route
  ▷ children: 15 mg/kg/d div PO BID
  ▷ adults: 250–500 mg PO BID
▶ how supplied
  ▷ susp 125 or 250 mg/5 ml
  ▷ tabs 250 mg, 500 mg

Clindamycin (Cleocin)

▶ class
  ▷ antibiotic, lincomycin
▶ precautions/contraindications
  ▷ pregnancy risk category B
  ▷ adverse effects include pseudomembranous enterocolitis (discontinue if diarrhea occurs) and pain with IM injection

- dosage/route
  - children under 1 mo: 15–20 mg/kg/d IV div QID; over 1 mo: 8–20 mg/kg/d PO div QID; 20–40 mg/kg/d IV div Q 6–8 °
  - adults: 150–450 mg PO QID; 600 mg IV/IM 8 h , max 1.8 g/d
- how supplied
  - caps 150 mg, 300 mg
  - sln 75 mg/5 ml
  - inj 650 mg/ml

Cloxacillin (Cloxapen, Tegopen)

- class
  - antibiotic, penicillinase-resistant penicillin
- precautions/contraindications
  - pregnancy risk category B
  - penicillin allergy
  - excreted in breast milk
- dosage/route
  - children: 50–100 mg/kg/d div PO QID
  - adults: 250–500 mg PO QID
- how supplied
  - sln 125 mg/5 ml
  - caps 250 mg, 500 mg

Cocaine

- class
  - local anesthetic, ester
- indication
  - topical anesthesia for mucous membranes
- pharmacodynamics/kinetics
  - mucosal application has onset of action within 1 min and peak effect in 5 min
  - ideal for treating epistaxis since achieves both anesthesia and vasoconstriction, which slows or stops bleeding
- precautions/contraindications
  - pregnancy risk category C
  - use cautiously when hypertension, severe cardiac disease, or thyrotoxicosis
  - adverse effects include hypertension, tachycardia, seizures
- dosage/route
  - use the lowest effective dose
  - do not exceed 1 mg/kg
- how supplied
  - sln 4%, 10%

Co-trimoxazole [trimethoprim/sulfamethoxazole] (Bactrim, Cotrim, SMZ-TMP, Sulfatrim, UroPlus, Septra)

▶ class
- ▶ antibiotic, sulfonamide/folate antagonist
▶ precautions/contraindications
- ▶ pregnancy risk category C (D near term)
- ▶ severe renal impairment
- ▶ porphyria
- ▶ breast-feeding
- ▶ G6PD deficiency
- ▶ megalobastic anemia
▶ dosage/route
- ▶ children under 2 mo: safe use not established
- ▶ children over 2 mo: by trimethoprim component, 8 mg/kg/d div PO BID or IV q 6–12 h
- ▶ adults: one double strength (DS) tab PO BID or equivalent dose IV q 6–12 h
▶ how supplied
- ▶ susp 40/200 mg/5 ml
- ▶ tabs regular, 80/400 mg; DS, 160/800 mg
- ▶ inj 80/400 mg/5ml

Cyclobenzaprine (Flexeril)

▶ class
- ▶ skeletal muscle relaxant
▶ pharmacodynamics/kinetics
- ▶ cyclic antidepressant derivative
▶ precautions/contraindications
- ▶ pregnancy risk category B
- ▶ do not use when there is hyperthyroidism or cardiac disease, or a monoamine oxidase (MAO) inhibitor has been used within 2 weeks
- ▶ caution in elderly and debilitated patients
- ▶ dispense small amounts in patients with depression or substance abuse since large overdoses are life-threatening
▶ dosage/route
- ▶ children: safe use not established
- ▶ adults: 10 mg PO BID to QID for up to 2 weeks
▶ how supplied
- ▶ tabs 10 mg

Cyclopentolate (AK-Pentolate, Cyclogyl, I-Pentolate, Minims, Pentolair)

▶ class
  ▶ anticholinergic, mydriatic/cycloplegic
▶ indication
  ▶ management of traumatic iritis
▶ pharmacodynamics/kinetics
  ▶ onset peak effect in 15–60 min
  ▶ recovery from cycloplegia in 6–24 h and from mydriasis in 24 h
  ▶ superior to homatropine since it has a shorter duration of action
▶ precautions/contraindications
  ▶ pregnancy risk category C
  ▶ do not use when there is elevated IOP, glaucoma
▶ dosage/route
  ▶ children and adults: 0.5–2% sln in eye, repeat in 5 min
▶ how supplied
  ▶ ophth sln 0.5%, 1%, 2%

Dexamethasone (AK-Dex, Decadron, Decaject, Dexasone, Dexon, Dexone, Hexadrol, Solurex)

▶ class
  ▶ glucocorticoid, anti-inflammatory, immunosuppressant
▶ indication
  ▶ management of cerebral edema
▶ precautions/contraindications
  ▶ pregnancy risk category C
▶ dosage/route
  ▶ children: 1–2 mg/kg/dose PO/IV/IM initially, followed by 1–1.5 mg/kg/dose div q 4–6 h; max 1.6 mg/24 h
  ▶ adults: 10 mg IV initially followed by 4 mg IM q 6 h for 2–4 d, then taper over 5–7 d
▶ how supplied
  ▶ inj variable concentrations

Dextran (Gentran, Macrodex)

▶ class
  ▶ volume expander, glucose polymer
▶ indication
  ▶ management of hemorrhagic shock
▶ pharmacodynamics/kinetics
  ▶ high molecular weight expands circulatory volume more than that infused
  ▶ duration: effect lasts about 12 h

► precautions/contraindications
  ► pregnancy risk category C
  ► do not use when cardiomyopathy, congestive heart failure, renal failure, edema, or coagulopathy
► dosage/route
  ► adults: bolus 500 ml; max 20 ml/kg/d
  ► children: bolus 5–10 ml/kg; max 20 ml/kg/d
► how supplied
  ► inj 10% dextran 40 (i.e., molecular weight 40,000), 6% dextran 70, 6% dextran 75

Diazepam (Valium)

► classes
  ► anticonvulsant, benzodiazepine
  ► sedative, benzodiazepine
  ► skeletal muscle relaxant
► indications
  ► status epilepticus
  ► sedation
  ► skeletal muscle relaxation
► pharmacodynamics/kinetics
  ► IM injection is not used since absorption is erratic
  ► onset 1–5 min IV, 30–60 min PO
  ► duration: effect lasts 3 h; up to several days in elderly or renal/hepatic dysfunction
  ► synergistic with opiates
► precautions/contraindications
  ► pregnancy risk category D, especially 1st trimester
  ► do not use when there is glaucoma, shock, coma
  ► adverse effects include CNS depression and hypoventilation
► dosage/route—sedation/muscle relaxation
  ► children: 0.05–0.1 mg/kg PO/IV q 6–8 h
  ► adults: 2–10 mg PO QID or IV q 6–8 h
► dosage/route—status epilepticus
  ► children: 0.2 mg/kg IV or 0.5 mg/kg PR q 10 min
  ► adults: 5–10 mg IV q 10 min, max dose 30 mg; repeat q 2–4 h prn
► how supplied
  ► tabs 2 mg, 5 mg, 10 mg
  ► caps 15 mg (extended release)
  ► sln 5 mg/5 ml or 5 mg/ml
  ► inj 5 mg/ml

Diclofenac Na (Voltaren) or Diclofenac K (Cataflam)

► class
  ► analgesic, NSAID

▶ indication
  ▶ relief of mild to moderate pain
▶ precautions/contraindications
  ▶ pregnancy risk category B
  ▶ avoid when peptic ulcer disease or renal insufficiency
  ▶ avoid in patients with history of asthma, or allergic reactions precipitated by ASA or other NSAIDS
  ▶ stop if abdominal pain, GI bleeding, or worsening of renal function
▶ dosage/route
  ▶ adults: 25–75 mg PO BID–QID; max 200 mg/d
▶ how supplied
  ▶ tab (Diclofenac Na) 25 mg, 50 mg, 75 mg
  ▶ tab (Diclofenac K) 50 mg

Dicloxacillin (Dycill, Dynapen, Pathocil)

▶ class
  ▶ antibiotic, penicillinase-resistant penicillin
▶ precautions/contraindications
  ▶ pregnancy risk category B, may cause transient elevations in LFTs, causing cholestastis or hepatitis
▶ dosage/route
  ▶ children: 25–50 mg/kg/d div PO QID, not to exceed adult dose
  ▶ adults: 250–500 mg PO QID
  ▶ take on empty stomach
▶ how supplied
  ▶ susp 62.5 mg/5 ml
  ▶ caps 125 mg, 250 mg, 500 mg

Diflunisal (Dolobid)

▶ class
  ▶ analgesic, NSAID, salicylate derivative
▶ indication
  ▶ relief of mild to moderate pain
▶ precautions/contraindications
  ▶ pregnancy risk category C
  ▶ avoid when peptic ulcer disease cholestasis, or renal insufficiency
  ▶ avoid in patients with history of asthma, or allergic reactions precipitated by ASA or other NSAIDS
  ▶ stop if abdominal pain, GI bleeding, or worsening of renal function
▶ dosage/route
  ▶ children: safe use not established
  ▶ adults under 70 years: 1 g initially then 250–500 mg PO BID–TID, max 1,500 mg/d
  ▶ adults over 70 years: half the usual adult dose

▶ how supplied
  ▶ tabs 250 mg, 500 mg

Diltiazem (Cardizem)

▶ class:
  ▶ calcium channel blocker
▶ indication
  ▶ rate control for atrial tachyarrhythmias
▶ precautions/contraindications
  ▶ pregnancy category C
  ▶ contraindicated in sick sinus syndrome or second- or third-degree AV block; WPW syndrome, LVF, hypotension, acute MI, pulmonary congestion.
  ▶ cautions in elderly, heart failure, concomitant beta-blockers.
▶ dosage/route
  ▶ adult: 0.25 mg/kg IV bolus over 2 min; repeat with 0.35 mg/kg IV bolus. If no response, then start IV infusion at 5–15 mg/h (up to 24 h)
▶ how supplied
  ▶ inj 5 mg/5 ml

Diphtheria and Tetanus Toxoids (dT, DT)

▶ class
  ▶ immunization, tetanus
▶ indication
  ▶ primary immunization
▶ precautions/contraindications
  ▶ pregnancy risk category C
  ▶ anaphylaxis
  ▶ may be ineffective in immunosuppressed patients
▶ dosage/route
  ▶ children under 6 years: DT, 0.5 ml IM
  ▶ children over 6 years and adults: dT, 0.5 ml IM
▶ how supplied
  ▶ inj DT = pediatric dose/0.5 ml
  ▶ inj dT = adult dose/0.5 ml

Dobutamine (Dobutrex)

▶ class
  ▶ inotrope
▶ indication
  ▶ management of cardiogenic shock
▶ pharmacodynamics/kinetics
  ▶ onset: effect within 2 min, peaks within 10 min
  ▶ duration 2 min after administration discontinued

▶ precautions/contraindications
  ▶ pregnancy risk category C
  ▶ correct hypovolemia before using
  ▶ do not use when known idiopathic hypertrophic subaortic stenosis
  ▶ adverse effects include tachycardia, ischemic chest pain, and ventricular arrhythmias
  ▶ do not mix with other drugs
▶ dosage/route
  ▶ children and adults: 2–20 mcg/kg/min
  ▶ titrate so that heart rate does not exceed 10% of baseline
▶ how supplied
  ▶ inj 12.5 mg/ml

Dopamine (Dopastat, Intropin)

▶ classes
  ▶ inotrope
  ▶ vasopressor
▶ indication
  ▶ adjunct in shock to increase CO, BP, and urinary output
▶ contraindications
  ▶ pheochromocytoma
▶ pharmacodynamics/kinetics
  ▶ peak effect within 10–20 min
  ▶ half-life 2 min
  ▶ specific effects are dose-related (see below)
▶ precautions/contraindications
  ▶ pregnancy risk category C
  ▶ adverse effects include tachycardia, ischemic chest pain, and ventricular arrhythmias
  ▶ do not mix with other drugs
  ▶ caution with monoamine oxidase inhibitors
  ▶ if extravasation occurs infiltrate with phentolamine (if available) or apply nitroglycerin ointment to site
▶ dosage/route
  ▶ children and adults:
    ▹ 2–5 mcg/kg/min increases GFR
    ▹ 5–10 mcg/kg/min beta-agonist effect and increases kidney perfusion
    ▹ over 10 mcg/kg/min alpha- and beta-agonist effect and increases kidney perfusion.
  ▶ titrate so that heart rate does not exceed 10% of baseline
▶ how supplied
  ▶ inj variable concentrations

Dorzolamide (Truspot)

▶ class
  ▶ topical carbonic anhydrase inhibitor

- indication
  - eye trauma associated with IOP over 20 mm Hg
- pharmacodynamics/kinetics
  - peak effect at 2 h
  - duration 8–12 h
- precautions/contraindications
  - pregnancy risk category C
  - avoid when electrolyte imbalance, renal or hepatic insufficiency as systemic absorption occurs
  - adverse effects include acidosis
- dosage/route
  - children: safe use not established
  - adults: 1 gtt in effected eye
- how supplied
  - ophth 2% sln

Doxacurium (Nuromax)

- class
  - paralytic, nondepolarizing
- indication
  - paralysis for intubation, mechanical ventilation, procedures
- pharmacodynamics/kinetics
  - onset within 2 min, max occurs in about 3–6 min
  - duration 100 min
- precautions/contraindications
  - pregnancy risk category C
  - use cautiously in neuromuscular disease
- dosage/route
  - children under 2 yr: safe use not established
  - children over 2 yr and adults: 0.05 mg/kg initially, then 0.005–0.01 mg/kg prn to maintain paralysis; use ideal body weight for obese patients.
- how supplied
  - inj 1 mg/ml

Droperidol (Inapsine)

- classes
  - sedative, antipsychotic, butyrophenone
  - antiemetic
- indications
  - sedation, management of acute psychosis
  - anesthetic premedication
  - antiemetic
- pharmacodynamics/kinetics
  - onset within 3–10 min, peaks in 30 min (IM)
  - duration 2–4 h

- ▶ more profound sedation than other butyrophenone
- ▶ powerful antiemetic effect is advantageous
- ▶ precautions/contraindications
  - ▶ pregnancy risk category C
  - ▶ may potentiate effects of other CNS depressants
  - ▶ adverse effects include orthostatic hypotension and dystonic reactions (treated with diphenhydramine or benztropine)
- ▶ dosage/route
  - ▶ children (over 2 yr old): 0.1–0.15 mg/kg, repeat in 30 min if necessary, max dose 2.5 mg
  - ▶ adults: 2.5–10 mg IV/IM, repeat in 30 min if necessary
- ▶ how supplied
  - ▶ inj 2.5 mg/ml

Ephedrine (Bofedrol, Efedron)

- ▶ class
  - ▶ vasopressor
- ▶ indication
  - ▶ management of hypotension associated with neurogenic shock (spinal cord injury)
- ▶ pharmacodynamics/kinetics
  - ▶ duration 1 h
  - ▶ alpha- and beta-adrenergic effects
- ▶ precautions/contraindications
  - ▶ pregnancy risk category C
  - ▶ use cautiously when elderly, hypertensive, underlying cardiac or hyperthyroid disease, or for those taking MOA inhibitors
  - ▶ adverse effects include anxiety, agitation, urinary retention, hypertension, and tachycardia
  - ▶ necessary to correct volume depletion before using any vasopressor
- ▶ dosage/route
  - ▶ children: 0.01 mg/kg slowly q 5–10 min prn; max 0.5 mg
  - ▶ adults: 10–25 mg IV slowly q 5–10 min prn; max 150 mg/d
- ▶ how supplied
  - ▶ inj variable concentrations

Epinephrine (Adrenaline)

- ▶ classes
  - ▶ vasopressor
  - ▶ inotrope
- ▶ indications
  - ▶ management of cardiac arrest: venticular fibrillation (VF), pulseless ventricular tachycardia (VT), asystole, pulseless electrical activity (PEA)
  - ▶ adjunct to local anesthetic to reduce bleeding and prolong anesthetic effect

- ▶ precautions/contraindications
    - ▶ pregnancy risk category C
    - ▶ do not use with local anesthetic in poorly perfused tissue or acral areas (i.e., fingers, toes, ears, nose, penis)
- ▶ dosage/route—for cardiac arrest
    - ▶ children: first dose 0.01 mg/kg (or 0.1 ml/kg of 1:10,000 sln)
    - ▶ adults: first dose 1 mg
    - ▶ doses repeated every 3–5 min during the arrest
    - ▶ higher doses have no proven advantage
- ▶ dosage/route—with local anesthetic
    - ▶ 1:500,000 to 1:50,000 premixed with local anesthetic or add 0.1 mg to 10 ml plain local anesthetic; max is 0.005 mg/kg
- ▶ how supplied
    - ▶ inj 1:1,000 (1 mg/ml); 1:10,000 (0.1 mg/ml); 1:100,000 (0.01 mg/ml)
    - ▶ syringes 1 mg/10 ml
    - ▶ premixed with various local anesthetics

Erythromycin Base (E-mycin, Eryc, Eryfed, Erithril 500, Robimycin), Estolate (Ilosone), Ethylsuccinate (E.E.S., E-Mycin E, EryPed, Pediamycin, Pediazole, Wyamycin E), and Lactobionate (parenteral)

- ▶ class
    - ▶ antibiotic, macrolide
- ▶ pharmacodynamics/kinetics
    - ▶ some oral forms are enteric-coated to prevent destruction by gastric acids
    - ▶ take base form on an empty stomach
- ▶ precautions/contraindications
    - ▶ pregnancy risk category B (avoid estolate)
    - ▶ interacts with theophylline and carbamazepine by increasing levels, with oral anticoagulants by increasing prothrombin time
    - ▶ adverse effects include vomiting, abdominal cramping, and hepatic toxicity (reversible cholestatic jaundice)
- ▶ dosage/route
    - ▶ children: 20–40 mg/kg/d div PO/IM/IV QID or q 6 h, max 4 g/d
    - ▶ adults: 250–500 mg PO QID or IM/IV q 6 h
- ▶ how supplied—base
    - ▶ tabs 250 mg, 333 mg, 500 mg
    - ▶ pellets 125 mg, 250 mg
- ▶ how supplied—ethylsuccinate
    - ▶ susp 200 or 400 mg/5 ml
    - ▶ chewable tabs 200 mg
- ▶ how supplied—estolate
    - ▶ drops 100 mg/ml
    - ▶ susp 50 or 125 or 250/5 ml
    - ▶ tabs 500 mg

- chewable tabs 125 mg, 250 mg
- caps 250 mg
▶ how supplied—ophthalmic oint
  - 5 mg/g

Esmolol (Brevibloc)

▶ classes
  - antihypertensive
  - antiarrhythmic
▶ indications
  - hypertension associated with traumatic aortic rupture
  - supraventricular tachycardia
▶ pharmacodynamics/kinetics
  - beta-adrenergic blockade
  - onset within 2 min
  - duration: effect stops within 9 min when drug discontinued
  - primary advantage over other beta-adrenergic blockers is the ability to terminate the effect rapidly should any significant adverse effects occur
▶ precautions/contraindications
  - pregnancy risk category C
  - do not use when there is bradycardia, hypotension, second- or third-degree AV block, CHF
  - use cautiously when there is asthma, COPD, or diabetes
  - adverse effects include bradycardia, atrial–ventricular conduction delays, and hypotension
▶ dosage/route
  - children: safe use not established
  - adults: remove 20 ml fluid from a 500-ml IV (NS or D_5W) bag; then add 20 ml (5 g) esmolol (2 amps) to create 10 mg/ml sln, load 500 mcg/kg over 1 min and infuse 50 mcg/kg/min for 4 min; if inadequate response, repeat load and increase infusion by 50 mcg/kg/min; repeat similarly q 4 min prn; stop when desired hemodynamic effect is achieved or max 300 mcg/kg/min
▶ how supplied
  - amp 250 mg/ml (for creating maintenance drip)
  - inj 10 mg/ml

Ethyl Chloride

▶ class
  - local anesthetic, halogenated hydrocarbon
▶ indication
  - topical anesthesia for minor procedures
▶ pharmacodynamics/kinetics
  - repeated doses can cause significant epithelial damage
  - do not store or use near heat source since highly flammable and explosive

▶ precautions/contraindications
  ▶ pregnancy risk category C
  ▶ do not inhale or use near eyes, broken skin, or mucous membranes
▶ dosage/route
  ▶ children and adults: hold the nozzle about 12 inches from the area and spray briefly until a light frosting appears
▶ how supplied
  ▶ topical liquid spray

Etodolac (Lodine)

▶ class
  ▶ analgesic, NSAID
▶ indication
  ▶ relief of mild to moderate pain
▶ precautions/contraindications
  ▶ pregnancy risk category C (D in third trimester)
  ▶ avoid when peptic ulcer disease or renal insufficiency
  ▶ avoid in patients with asthma or allergic reactions precipitated by ASA or other NSAIDS
  ▶ stop if abdominal pain, GI bleeding, or worsening of renal function
▶ dosage/route
  ▶ children: safe use not established
  ▶ adults: 200–400 mg PO TID or QID prn; max 1200 mg/d
▶ how supplied
  ▶ caps 200 mg, 300 mg
  ▶ tabs 400 mg
  ▶ extended release caps 400 mg, 1000 mg

Etomidate (Amidate)

▶ class
  ▶ sedative, nonspecific
▶ indication
  ▶ sedation, induction for intubation
▶ pharmacodynamics/kinetics
  ▶ onset with 60 s
  ▶ duration 3–5 min
  ▶ minimal hemodynamic alteration compared with thiopental
▶ precautions/contraindications
  ▶ pregnancy risk category C
  ▶ monitor signs, symptoms of adrenal insufficiency with prolonged use
  ▶ adverse effects include transient skeletal muscle movements
▶ dosage/route
  ▶ children under 10 years: safe use not established
  ▶ children over 10 years and adults: 0.3 mg/kg (range 0.2–0.6 mg/kg) IVP slowly over 1 min
▶ how supplied
  ▶ inj 2 mg/ml

Fenoprofen (Nalfon)

▶ class
  ▶ analgesic, NSAID
▶ indication
  ▶ relief of mild to moderate pain
▶ precautions/contraindications
  ▶ pregnancy risk category C (D in third trimester)
  ▶ avoid in patients with asthma or allergic reactions precipitated by ASA or other NSAIDS
  ▶ avoid when peptic ulcer disease or renal insufficiency
  ▶ stop if abdominal pain, GI bleeding, or worsening of renal function
▶ dosage/route
  ▶ children: safe use not established
  ▶ adults: 200–600 mg PO TID or QID prn
▶ how supplied
  ▶ caps 200 mg, 300 mg
  ▶ tabs 600 mg

Fentanyl (Sublimaze)

▶ class
  ▶ analgesic, opioid
▶ indication
  ▶ relief of severe pain, analgesia during a procedure, adjunct to anesthesia
▶ pharmacodynamics/kinetics
  ▶ onset IV, immediate
  ▶ duration 30–60 min
▶ precautions/contraindications
  ▶ pregnancy risk category C (D near term)
  ▶ adverse effects include vomiting, respiratory depression, bradycardia, and thoracic muscle rigidity (associated with rapid administration and high doses)
▶ dosage/route
  ▶ children: under 2 years: safe use not established
  ▶ children: over 2 years and adults: 1–2 mcg/kg IV for analgesia/sedation
  ▶ use half the loading dose every 5–10 min during procedure and titrate to pain and level of responsiveness
  ▶ push IV doses slowly over 1–2 min
▶ how supplied
  ▶ inj 50 mcg/ml

Flumazenil (Romazicon)

▶ class
  ▶ benzodiazepine reversal agent

▶ indication
  ▶ iatrogenic oversedation with benzodiazepine
▶ pharmacodynamics/kinetics
  ▶ onset effect within 1–2 min, peak within 6–10 min
  ▶ duration under 1 h
▶ precautions/contraindications
  ▶ pregnancy risk category C
  ▶ do not use when seizure disorder, benzodiazepine dependence, or mixed overdose
  ▶ adverse effects include seizures, pain at injection site
  ▶ since duration of flumazenil is shorter than that of benzodiazepines, patient must be monitored closely for at least 1 h after last dose to prevent unwitnessed respiratory arrest
▶ dosage/route
  ▶ children under 20 kg: 0.01 mg/kg over 15 s, repeat 0.005 mg/kg q 1 min prn to max 1 mg
  ▶ children over 20 kg and adults: 0.2 mg IV slowly over 15 s; repeat q 1 min prn to max 1 mg at a time
  ▶ redose total initial dose q 20 min if sedation reoccurs, may give up to 3 mg/h
▶ how supplied
  ▶ inj 0.1 mg/ml

Flurbiprofen (Ansaid)

▶ class
  ▶ analgesic, NSAID
▶ indication
  ▶ relief of mild to moderate pain
▶ precautions/contraindications
  ▶ pregnancy risk category B (D in third trimester)
  ▶ avoid when peptic ulcer disease or renal insufficiency
  ▶ stop if abdominal pain, GI bleeding, or worsening of renal function
▶ dosage/route
  ▶ children: safe use not established
  ▶ adults: 50–100 mg PO BID–QID prn, max 300 mg/d
▶ how supplied
  ▶ tabs 50/100 mg

Fosphenytoin (Cerebyx)

▶ class
  ▶ anticonvulsant, prodrug of phenytoin
▶ indication
  ▶ seizure control

- pharmacodynamics/kinetics
  - prodrug of phenytoin
  - water soluble
  - peak plasma concentration occurs 30 min after IM
  - conversion to phenytoin is about 15 min
  - serum concentrations of 10–20 mcg/ml are therapeutic
- precautions/cautions
  - less cardiovascular side effects then phenytoin
  - caution in patients with renal or hepatic impairment
  - pregnancy risk category D
- dosage/route
  - adults: loading dose: 15–20 mg/kg phenytoin equivalent (PE) at 100–150 mg PE/min IM or IV; maintenance dose: 4–6 mg/kg PE IM or IV
- how supplied
  - 150 mg PE/mL

Gatifloxacin (Tequin)

- class
  - antibiotic, quinolone
- precautions/contraindications
  - pregnancy risk category C
  - caution in patients with seizure disorders
  - contraindicated in children
  - renal clearance
  - may increase theophylline and warfarin toxicity
- dosage/route
  - adults: 200–400 mg PO or IV q d
- how supplied
  - tabs 200, 400 mg
  - inj 200, 400 mg

Gentamicin (Garamycin, Gentacidin)

- class
  - antibiotic, aminoglycoside
- precautions/contraindications
  - pregnancy risk category D
  - adverse effects include nephro- and oto-toxicity
  - use cautiously when prior hearing problems or renal insufficiency
  - concomitant with loop diuretics
- dosage/route—IV/IM
  - children: 2–2.5 mg/kg IV/IM q 8 h
  - adults: 2 mg/kg load IV/IM, then 1–1.7 mg/kg IV/IM q 8 h
  - in those with impaired renal function, dosing interval (h) = creatinine (mg/100 ml) times 8
  - loading dose is fixed but subsequent doses are lowered in renal insufficiency

> ► after the third dose, peak should be 4–10 mcg/ml and trough under 2 mcg/ml
► dosage/route—ophth
> ► children and adults: 1–2 gtt sln or apply oint in eye(s) q 4 h
► how supplied
> ► ophth 3 mg/g oint or 0.1% sln
> ► inj 40 mg/ml

Haloperidol (Haldol)

► class
> ► sedative, butyrophenone antipsychotic
► indication
> ► sedation, management of acute psychosis
► pharmacodynamics/kinetics
> ► onset peak effect in 30–45 min
> ► duration half-life 20 h
► precautions/contraindications
> ► pregnancy risk category C
> ► patients with seizure disorder
> ► adverse effects include orthostatic hypotension, dystonic reactions (treated with diphenhydramine or benztropine), and neuroleptic malignant syndrome
► dosage/route
> ► children: 1–3 mg IV/IM q 4–8 h, max 0.1 mg/kg/d
> ► adults: 2–10 mg IV/IM q 4–8 h; lower doses in elderly
► how supplied
> ► inj 5 mg/ml

Homatropine

► class
> ► anticholingeric, mydriatic/cycloplegic
► indication
> ► management of traumatic iritis
► pharmacodynamics/kinetics
> ► onset peak effect in 30–90 min
> ► recovery from cycloplegia in 10–48 h
► precautions/contraindications
> ► pregnancy risk category C
> ► do not use when elevated IOP
> ► use cautiously in patients with cardiac disease
► dosage/route
> ► children: 1 gtt 2% sln in eye, repeat if necessary in 5–10 min
> ► adults: 1–2 gtt 2-5% sln in eye, repeat if necessary in 5–10 min
► how supplied
> ► ophth sln 2 or 5%

Hydromorphone (Dilaudid)

▶ class
  ▶ analgesic, opiate
▶ indication
  ▶ relief of moderate to severe pain
▶ pharmacodynamics/kinetics
  ▶ onset effect in 15–30 min, peak in 30–60 min
  ▶ duration 4–5 h
▶ precautions/contraindications
  ▶ pregnancy risk category C (D near term)
  ▶ adverse effects include respiratory depression and vomiting
▶ dosage/route
  ▶ children: 0.01 mg/kg IV/IM q 4 h
  ▶ adults: 1–4 mg IV/IM q 4 h; lower doses in the elderly
  ▶ push IV doses slowly over 2–5 min
▶ how supplied
  ▶ inj variable concentrations

Ibuprofen (Advil, Medipren, Motrin, Nuprin, PediaProfen, Rufen, Trendar)

▶ class
  ▶ analgesic, NSAID
▶ indication
  ▶ relief of mild to moderate pain
▶ precautions/contraindications
  ▶ pregnancy risk category B (D in third trimester)
  ▶ avoid when peptic ulcer disease or renal insufficiency
  ▶ avoid in patients with asthma or allergic reactions precipitated by ASA or other NSAIDS
  ▶ stop if there is abdominal pain, GI bleeding, or worsening of renal function
▶ dosage/route
  ▶ children: 5–10 mg/kg q 6–8 h, max 40 mg/kg/d
  ▶ adults: 400–800 mg q 6–8 h; max 3,200 mg/d
▶ how supplied
  ▶ susp 100 mg/5 ml
  ▶ tabs 200 mg, 300 mg, 400 mg, 600 mg, 800 mg

Imipenem-cilastatin (Primaxin)

▶ class
  ▶ antibiotic, carbapenem
▶ precautions/contraindications
  ▶ pregnancy risk category C
  ▶ do not use when there is penicillin/cephalosporin allergy

- adverse effects include seizures; avoid in patients with history of seizure disorder or renal impairment
▶ dosage/route
  - children: 60–100 mg/kg/d IV div q 6 h although safe use not established
  - adults: 250 mg–1 g IV q 6–8 h, max is lower of 50 mg/kg/d or 4 g/d
  - less frequent dosing when there is renal insufficiency

Isoproterenol (Isuprel)

▶ classes
  - inotrope
  - vasopressor
▶ indications
  - bradycardia and hypotension refractory to atropine
  - low cardiac output states
▶ precautions/contraindications
  - pregnancy risk category C
  - do not use when there are preexisting ventricular arrhythmias or ischemic heart disease
  - adverse effects include tachycardia and ventricular arrhythmias
▶ pharmocodynamics/kinetics
  - onset immediate
  - duration: effect lasts only a few minutes after the drug discontinued
▶ dosage/route
  - children: 0.05–2 mcg/kg/min
  - adults: 2–20 mcg/min
  - start at lower dose and titrate up to desired response
▶ how supplied
  - inj 200 mcg/ml

Ketamine (Ketalar)

▶ class
  - dissociative anesthetic
▶ indication
  - induction for intubation, conjunction with benzodiazepine
▶ pharmacodynamics/kinetics
  - onset 60 s IV; 3–4 min IM
  - duration of unconsciousness, 5–10 min with IV, 12–25 min after IM
▶ precautions/contraindications
  - pregnancy risk category C
  - do not use when there are psychotic disorders (i.e., schizophrenia) or when sudden rise in BP may be harmful (e.g., elevated ICP, hypertension, cardiac disease, aneurysms)
  - adverse effects include hypertension, tachycardia, and hypersalivation (avoided by pretreatment with atropine)

- dosage/route—induction of general anesthesia
  - children and adults 2 mg/kg IV/IM; repeat in increments of half to full initial dose
- dosage/route—sedation
  - children and adults: 0.5–3 mg/kg IM or 1–2 mg/kg IV
  - often used in conjunction with a benzodiazepine
- how supplied
  - inj variable concentrations

Ketoprofen (Orudis)

- class
  - analgesic, NSAID
- indication
  - relief of mild to moderate pain
- precautions/contraindications
  - pregnancy risk category B (D in third trimester)
  - avoid when peptic ulcer disease or renal insufficiency
  - avoid in patients with asthma or allergic reactions precipitated by ASA or other NSAIDS
  - stop if there is abdominal pain, GI bleeding, or worsening of renal function
- dosage/route
  - children: safe use not established
  - adults: 50–75 mg PO TID or QID
- how supplied
  - caps 25 mg, 50 mg, 75 mg

Ketorolac (Toradol)

- class
  - analgesic, NSAID
- pharmacodynamics/kinetics
  - onset up to 1 h before peak effect, half-life 3.8–6 h, longer in patients with renal failure
- precautions/contraindications
  - pregnancy risk category C
  - avoid when peptic ulcer disease or renal insufficiency
  - avoid in patients with asthma or allergic reactions precipitated by ASA or other NSAIDS
  - stop if there is abdominal pain, GI bleeding, or worsening of renal function
- dosage/route
  - children: safe use not established
  - adults: 30 mg IV/IM initial dose then 15 mg IM/IV q 6 h; 10 mg PO QID prn
- how supplied
  - tabs 10 mg
  - inj 15 or 30 mg/ml

Labetalol (Normodyne, Trandate)

- ▶ class
  - ▶ antihypertensive, alpha- and beta-adrenergic blocker
- ▶ indication
  - ▶ management of hypertension with traumatic aortic rupture
- ▶ pharmacodynamics/kinetics
  - ▶ onset effect in 2–5 min, peaks in 5–15 min
  - ▶ duration 2–4 h
- ▶ precautions/contraindications
  - ▶ pregnancy risk category C
  - ▶ do not use when there is asthma, cardiomyopathy, bradycardia, or heart block
  - ▶ adverse effects include AV conduction disturbances
- ▶ dosage/route
  - ▶ children: safe use not established
  - ▶ adults: 20 mg IV slowly over 2 min, repeat 40–80 mg IV q 10 min until desired response or max of 300 mg; alternatively, 2 mg/min IV infusion until desired response or max of 300 mg; usual dose is 50–200 mg
- ▶ how supplied
  - ▶ inj 5 mg/ml

Levofloxacin (Levoquin)

- ▶ class
  - ▶ antiobiotic, quinolone
- ▶ precautions/contraindications
  - ▶ pregnancy category C
  - ▶ caution in patients with seizure disorders
  - ▶ contraindicated in children
  - ▶ may increase theophylline and warfarin toxicity.
- ▶ pharmacodynamics/kinetics
  - ▶ give 2 h apart between antacids, iron preparations, zinc products, and carafate
  - ▶ renal clearance
- ▶ dosage/route
  - ▶ adult: 250–500 mg q d
- ▶ how supplied
  - ▶ tab 250, 500 mg
  - ▶ inj 250, 500 mg

Lidocaine (Xylocaine)

- ▶ classes
  - ▶ local anesthetic, amide
  - ▶ antiarrhythmic, class Ib
- ▶ indications
  - ▶ local anesthesia
  - ▶ ventricular arrhythmias

- ► pharmacodynamics/kinetics
  - ► onset 60 s IV
  - ► duration 10–20 min IV; 30–60 min locally
- ► precautions/contraindications
  - ► pregnancy risk category B
  - ► do not use when heart block or sensitivity to other amide-type anesthetics
  - ► adverse effects include seizures
- ► dosage/route—antiarrhythmic
  - ► children or adults: 1–1.5 mg/kg IV/ET, repeat q 5–10 min to max 3 mg/kg; if desired response achieved, infuse 30–50 mcg/kg/min
- ► dosage/route—local anesthetic
  - ► infiltrate 1 or 2% sln locally
  - ► often used with epinephrine to prolong the anesthetic effect and to induce vasoconstriction
  - ► can buffer with bicarbonate to minimize the pain with infiltration
    - ► one part bicarbonate to ten parts lidocaine
- ► how supplied
  - ► inj variable concentrations
  - ► topical sln 2%, 4%, 10% (spray)
  - ► jelly 2%
  - ► oint 5%

Lorazepam (Alzapam, Ativan, Loraz)

- ► classes
  - ► sedative, benzodiazepine
  - ► anticonvulsant, benzodiazepine, antianxiety
- ► indications
  - ► sedation or anxiolysis
  - ► immediate seizure control
- ► pharmacodynamics/kinetics
  - ► onset 20 min
  - ► duration 6–8 h
  - ► dilute with equal volume of diluents for IV administration
  - ► IM absorption is rapid (unlike diazepam), but onset is slower (give 2 h before procedure)
- ► precautions/contraindications
  - ► pregnancy risk category D
  - ► do not use when there is severe hypotension or glaucoma
  - ► adverse effects include hypotension and respiratory depression
- ► dosage/route—sedation
  - ► newborns: safe use not established
  - ► children: 0.025 mg/kg IV/IM prn
  - ► adults: 1–2 mg IV/IM prn
  - ► push IV doses slowly over 2–5 min

- ▶ dosage/route—seizure control
  - ▶ children: 0.05 mg/kg IV/IM, repeat once if necessary in 15 min; be aware that safe use not established; max 4 mg/dose
  - ▶ adults: 4 mg IV/IM, repeat once if necessary in 15 min
- ▶ how supplied
  - ▶ inj 2 or 4 mg/ml

Mannitol (Osmitrol)

- ▶ class
  - ▶ osmotic diuretic
- ▶ indications
  - ▶ reduction of increased ICP
  - ▶ reduction of IOP
- ▶ precautions/contraindications
  - ▶ pregnancy risk category C
  - ▶ do not use when there is active intracranial bleeding, pulmonary edema, or anuria
  - ▶ adverse effects include pulmonary edema
- ▶ pharmacodynamics/kinetics
  - ▶ onset: decrease in ICP, under 15 min; diuresis, 1–3 h
  - ▶ duration: decrease in ICP, 3–6 h
  - ▶ increases intravascular volume and may temporize hemorrhagic shock until diuresis occurs
- ▶ dosage/route
  - ▶ children over 12 yr old or adults : 1.5–2 g/kg IV over 30–60 min
- ▶ how supplied
  - ▶ inj 15%, 20%, 25%

Meperidine (Demerol)

- ▶ class
  - ▶ analgesic, opioid
- ▶ indication
  - ▶ relief of moderate to severe pain
- ▶ pharmacodynamics/kinetics
  - ▶ onset peak in 10–45 min
  - ▶ duration 2–4 h
- ▶ precautions/contraindications
  - ▶ pregnancy risk category C (D near term)
  - ▶ patients who have received MOA inhibitors within the past 14 days
  - ▶ adverse effects include respiratory depression and seizures (with high doses), active metabolite nor-meperidine accumulates in renal impairment and potentially lower seizure threshold.
- ▶ dosage/route
  - ▶ children and adults: 1–2 mg/kg IV/IM q 3–4 h

▶ how supplied
  ▶ inj variable concentrations

Meropenem (Merrem)

▶ class
  ▶ therapeutic, carbapenem antibiotic
▶ pharmacodynamics/kinetics
  ▶ penetrates CSF
▶ precautions/contraindications
  ▶ pregnancy category B
  ▶ adjust dose for renal impairment
  ▶ do not use in penicillin/cephalosporin allergy
  ▶ caution in patients with seizure disorder
▶ dosage/route:
  ▶ adults: 1 g q 8 h
  ▶ children over 3 mo: 20–40 mg/kg q 8 h

Methylprednisolone (Solu-Medrol)

▶ class
  ▶ glucocorticoid, anti-inflammation
▶ indication
  ▶ management of sensory/motor defects caused by acute spinal cord injury; start within 8 h after trauma onset
▶ precautions/contraindications
  ▶ pregnancy risk category C
  ▶ use cautiously when peptic ulcer disease, renal disease, diabetes, or systemic fungal infections
▶ dosage/route (for spinal cord injury)
  ▶ children: safe use not established
  ▶ adults: 30 mg/kg IV over 15 min followed by infusion of 5.4 mg/kg/h IV for 23 h

Metronidazole (Flagyl)

▶ class
  ▶ antibiotic, unclassified
▶ pharmacodynamics/kinetics
  ▶ disulfiram-type reaction with alcohol
  ▶ excellent anaerobic bacterial coverage
▶ precautions/contraindications
  ▶ pregnancy risk category B (controversial whether contraindicated in first trimester)
  ▶ use cautiously when there is hepatic insufficiency
  ▶ interacts with oral anticoagulants by increasing prothrombin time

▶ dosage/route
  ▶ children and adults: initially 7.5 mg/kg IV q 6 h; max 4 g/d

Mezlocillin (Mezlin)

▶ class
  ▶ antibiotic, antipseudomonal penicillin
▶ pharmacodynamics/kinetics
  ▶ minimal CSF penetration
▶ precautions/contraindications
  ▶ pregnancy risk category B
  ▶ use cautiously when renal insufficiency
▶ dosage/route
  ▶ children and adults: 100–350 mg/kg/d IV/IM div q 4–6 h

Midazolam (Versed)

▶ class
  ▶ sedative, benzodiazepine
▶ indications
  ▶ pre-procedure sedation/anxiolysis
  ▶ induction of general anesthesia for intubation
▶ pharmacodynamics/kinetics
  ▶ onset 2–5 min IV, 15 min IM/PO
  ▶ duration 1–4 h, mean 2 h
▶ precautions/contraindications
  ▶ pregnancy risk category D
  ▶ do not use when severe hypotension/shock
▶ dosage/route—sedation/anxiolysis
  ▶ children: 0.05–0.15 mg/kg/dose IV/IM/intranasal repeat q 2 min prn
    for sedation to max 0.6 mg/kg; dose of 0.5–1.0 mg/kg PO in juice
  ▶ adults: 1–2 mg IV/IM q 2 min prn sedation
▶ dosage/route—induction for general anesthesia
  ▶ adults: 0.3 mg/kg IV over 20–30 s, repeat 0.1 mg/kg IV prn q 2 min to
    max 0.6 mg/kg
▶ how supplied
  ▶ inj 1 or 5 mg/ml
  ▶ oral sln 2.5 mg/ml, 3 mg/ml, syrup 2 mg/ml

Mivacurium (Mivacron)

▶ class
  ▶ neuromuscular blocking, nondepolarizing
▶ indication
  ▶ paralysis for intubation, procedures

- pharmacodynamics/kinetics
  - onset max 3 min, duration 15–20 min
- precautions/contraindications
  - pregnancy category C
  - do not use in neuromuscular disease, in myasthenia gravis, or in elderly or debilitated patients
  - respiratory depression
- dosage/route
  - adults: 0.15 mg/kg IV
  - children: 2–12 yr old: 0.2 mg/kg IV
  - reduce dose by 50% in renal and hepatic diseases

Morphine (MS)

- class
  - analgesic, opioid
- indication
  - relief of moderate to severe pain
- pharmacodynamics/kinetics
  - onset peak effect in 20 min IV, 30–60 min IM
  - duration 4–5 h
- precautions/contraindications
  - pregnancy risk category C (D near term)
  - histamine release
  - caution in asthmatics
- dosage/route
  - children and adults: 0.1–0.2 mg/kg/dose IV/IM q 15 min prn until desired response then q 3–4 h for maintenance
- how supplied
  - inj variable concentrations

Nafcillin (Nafcil, Unipen)

- class
  - antibiotic, penicillinase-resistant penicillin
- precautions/contraindications
  - pregnancy risk category B
  - adverse effects include necrosis with extravasation, hypokalemia, and neutropenia
- dosage/route
  - children: 100–200 mg/kg/d IV/IM div q 4–6 h
  - adults: 500 mg–2 g IV q 4–6 h

Naloxone (Narcan)

- class
  - opioid antagonist

- indications
  - treatment for hypoventilation due (at least partially) to opiates
  - diagnosing opiate intoxication
- pharmacodynamics/kinetics
  - onset 1–2 min IV, 2–5 min IM
  - may appreciate brief, minimal arousal when no opiates are present
- precautions/contraindications
  - pregnancy risk category B
  - adverse effects include pulmonary edema, acute opiate withdrawal, and combativeness
  - avoid in patients with asthma or allergic reaction precipitated by ASA or other NSAIDS
  - use cautiously in opiate-dependent pregnant woman
- dosage/route
  - children: 0.01 mg/kg IV/IM, repeat q 2–3 min prn
  - adults: 0.4–2 mg IV/IM; repeat q 2–3 min prn to max of 10 mg
  - consider a small dose (e.g., 1 mcg/kg) in patients without hypoventilation in whom naloxone is being used diagnostically to avoid acute withdrawal symptoms and combativeness
- how supplied
  - inj 0.4 or 1 mg/ml

Naproxen (Aleve, Anaprox, Naprosyn)

- class
  - analgesic, NSAID
- indication
  - relief of mild to moderate pain
- pharmacodynamics/kinetics
  - 275 mg naproxen sodium (Aleve, Anaprox) = 250 mg naproxen (Naprosyn)
- precautions/contraindications
  - pregnancy risk category B
  - avoid when peptic ulcer disease or renal insufficiency
  - stop if abdominal pain, GI bleeding, or worsening renal function
- dosage/route
  - children under 2 yr: safe use not established
  - children over 2 yr: 5 mg/kg PO BID
  - adults: 250–500 mg PO BID
- how supplied
  - susp 125 mg/5 ml for naproxen
  - tabs 250 mg, 375 mg, 500 mg for naproxen; 275 mg, 550 mg for naproxen sodium

Nicardipine (Cardene)

- class
  - calcium channel blocker, antihypertensive

- indication
  - antihypertensive
- pharmacodynamics/kinetics
  - onset within minutes
  - peak 20 min
  - titrate q 15 min if goal BP is not attained
- precautions/contraindications
  - pregnancy category C
  - do not used with advanced aortic stenosis
  - do not use in patients with conduction disturbance, CHF
- dosage/route
  - initially 5 mg/h then increase by 2.5 mg/h q 15 min, max 15 mg/h

Nitroprusside (Nipride, Nitropress)

- class
  - antihypertensive
- indication
  - management of hypertension with thoracic aortic rupture (with concomitant beta-adrenergic blocker)
- pharmacodynamics/kinetics
  - onset within 2 min
  - duration: BP returns to baseline 1–10 min after discontinued
  - wrap IV bag containing the drug with foil to prevent exposure to light
- precautions/contraindications
  - pregnancy risk category C
  - do not use when there is decreased cerebral perfusion or increased ICP
  - adverse effects include potential cyanide/thiocyanate toxicity (especially when there is renal insufficiency) and high doses
- dosage/route
  - children and adults: 0.5–10 mcg/kg/min; titrate to response; avg 3 mcg/kg/min
  - check BP at least q 5 min while titrating, then q 15 min thereafter
- how supplied
  - inj 10 mg/ml

Norepinephrine (Levophed)

- classes
  - vasopressor
  - inotrope
- indication
  - maintain BP in severe hypotensive states
- pharmacodynamics/kinetics
  - onset within 1 min

- ▶ duration: BP returns to baseline 1–2 min after discontinued
- ▶ stimulates beta$_1$ and alpha-adrenenergic receptors
- ▶ precautions/contraindications
  - ▶ pregnancy risk category D
  - ▶ adverse effects include myocardial ischemia (since myocardial oxygen requirement is increased) and tissue necrosis with extravasation
- ▶ dosage/route
  - ▶ titrate to desired effect
  - ▶ children: start at 0.05–0.1 mcg/kg/min, titrate to desired response; max dose 2 mcg/kg/ml
  - ▶ adults: start at 4 mcg/min, titrate to desired response
- ▶ how supplied
  - ▶ inj 1 mg/ml

Ofloxin (Floxin)

- ▶ class
  - ▶ antibiotic, quinolone
- ▶ precautions/contraindications
  - ▶ pregnancy risk category C
  - ▶ contraindicated in children
  - ▶ caution in patients with seizure disorder
- ▶ pharmacodynamics/kinetics
  - ▶ may increase theophylline level and increase warfarin toxicity
  - ▶ give 2 h apart with antacids, iron preps, zinc products, and sucralfate
- ▶ dosage/route
  - ▶ children: contraindicated
  - ▶ adults: 200–400 mg PO BID or 400 mg IV q 12 h
- ▶ how supplied
  - ▶ tabs 200 mg, 300 mg, 400 mg
  - ▶ inj 200 mg, 400 mg

Oxacillin (Bactocill, Prostaphlin)

- ▶ class
  - ▶ penicillinase-resistant penicillin
- ▶ precautions/contraindications
  - ▶ pregnancy risk category B
  - ▶ adverse effects include reversible hepatic dysfunction
- ▶ dosage/route
  - ▶ children over 1 mo: 50–100 mg/kg/d PO div QID or IV/IM div q 6 h
  - ▶ adults: 500 mg–1 g PO QID or 250 mg–2 g IV/IM q 4–6 h
- ▶ how supplied
  - ▶ caps 250 mg, 500 mg
  - ▶ sln 250 mg/5 ml
  - ▶ inj 250 mg, 500 mg, 1 g, 2 g, and 4 g

Oxymetazoline (Afrin)

▶ class
  ▶ nasal decongestant
▶ indications
  ▶ prevention of nasal congestion associated with sinus fractures
  ▶ epistaxis control
  ▶ pretreatment for nasal intubation to prevent epistaxis
▶ pharmacodynamics/kinetics
  ▶ vasoconstriction via alpha-adrenergic receptors
  ▶ onset 5–10 min, duration 5–6 h
▶ precautions/contraindications
  ▶ pregnancy risk category C
  ▶ use cautiously when hypertension, hyperthyroidism, or cardiac disease, or if MOA inhibitors have been taken within last 14 d
  ▶ adverse effects include rebound nasal congestion (when used over 3 d)
▶ dosage/route
  ▶ children: under 6 years: 0.025% sln, 2–3 gtt each nostril BID
  ▶ children: over 6 yr and adults: 0.05% sln, 2–3 gtt each nostril BID
  ▶ limit use to 3 d
▶ how supplied
  ▶ sln 0.025% drops (children)
  ▶ nasal drops or spray 0.05% (adults)

Pancuronium (Pavulon)

▶ class
  ▶ paralytic, nondepolarizing
▶ indication
  ▶ paralysis for intubation, mechanical ventilation, procedures
▶ pharmacodynamics/kinetics
  ▶ onset 3–5 min
  ▶ duration 45–60 min
  ▶ onset and duration are dose-related
  ▶ causes little or no histamine release
▶ precautions/contraindications
  ▶ pregnancy risk category C
  ▶ patients with neuromuscular disease, debilitated patients or elderly patients
  ▶ do not use when adequate airway/ventilatory support is unavailable
▶ dosage/route
  ▶ children and adults: 0.1 mg/kg IV for induction; subsequent dose of 0.01 mg/kg IV provides 45–60 min paralysis for maintenance
▶ how supplied
  ▶ inj 1 or 2 mg/ml

Penicillin G potassium (Cryspen, Deltapen, Lanacillin, Parcillin, Pensorb, Pentids) or Penicillin G procaine (Crysticillin, Duracillin, Pfizerpen, Wycillin)

► class
  ► antibiotic, natural penicillin
► precautions/contraindications
  ► pregnancy risk category B
  ► 1 in 2,000 develop anaphylaxis; of these up to 10% die
► dosage/route
  ► children: 25,000–100,000 U/kg IV/IM div q 4–6 h
  ► adults: 12–24 million units divided q 4–6 h

Penicillin V Potassium (Beepen-VK, Pen-Vee K, Veetids)

► class
  ► antibiotic, natural penicillin
► pharmacodynamics/kinetics
  ► give 1 h before or 2 h after meals
► precautions/contraindications
  ► pregnancy risk category B
► dosage/route
  ► children: 25–50 mg/kg/d div PO QID
  ► adults: 250–500 mg PO QID
► how supplied
  ► susp 125 or 250 mg/5 ml
  ► tabs 125 mg, 250 mg, 500 mg

Pentobarbital (Nembutal)

► class
  ► sedative, barbiturate
► indication
  ► barbiturate coma for increased ICP or uncontrollable seizures
► pharmacodynamics/kinetics
  ► onset within 1 min IV
  ► duration 3–4 h
► precautions/contraindications
  ► pregnancy risk category D
  ► use cautiously in all patients and always assess risk versus benefit
  ► patient must be intubated
► dosage/route
  ► children and adults: 1–3 mg/kg IV initially, then 1–3 mg/kg/h IV thereafter
► how supplied
  ► inj 50 mg/ml

Phenobarbital (Barbita, Solfton)

▶ class
  ▶ anticonvulsant, barbiturate
▶ indication
  ▶ seizure control
▶ pharmacodynamics/kinetics
  ▶ onset: effect within 5 min, peaks within 30 min
  ▶ duration 4–10 h
  ▶ serum concentrations of 20–40 mcg/ml are therapeutic
▶ precautions/contraindications
  ▶ pregnancy risk category D
  ▶ adverse effects include hypotension, respiratory depression, and decreased level of consciousness
▶ dosage/route for status
  ▶ children and adults: 10–20 mg/kg no faster than 50 mg/min
▶ how supplied
  ▶ inj variable concentrations

Phenylephrine (Allerest, Sinex)

▶ class
  ▶ nasal decongestant
▶ indication
  ▶ prevention of nasal congestion associated with sinus fractures
▶ pharmacodynamics/kinetics
  ▶ vasoconstriction via alpha-adrenenergic receptors
▶ precautions/contraindications
  ▶ pregnancy risk category C
  ▶ adverse effects include rebound nasal congestion (when used over 3 d)
▶ dosage/route
  ▶ do not use for more than 3 d
  ▶ children under 6 yr: 0.12% sln, 2–3 gtt each nostril q 4 h
  ▶ children over 6 yr and adults: 0.25–1% sln, 2–3 gtt each nostril q 4 h
▶ how supplied
  ▶ nasal spray 0.12%, 0.25%, 0.5%, 1%

Phenytoin (Dilantin)

▶ class
  ▶ anticonvulsant, hydantoin
▶ indication
  ▶ seizure control
▶ pharmacodynamics/kinetics
  ▶ serum concentrations of 10–20 mcg/ml are therapeutic
  ▶ observe cardiac monitor and frequently measure blood pressure during loading dose

- ▶ precautions/contraindications
  - ▶ pregnancy risk category D
  - ▶ adverse effects include hypotension and arrhythmias (associated with rapid IV loading)
- ▶ dosage/route
  - ▶ children and adults: load 15–20 mg/kg IV at a rate no greater than 50 mg/min (i.e., 1 gm over 20 min)
- ▶ how supplied
  - ▶ inj 50 mg/ml

Pilocarpine (ophthalmic)

- ▶ class
  - ▶ miotic, cholinergic
- ▶ indication
  - ▶ management of eye trauma associated with intraocular pressure (IOP) over 20 mm Hg (e.g., retrobulbar hemorrhage, complication of hyphema)
- ▶ precautions/contraindications
  - ▶ pregnancy risk category C
  - ▶ do not use when there is possible iritis
- ▶ dosage/route
  - ▶ children and adults: 1–2 gtt of 2% sln in eye q 5 min for up to 3–6 doses (stop when IOP is controlled); follow by 1 gtt q 1–3 h to maintain control of IOP
- ▶ how supplied
  - ▶ ophth sln 2%

Piperacillin (Pipracil)

- ▶ class
  - ▶ antibiotic, antipseudomonal penicillin
- ▶ precautions/contraindications
  - ▶ pregnancy risk category B
  - ▶ bleeding tendencies, uremia, or hypokalemia
  - ▶ high dose lowers seizure threshold
- ▶ dosage/route
  - ▶ children and adults: 100–300 mg/kg/d IV/IM div q 4–6 h; safe use not established for children under 12 years old

Piperacillin/Tazobactam (Zosyn)

- ▶ class
  - ▶ antibiotic, antipseudomonal penicillin with beta-lactamase inhibitor
- ▶ precautions/contraindications
  - ▶ pregnancy risk category B
  - ▶ bleeding tendencies, uremia, or hypokalemia
  - ▶ high dose lowers seizure threshold

▶ dosage/route
  ▶ children: safe use not established
  ▶ adults: 3.375 g IV over 30 min q 6 h

Prednisolone (ophthalmic)

▶ class
  ▶ corticosteroid, anti-inflammatory
▶ indication
  ▶ management of traumatic iritis
▶ precautions/contraindications
  ▶ pregnancy risk category C
  ▶ do not use when possible eye infection
▶ dosage/route
  ▶ children and adults: 1–2 gtt in eye QID
  ▶ may use hourly in severe conditions
▶ how supplied
  ▶ ophth sln 0.125%, 0.5%, 1%

Procainamide (Procan, Pronestyl)

▶ class
  ▶ antiarrhythmic, class Ia
▶ indication
  ▶ ventricular and supraventricular arrhythmias
▶ precautions/contraindications
  ▶ pregnancy risk category C
  ▶ do not use when heart block or OT prolongation
  ▶ adverse effects include hypotension (associated with rapid infusion)
▶ dosage/route
  ▶ children or adults: bolus 17 mg/kg IV at 25–50 mg/min until arryhth-mia terminates followed by maintenance (in adults) of 1–4 mg/min
▶ how supplied
  ▶ inj 100 mg/ml, 500 mg/ml

Prochlorperazine (Compazine)

▶ classes
  ▶ sedative, phenothiazine
  ▶ antiemetic
▶ indication
  ▶ management of vomiting
▶ pharmacodynamics/kinetics
  ▶ onset 3–5 min IV, 20 min IM
  ▶ duration 4–6 h
▶ precautions/contraindications
  ▶ pregnancy risk category C

- adverse effects include orthostatic hypotension and dystonic reactions (treated with diphenhydramine or benztropine)
- dosage/route
  - children: 0.1–0.15 mg/kg IV/IM q 6 h prn
  - adults: 5–10 mg IV/IM q 6 h prn
- how supplied
  - inj 5 mg/ml

Promethazine (Phenergan)

- classes
  - sedative, phenothiazine
  - antiemetic
- indication
  - management of vomiting
- pharmacodynamics/kinetics
  - onset 3–5 min IV, 20 min IM
  - duration 4–6 h
- precautions/contraindications
  - pregnancy risk category C
  - adverse effects include orthostatic hypotension and dystonic reactions (treated with diphenhydramine or benztropine)
- dosage/route
  - children: 0.25–0.5 mg/kg IM q 6 h prn
  - adults: 12.5–50 mg IV/IM q 6 h prn
- how supplied
  - inj 25 or 50 mg/ml

Propofol (Diprivan)

- class
  - sedative, phenol derivative
- indication
  - induction of general anesthesia before intubation, sedation
- pharmacodynamics/kinetics
  - duration half-life 2–8 min
- precautions/contraindications
  - pregnancy risk category B
  - do not use when there is increased ICP
  - do not use in patients with egg allergy, hypotension with rapid IV infusion and bradycardia
- dosage/route
  - children: safe use not established
  - adults: 2–2.5 mg/kg IV q 10 s until desired response occurs; use half dose for elderly or hypovolemic
- how supplied
  - inj 10 mg/ml

Propoxyphene Napsylate (Darvon-N)

▶ class
  ▶ analgesic, opioid
▶ indication
  ▶ relief of moderate pain
▶ pharmacodynamics/kinetics
  ▶ onset 20–60 min; peaks in 2 h
  ▶ duration 4–6 h
▶ precautions/contraindications
  ▶ pregnancy risk category C
▶ dosage/route
  ▶ adults: 100 mg PO q 4 h prn
▶ how supplied
  ▶ caps 50 mg, 100 mg
  ▶ tabs 50 mg, 100 mg
  ▶ susp 50 mg/5 ml

Refocoxib (Vioxx)

▶ class
  ▶ NSAIDS, analgesic, Cox-2 inhibitor
▶ indication
  ▶ relief of moderate pain
▶ pharmacodynamics/kinetics
  ▶ Al/Mg and $CaCO_2$, contained in antacids, decrease absorption
  ▶ potential drug interactions with rifampin, warfarin, cimetidine since affects liver metabolism
▶ precautions/contraindications
  ▶ pregnancy risk category C
  ▶ avoid in hepatic insufficiency, peptic ulcer disease, or renal insufficiency
  ▶ stop if there is abdominal pain, GI bleeding
  ▶ avoid in pregnancy (premature closure of ductus arteriosis)
▶ dose/route
  ▶ adults: osteoarthritis: 12.5–25 mg q d; acute pain: 50 mg q d × 5 days
▶ how supplied
  ▶ tabs 12.5 mg, 25 mg
  ▶ susp 12.5 mg/5 ml; 25 mg/5ml

Rocuronium (Zemuron)

▶ class
  ▶ paralytic, nondepolarizing
▶ indication
  ▶ paralysis for intubation, mechanical ventilation, procedures
▶ pharmacodynamics/kinetics
  ▶ onset within 2 min
  ▶ duration 30 min

▶ precautions/contraindications
  ▶ pregnancy risk category B
  ▶ do not use when adequate airway/ventilatory support is unavailable
  ▶ caution in patients with neuromuscular disease or myasthenia gravis, or elderly or debilitated patients
▶ dosage/route
  ▶ children over 3 months and adults: 0.6–1.2 mg/kg IV for induction; subsequent dose of 0.6 mg/kg IV provides 30 min paralysis for maintenance
▶ how supplied
  ▶ inj 10 mg/ml, store in refrigerator

Sodium Bicarbonate

▶ class
  ▶ alkalinization agent, systemic and urinary
▶ indication
  ▶ adjunct for severe metabolic acidosis due to extended CPR
▶ precautions/contraindications
  ▶ pregnancy risk category C
  ▶ do not use when there is acidosis due to hypoventilation
▶ dosage/route
  ▶ children and adults: 1 mEq/kg q 10 min, depending on ABG results
▶ how supplied
  ▶ sln 8.4% (50 mEq/50 ml), 4% (2.4 mEq/5ml)

Succinylcholine (Anectine, Quelicin, Sucostrin)

▶ class
  ▶ paralytic, depolarizing
▶ indication
  ▶ paralysis for intubation
▶ pharmacodynamics/kinetics
  ▶ onset: effect in 30 s, peak in 60 s; delayed if patient hypotensive
  ▶ duration 4–6 min
  ▶ causes histamine release
▶ precautions/contraindications
  ▶ pregnancy risk category C
  ▶ use cautiously in patients with neuromuscular disease, elderly, or debilitated
  ▶ adverse effects include muscle fasciculations, which can increase intracranial and intraocular pressure as well as cause transient elevation of the serum potassium
    ▶ fasciculations can be prevented by the preadministration of a small dose of a nondepolarizing paralytic
    ▶ do not use when there is penetrating globe injury or preexisting glaucoma
    ▶ do not use with subacute (i.e., between 48 h and 6 wk) burn, spinal cord injury, or crush mechanism, as dangerously high potassium levels can result

- dosage/route
  - children and adults: 1–2 mg/kg IV for induction
- how supplied
  - inj variable concentrations
  - stored in refrigerator

Sufentanil (Sufenta)

- class
  - analgesic, opioid
- indication
  - induction of general anesthesia
- pharmacodynamics/kinetics
  - onset 2–3 min
  - duration half-life 2.5 h
- precautions/contraindications
  - pregnancy risk category C (D at term)
  - do not use when there is increased ICP or respiratory depression
  - adverse effects include chest wall rigidity, hypotension, bradycardia, CNS depression, and vomiting
- dosage/route
  - children (over 2 years old) and adults: 8–30 mcg/kg for induction, then 3–5 mcg/kg incrementally
- how supplied
  - 50 mcg/ml

Thiopental Sodium (Pentothal)

- class
  - anesthetic, barbiturate
- indication
  - induction of general anesthesia for intubation, especially when the head is injured
- pharmacodynamics/kinetics
  - onset 20–40 s
  - duration 5–10 min
  - extravasation causes necrosis since pH or thiopental sodium is 10.6 (never given IM)
- precautions/contraindications
  - pregnancy risk category C
  - adverse effects include hypotension, myocardial depression, arrhythmias
  - caution in status asthmatics
- dosage/route
  - children: 2–3 mg/kg IV
  - adults: 3–5 mg/kg IV; use lower dose when elderly or hypotensive
- how supplied
  - inj variable concentrations

Ticarcillin (Ticar)

▶ class
  ▶ antibiotic, antipseudomonal penicillin
▶ precautions/contraindications
  ▶ pregnancy risk category B
  ▶ adverse effects include coagulopathy
  ▶ caution in hemorrhagic condition, hypokalemia
  ▶ cautions in patients with seizure disorder
▶ dosage/route
  ▶ children and adults: 200–300 mg/kg/d IV/IM div q 4–6 h; safe use not established for neonates

Ticarcillin/Clavulanate (Timentin)

▶ class
  ▶ antibiotic, antipseudomonal penicillin
▶ precautions/contraindications
  ▶ pregnancy risk category B
  ▶ adverse effects include coagulopathy
  ▶ caution in hemorrhagic condition, hypokalemia
  ▶ cautions in patients with seizure disorder
▶ dosage/route
  ▶ neonates: safe use not established
  ▶ children and adults: 200–300 mg/kg/d IV/IM div q 4–6 h (based on ticarcillin)

Timolol (Blocadren, Timoptic)

▶ class
  ▶ anti-glaucoma agent, beta-blocker
▶ indication
  ▶ decreases IOP
▶ precautions/contraindications
  ▶ pregnancy risk category C
  ▶ do not use when there is bradycardia, heart block, or CHF
▶ dosage/route
  ▶ children and adults: 0.25% sln, 1 gtt BID; increase to 0.5% sln if necessary
▶ how supplied
  ▶ ophth sln 0.25%, 0.5%

Tobramycin (Nebcin)

▶ class
  ▶ antibiotic, aminoglycoside
▶ precautions/contraindications
  ▶ pregnancy risk category D
  ▶ adverse effects include nephro- and oto-toxicity

- ▶ pharmacodynamics/kinetics
  - ▶ lower dosing as necessary based on peak/trough levels measured after the third dose; peak should be 4–10 mcg/ml and trough, 1–2 mcg/ml
- ▶ dosage/route—parenteral
  - ▶ children and adults 2 mg/kg IV/IM load then 1.7 mg/kg IV/IM q 8 h
  - ▶ loading dose is fixed, but subsequent doses are lowered further when there is renal insufficiency
  - ▶ obtain peak and trough measurements after the third dose in order to determine further doses and frequency
- ▶ dosage/route—ophth
  - ▶ children and adults: 1–2 gtt 0.3% sln (or oint) to affected eye q 4 h
- ▶ how supplied
  - ▶ ophth sln or oint 0.3%
  - ▶ inj 40 mg/ml

Tramadol (Ultram)

- ▶ class
  - ▶ analgesic, opioid-like
- ▶ indication
  - ▶ relief of moderate to severe pain
- ▶ precautions/contraindications
  - ▶ pregnancy risk category C (D near term)
  - ▶ avoid when concurrent monoamine oxidase (MAO) inhibitor use
  - ▶ adverse effects include CNS depression, vomiting, and respiratory depression
- ▶ dosage/route
  - ▶ children: safe use not established
  - ▶ adults: 1–2 tabs PO q 4–6 h prn, not to exceed 400 mg/d
- ▶ how supplied
  - ▶ tab 50 mg

Vancomycin (Vancocin)

- ▶ class
  - ▶ antibiotic, glycopeptide
- ▶ precautions/contraindications
  - ▶ pregnancy risk category C
  - ▶ do not use in patients with hearing loss
  - ▶ adverse effects include erythemic, pruritic rash on face/neck/shoulders ("red man syndrome") and nephro- and oto-toxicity
- ▶ dosage/route
  - ▶ children: 4 mg/kg/d IV div q 6 h
  - ▶ adults: 1 g IV q 12 h or 15 mg/kg. Adjust dose for renal impairment

Vasopressin (Pitressin)

▶ class
  ▶ vasopressor
▶ indication
  ▶ management of VF/pulseless VT
▶ pharmacodynamics/kinetics
  ▶ duration 2–8 h
  ▶ causes smooth muscle paristalsis and antidiuretic effect at renal tubule
▶ precautions/contraindications
  ▶ pregnancy risk category B
▶ dosage/route
  ▶ children: safe use not established
  ▶ adults: 40 U IV once
▶ how supplied
  ▶ inj 20 U/ml

Vecuronium (Norcuron)

▶ class
  ▶ paralytic, nondepolarizing
▶ indications
  ▶ paralysis for intubation, mechanical ventilation, and procedures
  ▶ preferred nondepolarizing paralytic agent in patients with renal in-sufficiency
▶ pharmacodynamics/kinetics
  ▶ onset 3–5 min
  ▶ duration 25–40 min
▶ precautions/contraindications
  ▶ pregnancy risk category C
  ▶ caution in patients with neuromuscular disease, elderly, and debilitated patients
  ▶ do not use when adequate airway/ventilatory support is unavailable
▶ dosage/route
  ▶ children over 10, adults: 0.15–0.25 mg/kg IV for induction; subsequent dose of 0.1 mg/kg IV provides 25–40 min paralysis for maintenance
▶ how supplied
  ▶ inj 10 mg

Appendix 45-1 Major Drug Categories

Analgesics

Non-opioid

Acetaminophen
Aspirin
Celecoxib
Diclofenac
Diflusinol
Etodolac
Fenoprofen
Fluribiprofen
Ibuprofen
Ketoprofen
Ketorolac
Naproxen
Piroxicam
Refocoxib
Sulindac
Tolmetin

Opioid

Acetaminophen/Codeine
Acetaminophen/Hydrocodone
Acetaminophen/Oxycodone
Alfentanil
Aspirin/Codeine
Fentanyl
Hydromorphone
Meperidine
Morphine
Propoxyphene
Sufentanil
Tramadol (opioid-like)

Anesthesia Agents

Local

Bupivicaine
Cocaine
Ethyl Chloride
Lidocaine

Paralytic

Atracurium
Doxacurium
Mivacurium
Pancuronium
Rocuronium
Succinylcholine
Vecuronium

Sedative, Barbiturate

Pentobarbital
Thiopental

Sedative, Benzodiazepine

Diazepam
Lorazepam
Midazolam

Sedative, Phenothiazine

Chlorpromazine
Droperidol
Haloperidol
Prochlorperazine
Promethazine

Sedative, Other

Chloral Hydrate
Etomidate
Ketamine
Propofol

Cardiac Agents

Antiarrhythmics

Adenosine
Amiodarone (class III)
Atropine

Diltiazem
Esmolol
Lidocaine (class Ib)
Procainamide (class Ia)

Inotropes

Dobutamine
Dopamine
Epinephrine
Isoproterenol
Norepinephrine

Vasopressors

Dopamine
Ephedrine
Epinephrine
Isoproterenol
Norepinephrine
Vasopressin

Antibiotics

Aminoglycoside

Amikacin
Gentamycin
Kanamycin
Tobramycin

Aminopenicillin

Amoxicillin
Amoxicillin/Clavulanate
Ampicillin
Ampicillin/Sulbactam
Bacampicillin

Antipseudomonal

Mezlocillin
Piperacillin
Piperacillin/Tazobactam

Ticarcillin
Ticarcillin/Clavulonate

Cephalosporin, 1st generation

Cefadroxil
Cefazolin
Cephalexin
Cephradine

Cephalosporin, 2nd generation

Cefaclor
Cefamandole
Cefmetazole
Cefonocid
Cefotetan
Cefoxitin
Cefpodoxime
Cefprozil
Cefuroxime

Cephalosporin, 3rd generation

Cefixime
Cefoperazone
Cefotaxime
Ceftazadime
Ceftizoxime
Ceftriaxone

Quinolone

Ciprofloxacin
Gatifloxacin
Levofloxacin
Norfloxin
Ofloxin

Macrolide

Azithromycin
Clarithromycin
Erythromycin

Natural Penicillin

Penicillin G
Penicillin V

Penicillinase-Resistant Penicillin

Cloxacillin
Dicloxacillin
Methicillin
Nafcillin
Oxacillin

Other

Aztreonam (monobactam)
Chloramphenicol
Clindamycin
Co-trimoxazole (trimethoprim/
   sulfamethoxazole)
Imipenem-cilastatin (carbapenem)
Lincomycin
Metronidazole
Vancomycin (glycopeptide)

46

Management Algorithms

Head Trauma

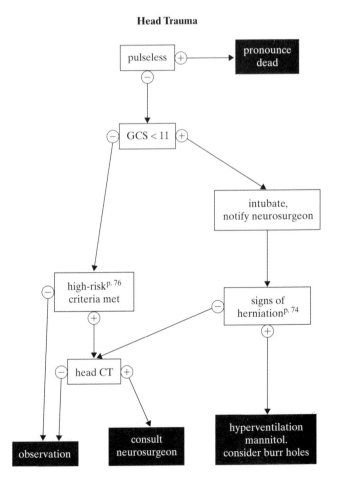

Penetrating Neck Trauma

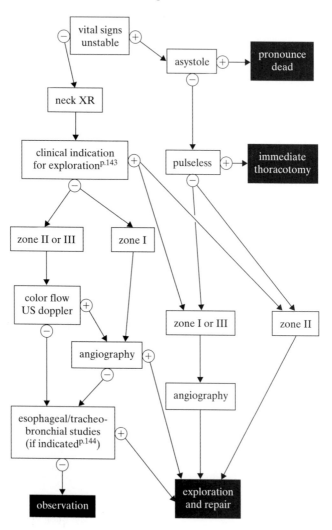

Blunt Chest Trauma

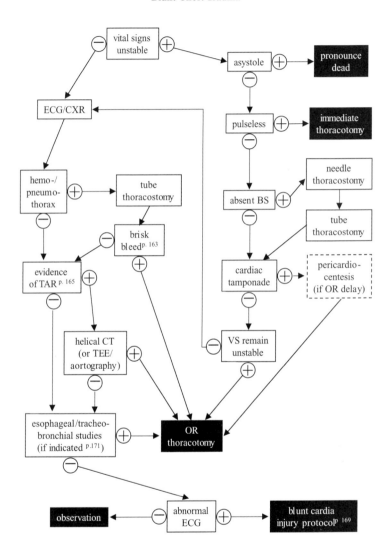

Penetrating Chest Trauma

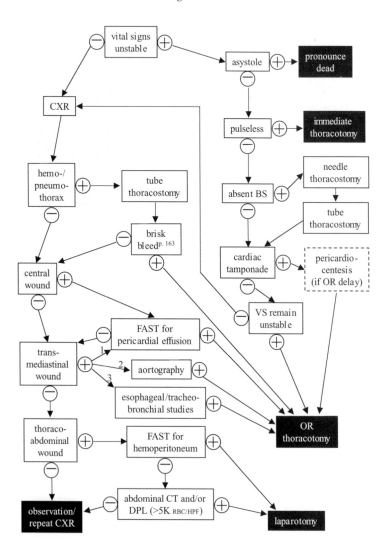

Blunt Abdominal Trauma

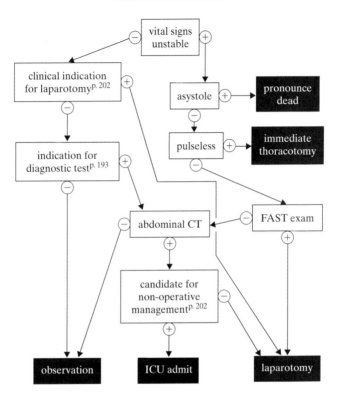

Penetrating Abdominal Trauma

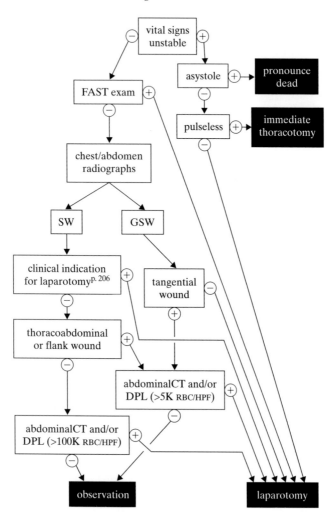

Severe Pelvic Trauma

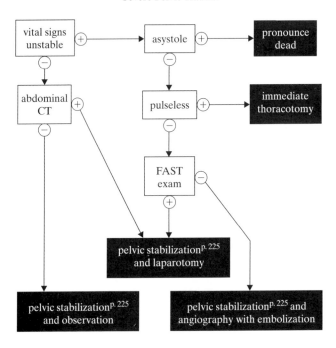

Genitourinary Trauma

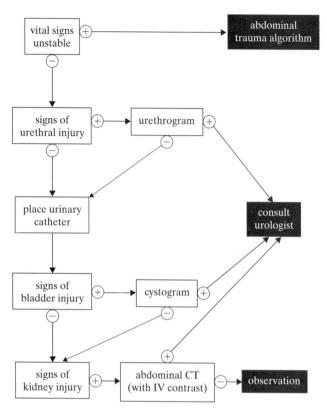

BIBLIOGRAPHY

Adler J (Chief Ed.), *Emergency Medicine,* eMedicine.com, 2000

American Academy of Neurology, Practice Parameters for Determining Brain Death in Adults, *Neurology* 45:1012–1014, 1995

American College of Surgeons, *Advanced Trauma Life Support Instructor Manual,* 6th ed.,1997

American Heart Association, Introduction to ACLS 2000, *Circulation* 102 (Supplement 1), 2000

American Heart Association, *Pediatric Advanced Life Support,* 1994

American Heart Association, *Textbook of Advanced Cardiac Life Support,* 1994

American Medical Association, *A Guide to the Hospital Management of Injuries Arising from Exposure to or Involving Ionizing Radiation,* January 1984

American Society for Surgery of the Hand, *The Hand,* 1st ed., 1985

Bukata WR, Rabies—Essential Facts for Primary Care Physicians, *Emergency Medicine & Acute Care Essays,* 23(8), 1999

Cullom RD, Chang B (Eds.), *The Wills Eye Manual—Office and Emergency Room Diagnosis and Treatment of Eye Disease,* 2nd ed., Lippincott-Raven, 1994

Dailey RH, Simon B, Young GP, Stewart RD, *The Airway—Emergency Management,* Mosby-Year Book, 1992

Fleckenstein P, Tranum-Jensen J, *Anatomy in Diagnostic Testing,* W.B. Saunders, 1993

Franz DR, Jahrling PB, Friedlander AM, et al., Clinical Recognition and Management of Patients Exposed to Biological Warfare Agents, *JAMA* 278(5):399–411, 1997

Galli RL, Spaite DW, Simon RR, *Emergency Orthopedics—The Spine,* Appleton & Lange, 1989

Gean AD, *Imaging of Head Trauma,* Raven Press, 1994

Harris JH, Harris WH, *The Radiology of Emergency Medicine,* 2nd ed., Williams, Wilkins, 1981

Hart RG, Rittenberry TJ, Uehara DT, *Handbook of Orthopaedic Emergencies,* Lippincott-Raven, 1999

Harwood-Nuss AL, *The Clinical Practice of Emergency Medicine,* 2nd ed., Lippincott-Raven, 1996

Haughey M, Calderón Y, Trauma in Pregnancy: Optimizing Maternal and Fetal Outcomes, *Emergency Medicine Reports* 21(16) 177–186, 2000

Keats TE, *Emergency Radiology,* Year Book Medical Publishers, 1984

Levitin H, *Improving Hospital Provider Response to NBC Terrorism,* Metropolitan Chicago Healthcare Commission, 1998

Marx JA (Guest Ed.), *Advances in Trauma* (Emergency Medicine Clinics of North America) Saunders, February, 1993

McCort JJ, *Trauma Radiology,* Churchill Livingstone, 1990

Moore EE, Mattox KL, Feliciano DV, *Trauma,* 3rd ed., Appleton & Lange, 1999

Norton ML, Brown ACD, *Atlas of the Difficult Airway,* Mosby-Year Book, 1991

Perry CR, Elstrom JA, Pankovich AM, *Handbook of Fractures,* McGraw-Hill, 1995

Physician's Drug Handbook, 8th ed., Springhouse, 1999

Raby N, Berman L, deLacey G, *Accident and Emergency Radiology,* W.B. Saunders, 1995

Reisdorff EJ, *Pediatric Emergencies* (Emergency Medicine Clinics of North America), Saunders, May, 1995

Richards C, Suter R, Waeckerle J, *ED Management,* November 1999

Roberts JR, Hedges JR, *Clinical Procedures in Emergency Medicine,* 3rd ed., W.B. Saunders, 1998

Rockwood CA, Green DP, Bucholz RW, *Fractures in Adults,* 4th ed., J.B. Lippincott, 1996

Rodriguez A, Maull K, Feliciano D (Guest Eds), *Trauma Care in the New Millennium* (Surgical Clinics of North America 79(6)), W.B. Saunders, 1999

Rose C, *Emergency Care of the Elderly* (Emergency Medicine Clinics of North America), W.B. Saunders, May, 1990

Rosen P, Barkin RM, et al., *Emergency Medicine–Concepts and Clinical Practice,* 4th ed., Mosby-Year Book, 1998

Rosenthal MA, Ellis JI, Cardiac and mediastinal trauma. In: *Advances and Updates in Cardiovascular Emergencies* (Emergency Medicine Clinics of North America), Wellford LA, Young GP (Guest Eds.), W.B. Saunders, November 1995

Scott JL, Ghezzi KT, *Emergency Treatment of the Eye,* (Emergency Medicine Clinics of North America), W.B. Saunders, August, 1995

Scott JR, DiSain PJ, Hammond CB, Spellacy WN (Eds.), *Danforth's Obstetrics and Gynecology,* 8th ed., Lippincott, Williams & Wilkins, 1999

Simon RR, Brenner BE, *Emergency Procedures and Techniques,* 3rd ed., Williams & Wilkins, 1994

Simon RR, Koenigsknecht SJ, *Emergency Orthopedics—The Extremities,* 3rd ed., Appleton & Lange, 1995

Snell RS, Smith MS, *Clinical Anatomy for Emergency Medicine,* Mosby 1993

Stern EJ (Ed.), *Trauma Radiology Companion,* Lippincott-Raven, 1997

Tintinalli JE, Krome RL, Ruiz E, *Emergency Medicine—A Comprehensive Study Guide,* 4th ed., McGraw-Hill, 1999

Touloukian RJ, *Pediatric Trauma,* 2nd ed., Mosby-Year Book, 1990

VanderSalm TJ, Cutler BS, Austen WG, *Atlas of Bedside Procedures,* Little, Brown, and Company, 1979

Weir J, Abrahams PM (Eds.), *An Imaging Atlas of Human Anatomy,* Wolfe Publishing Ltd., 1992

Wilson RF, Walt AJ (Eds.), *Management of Trauma—Pitfalls and Practice,* 2nd ed., Williams & Wilkins, 1996

INDEX